ANCIENT HINDU MEDICINE

AN INTERPRETATION
OF
ANCIENT HINDU MEDICINE

BY

CHANDRA CHAKRABERTY

LOW PRICE PUBLICATIONS
DELHI-110052

Published by
Low Price Publications
A-6, Nimri Commercial Centre,
Near Ashok Vihar Phase-IV,
Delhi-110052
Phones: 011-27302453
e-mail: info@Lppindia.com
url: www.Lppindia.com

First Published 1923
Reprinted in **LPP** 1993, 1997, 2008
ISBN 978-81-7536-446-2

Printed at
D K Fine Art Press P Ltd.
Delhi-110052

PRINTED IN INDIA

TO

SRIJUKTA LAKSHMIKANTA CHAKRABERTY

THIS BOOK IS AFFECTIONATELY DEDICATED

CONTENTS.

Foreword

I started this Book with the idea of making it a comparative study of the ancient Hindu and Greek systems of Medicine in the light of modern knowledge. But I soon realized that the Hindu students for whom this book is chiefly intended, would not be interested in the Greek Medicine, and as there are excellent translations of the works of Hippocrates,* I hve confined myself to the interpretation of the Ancient Hindu Medicinealonu.

I was forced to the conclusion that the Ancient Greek Schools of Medicine were indebted to the Hindu Systems for the following reasons :—(1) *Indigenous Indian drugs* are found in the works of *Hippocrates* as (a) *Kardamomon* from Sk. '*kardama*' (cardamon) as an emmenagogue in

---

* I. E. Littre : *Oevres Complete D' Hippocrate* (Text and translation) 10 Vols. J. B. Bailier et Fils, Paris, 1839-1861. I have used this edition for my reference.

2. Robert Fuchs : *Hippokrates Sammtliche Werke,* 3 Vols. München, 1895-1900.

3. F. Adams : *Genuine Works of Hippocrates* (partial), Sydenham Society.

Vol. VII. p 358 ; in dyspnea in Vol. VIII. p. 80 ; (b) *Amomon* from Sk. *'elā'* (Elettaria cardamomum) as an emmenagogue in Vol. VII. p. 358 ; (c) *Peperi* from Sk. *'pippalī'* (Piper longum) as an expectorant, mixed with honey-water in Vol. II. p. 464 ; in nasal catarrh in Vol. V. p. 183 ; in gingivitis in Vol. V. p. 244 ; as an errhine in Vol. V. p. 328 ; as a drink with honey, vinegar and water in Vol. VII. p. 150 ; with wine and oil in a pessary in Vol. VII. p. 364 ; in quartan fever in Vol. VIII. p. 654 ; *Dia-trion piperidon*, from Sk. *trikaṭu*,' a preparation made from three species of *'Piper'* (nigrum, longum and album) ; (d) *Kinnamomos* from Sk. *'tvak'* (Cinnamomum zeylonacum) with myrrha, and safran in fumigation in Vol. VII. p. 372 ; simple fumigation in Vol. VIII. p. 364 ; (e) *Akoros* from Sk. *'vacha'* (Acorus colamus) with myrrha as antiseptic injection in Vol. VII. p. 368 ; made infusion with dry pomegranate skin in wine for astringent injection in Vol. VIII, p. 860 ; (f) *Nardon* from Sk. *'jaṭāmāṃsī'* (Nardostachys valeriana) as antiseptic fumigation with cinnamon, myrrha and rose perfume in Vol. VII. p. 372 ; as an astringent antiseptic wash in lochia in Vol. VII. p. 04 ; (g) *Sesamon* from Sk. *'tila'* (Sesamum indicum) as a vulnerary in empyema—suppurative abscess in Vol. II. p. 518 ; in the treatment of adiposis in Vol. VI. p, 76; as a plaster in long-standing catarrh in Vol. V. p. 432 ; as a fattening food in .Vol. VI, p. 258. ; as a nutritive food in Vol. VI. p. 544 ; as a substitute for cheese in Vol. VII. p. 78; in coughing of the children in Vol. VIII. 82 ; (h) *Ziggiberis* from Sk. *'śṛṅgavera'* (Zingiber officinale) ; *Kostos* srom Sk. *'kuṣṭha'* (Costus speciosus) ; *Sakcharon* from Sk. *'śarkarā'* (Saccharum officinarum) ; Pepereos riza from Sk. *'pippalī-mūla'* (radix Piper longum) ; *Kupeiros* from Sk. *'mustaka* (Cyperus rotundus);' *Bdellion* from Sk. *'guggula'* (Aquilaria agallocha) ; etc.

(2) *Humoral Pathology* : In *'Peri Physios Anthropoy'* (On the Nature of Man) Vol. VI. p. 32-69, Hippocrates advances arguments of superiorty of the principles of the four humors whose equilibrium in the body preserves the normal health and whose derangements are the etiological factors of disease, as the *'cima'* (blood : Sk. *'rudhira'*), *'phlegma'* (phlegm : Sk. *'śleṣmā,)'* *'cholen xanthen'* (yellow bile : Sk. *'pitta'*), and *'cholen melainam'* (black bile : as a substitute for Sk. *'vāyu'*), which he for the first time introduced into Greece over the ancient doctrine

of '*hot*' (from fire) '*cold*' (from earth), '*dry*' (from air) and '*moist*' (from water) qualities which were supposed to be the basic factors of health and disease, and which he also argues in his book '*Peri Archaies Ietriches*' (Ancient Medicine), Vol. I. pp. 570-637. In his '*Peri Gones*' (Generation, 3), Vol. VII. p. 474, '*aima, chole, udor, phlegma*' are mentioned as the four humors, using '*bile*' without any qualification, and in the place of one, '*udor*' (Sk. *udaka* = serous fluid) is substituted, thus proving that the humoral question was still in transitional flux, and was not settled or fixed. In '*Peri Chymon*' (Humors, 8, 14), Vol. V. p, 488, 496, seasonal changes are mentioned to cause the increase and the decrease of the humors, as the increase af the bile in the summer, and thus organisms are predisposed to certain diseases in particular seasons in which their controling humors are predominant, in a very strikingly similar language as described in *Suśruta* (I. 6) on '*ṛtu-charyyā*''. In '*Pery Physios Anthropoy*' (The Nature of Man, 7), Vol. VI. p. 46, it is argued that '*phlegma*' is dominant in the winter, for the reason that man conforms to the laws of nature, and as everything is cold in the winter, and as phlegma is the coldest of all the humors in tactile sensation, it naturally therefore is in excess over other humors ; in the spring, the blood is dominant, as the phlegma is still strong, owing to the plenty of rain and sap in the soil and plant, but it becomes desiccated by the warm sun ; in the summer, the blood is still strong, but the bile is formed by the strong sun. and the phlegma is in the minimum owing to the hot, desiccant sun ; in the autumn the blood is in the minimum, but the black bile is formed in abundance, as the season is dry and the nature tends to cool itself. In '*Peri Noyson to Tetarton*' (The fourth Book of Maladies, 33), Vol. VII. p. 542, it is described how the humors are in excess or in deficiency : "I shall describe now, how the bile, the blood, the '*udrops*' (serous fluid) and the phlegma are in excess or in deficiency ; it is through the food and the drink, in this way : the full stomach is the source of all things ; but when empty, it profits at the cost of the body which it disintegrates. Moreover, there are other four sources from which each of the humors can come to the organs ; they come to the stomach, and when the stomach is empty, they go to the organs (superficial), but they come back, when the stomach has something (ingesta). The source for the blood, is the heart, for the phlegma—the brain, for the *'udrops'* (serous fluid)—the spleen, and for the bile, the part that is in the liver (bile-duct)." And in the same book (34—38), it is mentioned that as the plant can select its food from the soil it needs, so each humor can get its nourishment from all kinds of food ; but phlegma is particularly increased by the ingestion of cheese, acrid substance, or phlegmatic food or drink ; the bile is increased by bitter food and drink, or bilious substance ; *'udrops'* (serous fluid) is increased by the water one drinks, and is pumped by the spleen to itself and other parts of the body ; the blood is increased by the bloody food one takes, and which is attracted to all parts of the body, and especially by the heart. As the disease is caused by the excessive increment of one humor over the rest, its cure lies in bringing out the coction (*pāchana*) of the said humor, and cause its evacuation and expulsion from the body ; the crisis of a disease is the turning point when the coction of the deranged humor begins, and the coction produces the periods in fever (Vol. I. p. 617 ; Vol. II. p. 635 ; Vol. IV. p. 469 ; Vol. V. p. 485 ; Vol. VIII. p. 651).

(3) *India is directly mentioned in association*

with some of the drugs : (a) "Echochchous echlepsanta oson treis *indichoy pharmachoy* tou ton ophthalmon, o chaleetai peperi,chai tou stroggyloy, tria tauta leia tribein,chai oino palaio chliero dieis, balanion peri pteron ornithos tithenai,chai ode prosagein."(Another : three decorticated grains, *Indian drug* which is for the eyes and is called 'pepper', the round grain—these three are to be pounded and moistened with warmed old wine, it is to be pasted round a plum, and to be introduced thus (as a pessary). *Gynaikeiion Proton* : (Female Diseases, 81 ; Vol. VIII. p. 202). (b) "E echlepsas chochchous pentechaidecha,esto de chai *indichoy poson*" (Or rather decorticate fifteen grains of Cnide, and add to it, the *Indian preparation* ; ibid 158 ; Vol. VIII. p. 336). (c) "Toyto to pharmachon odontas chathairei chai euodeas poieei chaleetai de *indichon* pharmachon." (This preparation cleanses the teeth, and imparts to them a fine aroma ; it is called Indian preparation ; ibid 185 ; Vol. VIII. p. 366). (d) "Eteron prostheton echlepsas chochchous triechonta, *to indichon*, o chaleousin oi Persai peperi." (Another pessary : thirty decorticated grains, and the *Indian substance* which the Persians call 'pepper'; ibid 205 ; Vol. VIII. p. 394).

(4) *Indirect Inference* : Urine of cow

go-mūtra) is recommended as a therapeutic agent in fistula, in Vol. VI. p, 453 ; as a disinfectant wash for the female genitals and in sterility in Vol. VII. p. 365 ; in fumigation and lotion in female diseases in Vol. VIII. p. 211. Cow-dung (*go-maya*) is recommended with aromatic substances as a fumigation in female diseases in Vol. VIII. p. 119. ; bovine desiccated bile (*go rochanā*) as a vulnerary preparation for wounds in Vol. VI. p. 415 ; in a purgative compound in Vol. VI. p. 419 ; in pessary with myrrh and honey in Vol. VIII. p. 59,157,203,395 ; as a laxative drink with wine in Vol. VII. p. 425. The cow being regarded as the sacred animal of the Hindus, it can be imagined that her excretory products may be used in India as therapeutic agents, but their use among the Greeks who had no such passions, indicates their foreign importation.

It may be said that all the writings that are now included in the Hippocratic Collection were not the genuine works of Hippocrates (460--377 B. C.). That may be so. We are not concerned with that problem. It suffices for our purpose to know that the Hindu thoughts influenced deeply the Greek medical literature in the fifth and the fourth century B. C. We do not yet definitely know how the Medical science reached

Hellas ; perhaps by the Persian intermediatories, or directly by the Hindu settlers in the Persian Empire. We know that in 606 B. C. the Median king Cyaxares conquered Assyria and annexed to it the territories up to the coasts in Asia Minor where there were many Hellenic settlers. Cyrus, (559—530 B. C.) the great Persian nation-builder, defeats Astyages and conquers Media in 550 B. C., defeats Croesus, the Lydian king, and captures Sardis in 547 B. C., conquers Babylon and Greek cities of Asia Minor in 546—539 B. C. His son Cambyses (529—522 B. C.) conquers Egypt in 527 B. C., by defeating the Egyptian ruler Psammetichus III or better known as Amasis, under whom were numerous Ionian and Cartan mercenaries. The empire of Darius I (522---486 B. C.) extends from Macedonia to the Indus, and from the Danube and the Black Sea to Nubia; while in 512 B. C. Darius invaded Scythia, to subdue the nomadic hordes, his general Megabazus reduced Thrace, and a few years later penetrated up to the river Peneus in Thessaly ; the Ionians revolted against the Persian domination, and with the assistance of Athenians and Eretrians, burnt Sardis in 499 B. C., which led to the Persian invasion of Northern Greece in 492 B. C. under the generalship of Mardonius, and of Attica in 490 B. C., which ended with the defeat of the Persians at the battle of Marathon on Sept. 12—490 B. C.

Siddhārtha Gautama (*the Buddha* 563—483 B. C.) entered into '*nirvāṇa*' in 483 B. C. after a strenuous life of may years' preaching. In Mahāvagga (1. 6 ; 1. 8) a very old Buddhist work of the fifth century B. C., we find desciiption of advanced medical treatment.

But the Hindu influence over Greece even goes beyond that period. There is every reason to believe that the Dionysos orgies were the imported Soma-Śiva cult from India. Dionysos is a Moon-god like Soma. He introduced wine-culture (and civilization) into Hellas. The bull, the goat and the serpent are sacred to him. And he is represented like Śiva, as accompanied by a leopard, and in Alexandrian time,riding on a tiger (*Encyc. Brit.* Vol. VIII. p. 287). The Orphic religion seems to be no less indebted to the same source. Abstinence from meat, fish etc., from animal sacrifices, the wearing of a special garment, the practice of austere asceticism, belief in the transmigration of soul, and the soul will attain perfection, passing through various beings, and when it attains it, it will be free from rebirth—

the circle of generation' (*kyklos geneseos*), as the body is the bondage of the soul (Ency Brit. Vol. XX. p. 328)—all these unmistakably indicate pre-Buddhistic Indian origin, where these doctrines have been indigenous, and are still believed by the multitude. Arthur Lille in his '*Rama and Homer*' argues that in the Rāmāyaṇa, Homer found his theme for his great epics for the following reasons: (1) Like the two inseparable brothers in the Rāmāyaṇa, Rāma and Lakṣmaṇa, in the story of Menelaus, there are also two inseparable Greek brothers. (2) Rāma and Lakṣmaṇa have been banished by the conspiracies of a stepmother while the Greek brothers are banished from Argos by their usurping uncle Thyestes. (3) Sîtā is born of a swan's egg (*Brahmā's emblem*) in a furrow, Helen is also born from a swan's egg left by her mother, Leda, the swan, and Helen emerged from her egg in a 'yperwon' which means a furrow. (4) At the '*svayṃvara*' Rāma defeats all the competing princes, and Sîtā chooses him as her husband, and in Greece, Menelaus is made to defeat all the competing princes, and wins Helen, though neither a competing tournament for winning a bride, nor the choosing of a husband (*svayaṃvara*) was customary in Greece, and they were time-honored institutions in India. (5) Whilst Rāma is away, Sîtā is carried away to Laṅkā across the sea ; likewise Helen is carried away across the sea to Troy. (6) Vibhîṣaṇa from a high hill points out to Rāma the principal warriors of the forces of Rāvaṇa ; Helen points out to Priam the chief Greek captains, after nine years of war and who came to rescue her. (7) The arrows of Rāvaṇa and the arrows of Hector come back to their hand after their flight. (8) As Hanumān with a mighty shout daunts the whole of the army of Rāvaṇa, so Achilles with a mighty shout daunts the whole of the Trojan army. (9) The heavens rain blood as an omen of the coming death of Rāvaṇa, and when the favorite son of Zeus, Sarpedon, is about to die, Zeus and Hera see a shower of blood falling on the battle-field. (10) The Hindu besiegers fare badly in the early encounters and Rāma proposes to bring the army back to India ; the Greek besiegers fare badly as well and Agamemnon proposes to carry the army back to Greece. (11) In the Rāmāyaṇa the Rākṣasas are depicted to be as big as mountains ; Mars, when thrown down by angry Pallus who flings a rock at him, covers seven acres with his gigantic body. (12) In the Hindu epic, the gods and the demons gather round to watch the crucial battles between the paramount chiefs Rāma and Rāvaṇa ; in the Iliad, the opposing gods also crowd round to watch the course of the battle, though the chiefs are not paramount, nor the encounter crucial. (13) Kuvera, the god of wealth, and Śiva, the god of death, throw dice ; in the Iliad, Jove suspends golden scales. (14) When Sîtā makes her determination to starve to death, Indra comes down and gives her the '*amṛta*'—the immortal food ; when Achilles is of the same frame of mind, though he was not a wronged party, Jove sends down Minerva with the ambrosia for him. (15) Vibhîṣaṇa is the wisest denizen in Laṅkā ; Antenor has the same reputation in Troy. When Rāvaṇa is about to kill Hanumān, the ambassador of Rāma, Vibhîṣaṇa remonstrates and saves his life ; when Menelaus and Odysseus came into Troy as ambassadors, they would have been killed, but for the intervention of Antenor. Vibhîṣaṇa advises Rāvaṇa to give up Sîtā ; Antenor advises Paris to give up Helen. Vibhîṣaṇa conspires against his country with the enemy, shows the enemies how to pass the sea, reveals the secrets of the '*chaitya*' of

Nikumbhilā ; Antenor also plots secretly against his own country, and advises Ulysses to seize the Trojan Palladium, and make the wooden horse. Vibhîṣaṇa, after the death of his brother and the capture of the city, becomes the crowned king of Laṅkā ; Antenor founded a new kingdom out of the ruins of the old. (16) Rāma is loaned by the supreme god, his chariot with the celestial charioteer—Mātali, and the terrible missile *'Brahmaśiras'* which alone can kill the ravisher of Sitā, and the fiend of the gods. Achilles, the avenging hero, not the wronged husband, is given the coat of arms from the anvils of Vulcan, the chariot with the deathless steeds of Jove, and the charioteer Automedon who alone can drive such steeds, but he lacks the terrible *'arrow of Philoctetes'* which alone can kill the ravisher of Helen, and instead of killing the foe, he is himself killed by that foe. (17) Inconsistency and the lack of unity of the Homeric plot, and the invulnerable logic and conclusion of Vālmîki's story : cattle-stealing and wife-stealing being then the prevailing custom in Hellas, and Helen being carried off by a fop, and not a fiend of the gods, it could not have precipitated a war between two peoples.

Then the question arises as to the age of Suśruta and Charaka Saṃhitās, and that is very hard to determine with any positive certainty. All that we know is that the great Buddhist scholar Nāgārjjuna revised the old Suśruta, and added to it the supplementary section (*uttara-tantra*). Nāgārjjuna was a leading director of Kaniṣka's Council that was held about 78 A. D.. He salutes Suśruta in the beginning of the work (*Suśruta* I. I) with Brahmā, Prajāpati, the Aśvins, Indra, and Dhanvantari. It must have taken centuries to have made Suśruta a mythical figure, and to be classified with the gods. Charaka is mentioned in the Chinese Buddhist chronicles, as the family-physician of the Indo-Scythian king Kaniṣka (about first century A. D.), and who attended at a difficult child-birth of his wife. But Charaka is a family name, and there is an old Vedic Charaka school, known as Kapiṣṭhala Charaka (I. 1. 3). The internal evidence of both the works indicates that they were composed in pre-Buddhistic times, though there are numerous interpolations of a later age. The '*Sūtra-sthāna*' (Section of General Principles) and the metrical portions which are more or less explanatory, seem to be later additions. Not only do the prose versions resemble the Brāhmaṇas in composition, but all the gods also are post-Vedic, and the common use of meat, especially beef (Charaka I. 2, 18 ; Suśruta I. 46. 89), points out to a pre-Buddhistic age. The osteological nomenclature used in Suśruta is almost identical with that used in Atharva Veda (X. 2), and in the Śatapatha Brāhmaṇa (S. B. E. Vol. XLIV. p. 164). It is possible that the sage Yājñavalkya whose name is mentioned in the Brāhmaṇas, and in association with the King Janaka, the reputed teacher of the '*Vājasaneyi Saṃhitā*' (the White Yajur-Veda), and the Law-book is the same person, and he lived about sixth century B. C. And the King Janaka of Mithilā might have been known as '*Kāśi-rāja*' and Divodāsa. It may be said that the Hindu medical science could not make such a rapid advancement from the primitive magic charms and sorceries of the Atharva-Veda period, which has been put at 1000 years B. C. It is true that the '*Āyurveda*' (medical science) claims to be a branch of the Atharva-Veda, as the priest is the successor of the magician, and the medicine-man is a magician priest. But the Atharva Veda contains many of the oldest superstitions of the Indo-Dravidian masses, and they did not become embodied in the Ṛg-Veda, simply because they represented the attitude of the masses rather than that of the nobility. And when they became hoary with age, they became entitled to respect, and became admitted in the sacred book. The Charaka is older than the Suśruta, for in anatomical description, physiological explanation, in the classification of subject-matter, in the form of language and in the therapeutic technique, it represents a more ancient school. As there are many passages that are common, it seems that they were borrowed by the latter from the former.

In the following pages, I have tried to interpret and explain the *Ancient Hindu Medicine*, principally based upon Charaka and Suśruta in modern medical terminology. Translation is an ungrateful task, especially of technical subjects, written nearly twenty-five centuries ago, their modes of expression being quite different from those of the present age. However, I have tried to be as careful and accurate as possible. The translation could be much improved by transposition of words, or outstretching their meanings. I have preferred accuracy to diction, and I have often sacrificed, whenever it has been necessary, a good literary form, to make it as true to the original as possible and to reflect its meaning.

Yet it is very likely that some of my interpretations may not find ready acceptance in many orthodox quarters. But sooner it is realized, it will be better for the communal health, that the ancient medical works can not serve us to-day any other useful purpose than to supply rich materials for the cultural history of the race. Its prolific vocabulary might be also profitably utilized to create a National School of Medicine, for continuity of historic consciousness activates and acts as a stimulus for progress. And it is well to know and remember that many of the medical books before they come from the press need revision to be up-to-date, and most of them, before they are ten years old, are almost antiquated. Bacteriology, micro-biology, chemistry, bio-chemistry, non-irritant antiseptics, prophylaxis, serum-therapy, organo-therapy, skiagrapy and the mechanical appliances have completely revolutionized during the last generation in method and technique '*the treatment and prevention of disease*,' which is the object of Medical Science (*Suśruta* I. 1. 12). Our very great achievements in the past, which we have every reason to be proud of, instead of inspiring us with the greatest efforts to lead in arts and sciences, should not mortgage our future to the *Dead Past*. For a race that does not take the utmost care and the most advanced methods for the prevention of disease and the preservation of health, can not effectively compete in the struggle for existence, with more forward races, and succeed in the survival of the fittest. Health is the foundation of all wealth and progress. We can not afford to cling to an empty shell, carry the dead weight of the past on our back, sacrificing our future, unless we want to be counted with the extinct races.

At the other extreme, there may be some who will contend that I have made a free ride on the wings of imagination, and there could not be such an advanced medical technique in the remote past. I want them to follow closely the original text. I suffer from no national hypnotism or megalomania. Exaggeration, on the other hand, I believe, is apt to lower the intrinsic value of a thing. Have I been subconsciously influenced by the sense of the grandeur of the country, as an expression of suppressed or subdued patriotism? I leave that for the readers to judge. I have always believed that in ancientness—Egypt, in social polity—China, in art—Greece, have nobler records of fundamental value than India can boast of. I admit, with all her faults, I love my country. I take pride and glory in her past achievements. Tremors of her new awakening from the slumber of centuries, have sent me joyous thrills, made me vibrant with emotions and intoxicating dreams. And I live to see that she will contribute her share, worthy of her past, promising of a bright and brighter future, to the advancement of Human Civilization, and take her leading place in science and culture, and in the Council of Nations. But when studying history, intellect should not and does not need to be influeneed by a gamut of sentiments and feelings, and can be left free to exercise its supreme prerogative to judge facts as they are on their own merit. I have tried to keep that attitude of my mind—not to corrupt my intellect with emotions. In studying the medical history of India, one should not be misled by the prevailing pathetic condition,—lack of hygiene, vicious dietary of the rich and the poor alike, ignorance and ineptitude of the medical practitioners, and the credulity of the public, for progress is not always steady and continuous. Except in the application of the mechanical developments and the appliances of machine power, modern nations have hardly made any further advancement in pure arts and literature than the Greeks. Medieval Europe, after the destruction of the Greek States and the downfall of the Roman Empire, sank deeper in superstition and ignorance. In medical science the name of Galen (Claudius Galenus 130—201 A. D.) remained as the only supreme authority in Europe up to the seventeenth century, and in the Saracen empire up to the fourteenth century. The Arabs formed an eclectic school of medicine out of the synthesis of the Greek and the Hindu systems. In India medical science had its highest expression under the Buddhist rule when the relief of pain, human as well as animal, was regarded as a state religious duty, and hospitals were built in every important locality for men as well as animals. In the famous Buddhist universities of Takṣaśilā and Nālanda, there were thousands of students from all parts of India and Outer-India who went there to study medicine alone. With the downfall of the Buddhist states, and the dispersion of the monks, whose principal duties were to administer to the sick, the acquired knowledge virtually disappeared from India, and healing became the profession of the mendicants by magic charms and incantations, or of the quacks, charlatans and barbers.

It is possible, however, that though I have

been careful in the selection of the equivalent scientific terms for the Sanskrit, a few minor ones may need revision. I have labored under great disadvantages. Though New York Libraries are splendid institutions, and grant liberal privileges and easy access to the books, there are very few books on Indian Medicine, and I have not been able to avail myself of any book on the subject. Moreover it is very hard to write competently for one individual on all subjects dwelt on in Charaka and Suśruta Saṃhitās, and as they are the product of a medical assemblage —the collected wisdom of the sages that gathered together from all parts of India, as the drugs clearly indicate, and Agniveśa and Suśruta might have simply acted as secretaries (Charaka I. 1. 3), so their interpretation could be best done by a medical association with competent departmental heads on all subjects dealt with in those works. Mine has been simply a pioneer attempt, knowing not whether this task has been undertaken by any efficient Indian medical organization, and I have had to work single-handed, without any advice from any source. This, I understand, can be no excuse or justification for any misleading statement or false conclusion, and I shall be grateful to my readers to have them pointed out.

For transliteration, I have used the following method :—

अ = a	क = k	ड = ḍ	म = m
आ = ā or á	ख = kh	ढ = ḍh	य = y
इ = i	ग = g	ण = ṇ	र = r
ई = ī ï, or î	घ = gh	त = t	ल = l
उ = u	ङ = ṅ	थ = th	व = v
ऊ = ū or ü	च = ch	द = d	श = ś
ए = e	छ = chh	ध = dh	ष = ṣ
ऐ = ai	ज = j	न = n	स = s
ओ = o	झ = jh	प = p	ह = h
औ = au	ञ = ñ	फ = ph	ं = ṃ
ऋ = ṛ	ट = ṭ	ब = b	: = ḥ
ऌ = ḷ	ठ = ṭh	भ = bh	

I regret very much that it will not be possible for me to add an index to this book. This work has already taken more than double of the time I anticipated it would require, and the pressure of other works does not permit me to devote more time to it. Under these circumstances, I beg leave to bring to a conclusion the arduous task, I so light-heartedly undertook.

July 22—1922
364, West 120th Street,
New York.

C. CHAKRABERTY

AN INTERPRETATION
OF
ANCIENT HINDU MEDICINE.

ANATOMY.

The ancient Hindu physicians lacked profound and accurate anatomical knowledge. They have left more or less superficial, vague and imaginary description of the human anatomy, as found in their treatises, except in osteology. There is nothing astonishing in this. The Hindu medical science developed in the Buddhistic period for alleviation of physical sufferings. The Buddhists regarded all life as sacred. They naturally regarded with horror the idea of inflicting pain, and of depriving an animal of life for experimental medicine. In a tropical climate, as a hygienic measure, cremation of the dead has been ordained as a religious duty from misty antiquity. So there was no regular chance for human dissection and to acquire the exact knowledge of human anatomy. Whatever knowledge they acquired, they obtained it from personal observation and experience, from caring for the wounded and disabled on the battle-fields, from a comparative study of the animal anatomy from the sacrificial animals in the pre-Buddhistic period. There is no record of the custom of human sacrifice, except the legend of Śunaḥśepa (*Aitareya Brāhmaṇa, VII.3*), as the act was repudiated by all presiding priests of the Rājasūya ceremony. If it was a mock-belief as a reminiscence of the remote past, it, however, clearly indicates that human sacrifice was no longer countenanced by the Vedic priesthood and was not practised in the post-Vedic Sūtra period. The students of surgery were taught the technique of instrumental operation on dead animals and vegetables, as water-melon, cucumber, pumpkin, gourds or skin-bags filled with water (*Suśruta, I. 9. 2-5)*. Under these circumstances, proficiency was not possible.

Neither in Greece was it better. In the time of Hippocrates, the anatomical knowledge was very defective and superficial. No differentiation was yet made between the arteries and the veins and both were called 'phleps'—blood-vessels.

However, this distinction was made by Polybus, but on the whole his anatomical and physiological knowledge was erroneous. But Aristotle (*B. C. 385-322*) by his comparative study of animals, laid the foundation of positive anatomy and physiology. In his '*History of Animals*,' he devotes two-fifths of the work, the first four books, to the structural constitution of animals. He synthesizes all the knowledge of the time on the subject and corrects many inaccurate and misleading impressions of his predecessors. But he confuses, like Charaka and Suśruta, bones with cartilage and ligaments. He had vague ideas about nerves (*neura*) and identified them with the tendons, arising from the heart and he regarded the aorta as the nervous vein (*neurodes phleps*). And the human anatomy was not studied with experimental observation and dissection before the famous Alexandrian schools attracted the best intellects of the age under the patronage of Ptolemy Soter (*B. C.323-282*). Erasistratus and Herophilus were both celebrated anatomists of antiquity. They acquired a tolerably sound knowledge of the organs and their functions, not only by animal but also by human dissection and experimentation. Erasistratus found out that the nerves originated from the brain and Herophilus distinguished them into those of sensation and voluntary motion. Herophilus also wrote a treatise on the liver, which Galen has transmitted among his writings. Galen (*130-200 A. D.*), the really accurate anatomist of antiquity, went to Alexandria to study medicine under the famous anatomist Heraclianus, and Claudius Galenus of Pergamum can be called the founder of exact medical science by his vast erudition, scholarly research and his accurate clinical observation, and no wonder, for generations, his writings have held unchallenged authority both in Europe and Asia. The Arabic schools of medicine regarded him almost as infallible.

Herodotus (*B. C. 484-427*) mentions in his history II. 85, that the Egyptian medical profession was very advanced and learned, and it specialized in different diseases. But there is nothing left but a fragment of papyrus of the sixteenth century B. C. to indicate the extent of the medical knowledge of the ancient Egyptians. In this papyrus, it is found that the heart, vessels, liver, spleen, kidneys, ureters and bladder were recognized and the blood-vessels came from the heart. Their vessels are described, some carrying air, some mucus, while two to the right ear are mentioned to carry the breath of life and to the left ear, the breath of death. (*Journal of Anatomy and Physiology, vol. XXXII. P. 775*). Even in the third millennium B. C. the Babylonians possessed quite to a praise-worthy extent the knowledge of the liver which they regarded as the seat of life. The Chaldeans used the liver of the sacrificed sheep for the divination of events. In the code of Hammurabi about 1900 B. C. it seems that the Babylonian medical art had already attained a marvellous efficiency, as the operation on the eye is mentioned with bronze lancet as a regular professional daily business. And a successful eye operation is not possible without a thorough anatomical knowledge of its structure.

1. OSTEOLOGY

Parts of the body.	Number of bones according to modern anatomical Text-books	Charaka	Suśruta	Hippocrates
I. Four Extremities.				
Phalanges (*aṅguli*) Bones of fingers and toes	14 × 4 = 56,	15 × 4 = 60,	15 × 4 = 60	
Metacarpus (*śalākā*) Long bones of the palm	5 × 2 = 10,	5 × 2 = 10,	5 × 2 = 10	
Metatarsus (*śalaka*) Long bones of the anterior portion of the foot	5 × 2 = 10,	5 × 2 = 10,	5 × 2 = 10	Hands 27
Carpus (*1. adhiṣṭhāna ; 2. kūrchcha ; 3. gulpha*) The wrist-bones	8 × 2 = 16,	5 × 2 = 10,	5 × 2 = 10	
Tarsus (*1. adhiśṭhana ; 2. kurchcha ; 3. gulpha*) Ankle-bones	7 × 2 = 14,	5 × 2 = 10,	5 × 2 = 10	Feet 24

Os calcis (*pārṣṇi*) Heel	*1 × 2 = 2,	1 × 2 = 2,	1 × 2 = 2	
Styloid processes of the wrist (*maṇika*)	—	2 × 2 = 4,	1 × 2 = 2	
Tibia and Febula (*iaṅghā*) The leg bones	2 × 2 = 4,	2 × 2 = 4,	2 × 2 = 4	
Radius and Ulna (*aratni*) Bones of the forearm	2 × 2 = 4,	2 × 2 = 4,	2 × 2 = 4	
Patella (*jānu*) Knee-cap	1 × 2 = 2,	1 × 2 = 2,	1 × 2 = 2	
Olecranon (*kūrpara*) Elbow process	—	1 × 2 = 2,	1 × 2 = 2	
Femur (*uru*) Thigh-bone	1 × 2 = 2,	1 × 2 = 2,	1 × 2 = 2	
Humerus (*bāhu*) The bone of the upper arm	1 × 2 = 2,	1 × 2 = 2,	1 × 2 = 2	
	120	122	120	51

* Included among the Tarsus bones.

II. The Trunk.

Parts of the body	Number of bones according to modern anatomical Text-books	Charaka	Suśruta	Hippocrates
Clavicle (*akṣaka*) Collar-bone	$1 \times 2 = 2$	$1 \times 2 = 2$	$1 \times 2 = 2$	
Scapula (*aṃsa*) Shoulder-blade	$1 \times 2 = 2$	$1 \times 2 = 2$	* $1 \times 2 = 2$	
Sternum (*bakṣa*) Breast bone	1	17	8	
Ribs [*pārśvaka*]	$12 \times 2 = 24$	$36 \times 2 = 72$	$36 \times 2 = 72$	
Vertebrae : [*spinal column*] 12 *Thoracic* } 5 Lumber } *pṛṣṭhe*	17	35	30	20

* Enumerated among '*bakṣha.*'

Pelvis: Sacrum (*trika*)	1	1	1	
Pelvis: Coccyx (*guda*)	1	1	1	5
Pelvis: Ilium ; Ischium (*śroṇi-phalaka*)	2	2	2 (*nitamba*)	
Pelvis: Pubis (*bhaga*)		1	1	
	50	133	117	25

III. The Neck and the Skull

Vertebra Cervix (*grīvā*)	7	15	9	7
Trachea and Bronchi (*jatru*)				
The Windpipe		1	4 (*kaṇṭhanalī*)	
Cranium: Frontal	1			
Cranium: Parietal	2 (*chakṣu*)	2		
Cranium: Occipital	1		(*mastaka*)	
Cranium: Sphenoid	1	4	6	skull
Cranium: Ethmoid	1			8

Parts of the body	Number of bones according to modern anatomical Text-books	Charaka	Suśruta	Hippocrates
OS Temporale (*Śaṅkha*)	2	2	2	
Superior maxillary	2 } (*hanu*)			
Inferior maxilla	1 }	2	2	
{Ossa faciei: Nasal(*nāsikā*)	2 }	3	3	
{Bones of the face. Vomer	1 }			
Palate *tālu*	2	2	1	
Lachrymal	2	—	—	
Inferior turbinated	2	—	—	
Malar (*gaṇḍa*)	2	—	2	
Hyoid	1 *			
The Ossicles of the ear :				
Malleus } Incus } Stapes }	$3 \times 2 = 6$		$1 \times 2 = 2$	

* Enumerated among the '*grīvā*.'

Teeth (*danta*)	—	32	32	
Sockets of teeth (*udūkhala*)	—	32	—	
Nails (*nakha*)	—	20	4	20
	36	105	63	35
I. The Four Extremities	120	122	120	51
II. The Trunk	50	133	117	25
III. The Neck and the Skull	36	105	63	35
The total number of the human bones	206	360(*1*)	300(*2*)	111

"With teeth, sockets of teeth and nails, there are altogether 360 bones in the whole of the (*human*) body. As the following :—sockets of teeth 32 ; nails 20 ; long bones of hand and feet 20 ; their bases 4 ; bones of fingers 60 ; heels 2 ; bases of the feet 2 ; wrist bones 4 ; ankle-bones 4 ; in the fore-arms 4 ; in the leg 4 ; knee-caps 2 ; elbow-pans 2 ; in the thighs 2 ; in the arms 2 ; collar bones 2 ; shoulder-blades 2 ; palate bones 2 ; the pelvic ring 2 ; ilium 1 ; sacrum 1 ; coccyx 1 ; back-bone 35 ; neck-bones 15 ; trachea 1 ; jaw bones 2 ; bases of the jaw bones 2 ; parietal 2 ; malar 2 ; nasal bones 3 ; ribs ; 24 ; thoracic ribs 24 and sockets of the ribs 24 and altogether on the sides 72 bones ; temporal bones 2 ; frontal craniun 4 ; breast bones 17 ; altogether three hundred and sixty bones." Charaka IV.7.4.[1]

---

1. Charaka IV. 7. 4 त्रीणि षष्ट्यधिकानि शतान्यस्थ्नां सह दन्तोलूखलनखैः । तद्यथा,—द्वात्रिंशद्दन्तोलूखलानि, द्वात्रिंशद्दन्ताः, विंशतिर्नखाः, विंशतिः पाणिपादशलाकाः, चत्वार्य्यधिष्ठानान्यासां, चत्वारि पाणिपादपृष्ठानि, षष्टिरङ्गुल्यस्थीनि, द्वे पार्ष्ण्योर्द्वे कूर्च्चाधश्चत्वारः पाण्योर्मणिकाश्चत्वारः पादयोर्गुल्फाः, चत्वार्य्यरत्न्योरस्थीनि चत्वारि जङ्घयोर्जानुनोर्द्वे कूर्परयोर्द्वे ऊर्व्वोर्द्वे वाह्वोः सांसयोः द्वावक्षकौ, द्वे तालुनि, द्वे श्रोणिफलके, एकं भगास्थि, पुंसां मेढ्रास्थि, एकं त्रिकसंश्रितमेकं गुदास्थि, पृष्ठगतानि पञ्चविंशत्, पञ्चदशास्थीनि ग्रीवायां, द्वे जत्रुण्येकं हन्वस्थि, द्वे हनुमूलबन्धने, द्वे ललाटे, द्वे अक्ष्णोर्द्वे गण्डयोर्नासिकायां त्रीणि घोणाख्यानि, द्वयोः पार्श्वयोश्चतुर्व्विंशतिश्चतुर्व्विंशतिः पञ्जरास्थीनि च पार्श्वकानि तावन्ति चैषां स्थालिकान्यर्व्वुदाकाराणि, तानि द्विसप्ततिर्द्वौ शङ्खौ, चत्वारि शिरःकपालानि वक्षसि सप्तदशेति त्रीणि षष्ट्यधिकानि शतान्यस्थ्नामिति ।

"According to the medical men, there are 360 bones, but in surgery 300 bones are enumerated. Of these 300 bones, in the branches, that is in both the arms and feet, there are 120; in the pelvic region, back and the breast, there are 120; and above the trunk 63: altogether there are 300 bones in the human body.

"Following are the 120 bones in the branches:—at every finger of the foot, there are 3—so 15; the foot-support (*metatarsus*), the ankle-bones and their base 10; heel 1; in the leg 2; in the knee-cap 1; in the thigh 1; so in one foot there are 30 bones: so in the other foot and arms.

"In the pelvis 5 as coccyx, ilium, pubis 4 and sacrum 1; ribs 32 one side and the same on the other; back-bones 30; in the breast 8; shoulder-blades 2.

"In the neck 9; in the wind-pipe 4; jaw-bones 2; teeth 32; in the nose 3; palate 1; malar, temporal and ear bones 2 each; in the cranium 6." Suśruta III. 5. 17-20. [2]

Suśruta III. 5. 17-20 त्रीणि सषष्टीन्यस्थिशतानि वेदवादिनो भाषन्ते। शल्यतन्त्रे तु त्रीण्येव शतानि। तेषां सविंशमस्थिशतं शाखासु। सप्तदशोत्तरं शतं श्रोणिपार्श्वपृष्ठोदरोरस्सु। ग्रीवां प्रत्यूर्द्धं त्रिषष्टिः। एवमस्थ्नां त्रीणि शतानि पूर्य्यन्ते॥ १७

एकैकस्यान्तु पादाङ्गुल्यां त्रीणि त्रीणि,—तानि पञ्चदश। तलकूर्चगुल्फसंश्रितानि दश। पार्ष्ण्यामेकम्। जङ्घायां द्वे। जानुन्येकम्। एकमूराविति त्रिंशदेवमेकस्मिन् सक्थनि भवन्ति। एतेनेतरसक्थिबाहू च व्याख्यातौ॥ १८

श्रोण्यां पञ्च, तेषां गुदभगनितम्बेषु चत्वारि, त्रिकसंश्रितमेकम्, पार्श्वे षट्त्रिंशदेवमेकस्मिन्; द्वितीयेऽप्येवम्। पृष्ठे त्रिंशत्। अष्टावुरसि। द्वे अक्षकसंज्ञे। १९

ग्रीवायां नवकम्। कण्ठनाड्यां चत्वारि। द्वे हन्वोः। दन्ता द्वात्रिंशत्। नासायां त्रीणि। एकं तालुनि। गण्डकर्णशङ्खेष्वेकैकम्। षट् शिरसि॥ २०

"The bones of the hand are 27 ; of the feet 4 ; of the neck up to the grand (*back-bone—shoulder blades*) 7 ; pelvis 5 ; back-bones 20 ; the head with eyes 8 ; in total 91 with the nails 111. As to man, the bones we have ourselves learnt to know are :—the back-bones above collar-bones with the grand (*shoulder-blades*) 7 ; the back-bones as well as those of the sides (*ribs 12 ; the back-bones that go farther the ribs in the pelvis 5.*") Hippocrates : *The Nature of Bones*, I. (*Peri osteon physios*).

From the above comparative table, it is evident that the Hindu anatomists, especially the Suśruta school, had a tolerably sound knowledge of **osteology**. The discrepancies in the figures are due to the fact that the Hindus counted the processes, cartilaginous structures and the teeth as bones. But they classified the bones into five kinds according to their nature of constitution. (*Suśruta III. 5. 21*). The nails—the epidermal formations were dismissed by Suśruta as bones. If the teeth were counted in the skeleton, it is because the teeth are bone-like, hard and strong. Histology is a recent science and it could not be known in ancient times that tooth is a calcified papilla of the mucous membrane. If the cartilages, especially the costal cartilages of the ribs have been counted as the bones, it is because in the embryonic state all the bones are in cartilaginous condition and in certain diseases, the costal cartilages become ossified. Suśruta counts 30 as the dorsal and the lumbar vertebrae, for the reasons that the spinal column really consists of 33 irregular bony segments of which the upper 24 are separated during life by discs of spinous cartilaginous articular processes, and are therefore called "true" or "movable" vertebræ, in distinction from the lower 9 which are called the "false" or "fixed" vertebræ, for they become consolidated into the sacrum and the coccyx. The Hindu anatomists counted the constituent bones of the sacrum and the coccyx as separate bones as well as the spinous processes, belonging to the vertebræ. While the modern anatomists designate as vertebræ the upper 24 loose bones, consisting of the 'cervical' 7, 'dorsal' or 'thoracic' the succeeding 12, and the 'lumbar' the lower 5. The Hindu anatomists enumerated the cervical vertibræ as the 'grîvā' or neck bones, adding also to it the hyoid bone. In the wind-pipe (*kaṇṭhanalī*) the four cartilages—cuneiform, arytenoid, thyroid and cricoid, were counted as bones. The breast-bone is given by Suśruta to be 8, for he includes among the breast-bones the 2 collar bones and as the sternum really consists of three parts, the 'manubrium' which usually remains separate throughout life from the rest of the bone, the cartilaginous 'metasternum' and the 'corpus sterni' or 'mesosternum' which is formed by the fusion in early life of four segments.

So if we try to identify the nomenclature and designation of the ancient Hindu and the modern systems of osteology, it becomes clear that the Hindus had acquired a sound knowledge of the human skeleton. And the term 'skeleton' (*from the Gr. skeletos=dried*) is applied to the parts which remain after the softer tissues of the body have been disintegrated or removed and includes not only the bones ,but also the cartilages and ligaments which bind them together (Cunningham : *Anatomy*, p. 67). In this generic sense the Hindus described their bony frame-work, but classified the bones into five kinds according to their composition as flat (*kapāla*), tooth (*ruchaka*), tender (*taruṇa*), strong (*balaya*) and hollow (*nalaka*) bones.

(3) "These bones are of five kinds as the following:—'flat' bones, 'tooth' bones, 'tender' bones,

'strong' bones and 'hollow' bones. The bones of the knee, pelvis, shoulder, malar, palate and the head are flat bones. The teeth are of 'tooth' bones; the nose, ear, neck and the eyesockets are of 'tender' bones. Those of the hand, foot, sides, back and breast are of 'strong' bones. The rest of the bones are 'hollow'." *Suśruta* III. 5. 21. [3]

11. Arthrology.

In *Arthrology*, that is, in the description of the articulations or joints (*Sandhi*), Suśruta shows also remarkable accuracy. "Joints are of two kinds—'movable' (*diarthroses*) and unmovable (*amphiarthroses.*). In the four branches (*hands and feet*), in the jaw-bones and the loin, the joints are movable and the rest of the joints, the wise should regard as permanent (that is, of partial or incomplete movement).

"There are 200 joints in the body. Of them 68 are in the four extremities, 59 in the trunk and 83 above the shoulder (that is, in the neck and the head).

---

(3) एतानि पञ्चविधानि भवन्ति। तद्यथा—कपालरुचकतरुणवलयनलकसंज्ञानि। तेषां जानुनितम्बांसगण्डतालुशङ्खशिरःसु कपालानि। दशनास्तु रुचकानि। घ्राणकर्णग्रीवाक्षिकोषेषु तरुणानि। पाणिपादपार्श्वपृष्ठोदरोरःसु वलयानि शेषाणि नलकसंज्ञानि॥ २१ Suśruta III. 5, 21.

"In every toe there are 3,except the great toe (corresponding to the thumb) which has two joints, thus 14 ($4 \times 3 + 2 = 14$). The knee, ankle and hip has each a joint. So one foot has 17 joints; the other foot likewise, as well as both the arms.

"In the pelvis 3; in the spinal column 24; in the sides (*ribs*) 24; in the breast 8; in the (*vertebral-cervical*) neck 8; in the trachea 3; in the conjunction joints of the heart and lungs 18(*hṛdayaklomanibaddha*); in the sockets of teeth 32; 1 in the thyroid cartilage (*kākalaka*) and one in the nose; 2 between the eye-sockets and the eyeballs (*dvau vartmamaṇḍalau netrāśrayau*). In the malar, temporal and the ears 6; in the jaw bones 2; on the top of the brows 2; in the craniun 5 and 1 in the forehead.

"These joints are of eight kinds as:—gynglymoid (*kora*—a hinge joint),enarthrodial (*udūkhala* = mortar-like in shape ball-and-socket joint), enarthrodial (*sāmudga* = cup-like), costo-vertebral (*pratara* = raft-like), circular (*maṇḍala*), sutural (*tunnasevanī* = sewing) and symphysic (*conch-shell like*) joints. Interphalangeal (*gynglymus*-simple hinge joints, surrounded by a capsule), radiocarpal (*condyloid-ellypsoidal*), the ankle-joint (*gynglymus*), the knee-joint (*gynglymus*), the elbow-joint (*gynglymus*) are all '*kora*'; the shoulder-joint (*enarthrodial-ball-and-socket-joint*), the hip-joint (*enarthrodial*), teeth-sockets (*synarthrodial-immovable* ?), are all '*udūkhala* ; the sterno-clavicular joint (*diarthrodial*-freely movable), sacro-iliac joint (*diarthrodial*), symphysis pubis (*amphidiarthrodial*—a combined gliding and hinge joint), and lumbo-sacral joints (*amphidiarthrodial*) are all (*sâmudga*); cervical, dorsal and lumbar vertebral joints (*limited amphidiarthrodial*) are '*pratara*' ; the temporal and the cranium joints (*sutural*) are *tunnasevanï* ; trachea, heart, eye and lung-joints are *maṇḍala* ; the ear and the nose joints (*symphysic*) are *śankhāvartta*. According to the shape of the joints nomenclature has been fixed. Only the joints of the bones have been described. The joints of the muscles, nerves and arteries are countless". *Suśruta* III. 5. 23-29[3a]

3a. शाखासु हन्वोः कट्यांञ्च चेष्टावन्तस्तु सन्धयः ।
शेषास्तु सन्धयः सर्व्वे विज्ञेया हि स्थिरा बुधैः ॥ २३

सङ्घातस्तु दशोत्तरे द्वे शते । तेषां शाखास्वष्टषष्टिः, एकोनषष्टिः कोष्ठे, ग्रीवां प्रत्यूर्द्ध त्र्यशीतिः ॥ २४

एकैकस्यां पादाङ्गुल्यां त्रयस्त्रयः, द्वावङ्गुष्ठे,—ते चतुर्द्दश । जानुगुल्फवङ्क्षणेष्वेकैकः । एवं सप्तदशैकस्मिन् सक्थनि भवन्ति । एतेनेतरसक्थिबाहू च व्याख्यातौ ॥ २५

त्रयः कटीकपालेषु । चतुर्व्विंशतिः पृष्ठवंशे । तावन्त एव पार्श्वयोः उदरस्याष्टौ । तावन्त एव ग्रीवायाम् । त्रयः कण्ठे । नाड़ीषु हृदयक्लोमनिबद्धास्वष्टादश । दन्तपरिमाणा दन्तमूलेषु । एकः काकलके नासायाञ्च । द्वौ वर्त्ममण्डलजौ नेत्राश्रयौ ।

III. Myology

In myology, the muscular system, though Suśruta at first appears to be fantastical and vague, yet by comparative study, it can be easily seen that notwithstanding imperfection and clumsiness, there is some fundamental truth in the statement. Suśruta mentions 500 muscles (*peśī*) while Steadman's Medical Dictionary gives the names of 427 muscles. It is possible that Suśruta duplicates many continuous muscles and omits many deep-underlying muscles, especially of the upper part of the body.

	Muscles according to Suśruta.		Muscles according to Cunningham's Anatomy.	
I. The Lower Exremity				
Toe	3 × 5 = 15		3	
Fore foot	10		7	
Ankle & Sole	10		9	
Heel	10	2 tendons and 2 ligaments.	–	Leg and foot 25
Leg	20		12	
Knee	5	3 tendons and 4 ligaments.	–	

गण्डकर्णशङ्खेष्वेकैकः। द्वौ हनुसन्धी। द्वावुपरिष्टाद्भ्रुवोः। शङ्खयोश्च। पञ्च शिरःकपालेषु। एको मूर्द्धि्न॥ २६।२७

त एते सन्धयोऽष्टविधाः। कोरोदूखलसामुद्गप्रतरतुन्नसेवनीवायसतुण्डमण्डलशङ्खावर्त्ताः। तेषामङ्गुलिमणिबन्धगुल्फजानुकूर्परेषु कोराः सन्धयः कक्षावङ्क्षणदशनेषूदूखलाः। अंसपीठगुदभगनितम्बेषु सामुद्गाः। ग्रीवापृष्ठवंशयोः प्रतराः। शिरःकटीकपालेषु तुन्नसेवनी। हन्वोरुभयतस्तु वायसतुण्डाः। कण्ठहृदयनेत्रक्लोमनाड़ीषु मण्डलाः श्रोत्रशृङ्गाटकेषु शङ्खावर्त्ताः। तेषां नामभिरेवाकृतयः प्रायेण व्याख्याताः॥ २८

अस्थ्नान्तु सन्धयो ह्येते केवलाः परिकीर्त्तिताः।
पेशीस्नायुशिराणान्तु सन्धिसङ्ख्या न विद्यते २९

Thigh	20		22	Thigh and buttock 25 and 2 ligaments.
Groin	10		8	
	———		———	
	100			

II. The Trunk of the Body

Pelvic region	3		2	Ischio-coccygeus anp Levator Ani; but the 'Levator ani' is divisible into 4 parts.
Penis	1	Erector penis	1	Perineum 12
Spermatic cord	1		1	Spermatic cord passing through 'cremaster' muscle.
Testes	2		1	Dartos muscle in scrotum.
Bladder	2		1	Compressor Urethrae
Stomach	5	Thorax 12		
Breast	10			Anterior muscles of the Trunk 19
Abdomen	6		3	
Navel	1		-	
Shoulder	7		5	
Back	16		16	There are 16 superficial and and 15 deeper muscles in the back.
Buttocks	2 × 5 = 10		8	

Heart and Colon	2	3	myocardium and masculi papillares tunica muscularis (colon).

III. The Neck and the Head.

The back neck	4	6	
Jaws	2 × 4 = 8	5	
Thyroid	1 × 2 = 2	3	Thyro-hyoid, Stylo-hyoid and Sterno-hyoid.
Tongue	1	2	or 8. The 'extrinsic muscles': genio-glossus, hyoglossus, styloglossus and palato-glossus. The 'intrinsic muscles': superior lingualis, inferior lingualis, transverse fibres and vertical fibres.
Cheeks	1 × 2 = 2	5	The mouth 11 (eleven)
Nose	2	5	
Front neck	2 + 2 = 4	10	
Eye	1 × 2 = 2	7	in the orbit and 4 in the eye-lids.
Forehead	4	Frontalis 1	The scalp 6
Palate	2	Occipitalis and Trapezius 2	
The top of the head	1	1	Epicranial Aponeurosis
Ear	2	3	

IV. The Female Reproductive Organs

Mammae	5 × 2 = 10	5	Pectoralis major, serratus magnus, ligaments of Cooper, aponeurosis and recto abdominis muscles.
Vagina	2 + 2 = 4	2 + 3 = 5	Tunica muscularis, rugae vaginales, and (common bulbo cavernesus, sphincter ani, externeus levator ani and erector clitoridis = erector penis).
Uterus	3	3	Ligamentum latum uteri (broad ligament), ligamentum teres uteri (round ligament) and the muscular 'corpus uteri'.
Fallopian tube	3	3	Tunica muscularis, ligamentum ovarium proprium and mesovarium.

"There are 500 muscles [*peśī*]. 400 of them are in the 4 extremities, 66 in the trunk, and 34 above the shoulder (in the neck and the head).

"The toes (*pādāṅguli*) of each foot have 15 muscles, having 3 muscles for each toe ; 10 in the fore-foot (*pādāgre*) ; 10 in the heel (*kūrch-cha*) ; in the ankle and the sole (*gulpha-talayoḥ*) 10 ; between the ankle and the knee (*gulpha-jānvantare = leg*) 20 ; 5 in the knee (*jānu*) ; 20 in the thigh (*uru*) ; 10 in the groin (*vaṅkṣaṇa*) : thus in one foot there are 100 muscles ; so in the other foot and the two arms.

"In the pelvis (*pāyu*) 3 ; in the penis (*meḍhre*) 1 ; in the spermatic cord (*sevanī*) 1 ; in the testes (*vṛṣaṇ*) 2 ; in the buttocks (*sphicha*) 5 each ; in the upper part over the bladder (*vasti-śirasi*) 2 ; 5 in the stomach (*udara*) ; in the navel (*nābhi*) 1 ; in the upper back (*pṛṣṭh-ordha*) 5 longitudinal (*muscles*) on each side ; in the sides(of the spinal column = *pārśva*)6 ; 10 in the breast (*Vakṣa*) ; in the shoulder (*akṣakāṃsa*) 7 ; 2 in the heart and colon (*hṛdayāmāśaya*) ; 6 in the spleen, liver and the lower intestine (*yakṛt-plīhā-uṇḍuka = abdomen*).

"In the back part of the neck (*grīvā*) 4 ; 8 in the jaws (*hanu*) ; in the thyroid cartilage (*kākalaka*) 2 ; in the palate (*tālu*) 2 ; in the tongue (*jihvā*) 1 ; in the cheeks 2 ; in the nose (*ghoṇa*) 2 ; 2 in the eyes (*netra*); in the front neck (*gaṇ a*) 4 ; in the two ears (*karṇa*) 2 ; 4 in the forehead (*lalāṭa*), and 1 (*one*) on the top of the head (*śirasi*).

"A woman has 20 more muscles than man: 10 in the two mammæ (*stana*) at 5 each, which are developed in adolescence; in the vagina (*apatyapatha*) 4, two in the entrance and two in the interior; in the uterus (*garbha-cchidra*) 3 and in the fallopian tubes (*śukrārttava-praveśa*), the muscles are 3.

"According to the position, the muscles are grouped together (*vahula*), isolated (*pelava*), thick (*sthūla*), thin (*sūkṣma*), extensive (*pṛthu*), globular (*vṛtta = tendon*), short (*hrasva*), long-cylindrical (*dīrgha*), hard (*sthira*), soft (*mṛdu*), smooth (*ślakṣṇa* = unstriated, that is primitive involuntary muscles), striated (*karkaśa*-voluntary muscles with transverse stripes), and they cover the joints, bones, arteries and nervous fibres according to their respective needs.

"The muscles that have been mentioned of men in their penis and testicles, cover in women their interior reproductive organs." *Suśruta* III. 5. 37-45.[4]

4. पञ्च पेशीशतानि भवन्ति। तासां चत्वारि शतानि शाखासु। कोष्ठे षट्षष्टिः। ग्रीवां प्रत्यूर्द्ध्वं चतुस्त्रिंशत्॥ ३७

एकैकस्यान्तु पादाङ्गुल्यां तिस्रस्तिस्रस्ताः पञ्चदश। दश प्रपदे। पादोपरि कूर्चसन्निविष्टास्तावत्य एव। दश गुल्फतलयोः गुल्फजान्वन्तरे विंशतिः। पञ्च जानुनि।

The difference between Suśruta's 500 muscles and Stedman's 427 muscles, which if counted separately like Suśruta on both sides of the body would amount to nearly 800 muscles, can be easily accounted for by the fact that not only the modern classification and nomenclature of the muscles are different from the

---

विंशतिरूरौ। दश वङ्क्षणे। शतमेवमेकस्मिन् सक्थनि भवन्ति। एतेनेतरसक्थिबाहू च व्याख्यातौ ॥ ३८

तिस्रः पायौ। एका मेढ्रे। सेवन्याञ्चापरा। द्वे वृषणयोः। स्फिचोः पञ्च पञ्च। द्वे वस्तिशिरसि। पञ्चोदरे। नाभ्यामेका। पृष्ठोर्द्ध्वसन्निविष्टाः पञ्च पञ्च दीर्घाः। षट् पार्श्वयोः। दश वक्षसि। अक्षकांसौ प्रति समन्तात् सप्त। द्वे हृदयामाशययोः। षट् यकृत्प्लीहोण्डुकेषु ॥ ३९

ग्रीवायां चतस्रः। अष्टौ हन्वोः। एकैका काकलकगलयोः। द्वे तालुनि। एका जिह्वायाम्। ओष्ठयोर्द्वे। घोणायां द्वे। द्वे नेत्रयोः। गण्डयोश्चतस्रः। कर्णयोर्द्वे। चतस्रो ललाटे। एका शिरसि इत्येवमेतानि पञ्च पेशीशतानि ॥ ४०

शिरास्नाय्वस्थिपर्व्वाणि सन्धयश्च शरीरिणाम्।
पेशीभिः संवृतान्यत्र बलवन्ति भवन्त्यतः ॥ ४१

स्त्रीणान्तु विंशतिरधिका। दश तासां स्तनयोरेकैकस्मिन् पञ्च पञ्च, यौवने तासां परिवृद्धिः। अपत्यपथे चतस्रः, तासां प्रसृतेऽभ्यन्तरतो द्वे, मुखाश्रिते वाह्ये च प्रवृत्ते द्वे। गर्भच्छिद्रसंश्रितास्तिस्रः। शुक्रार्त्तवप्रवेशिन्यस्तिस्र एव ॥ ४२

पित्तपक्वाशयमध्ये गर्भाशयो यत्र गर्भस्तिष्ठति ॥ ४३

तासां बहलपेलवस्थूलाणुपृथुवृत्तह्रस्वदीर्घस्थिरमृदुश्लक्ष्णकर्कशभावाः सन्ध्यस्थिशिरास्नायुप्रच्छादका यथादेशं स्वभावत एव भवन्ति ॥ ४४

भवति चात्र—पुंसां पेश्यः पुरस्ताद्याः प्रोक्ता लक्षणमुष्कजाः।
स्त्रीणामावृत्य तिष्टन्ति फलमन्तर्गतं हि ताः ॥ ४५ ॥

ancient Hindu system, but Suśruta did not include the tendons (*māṃsa-rajju*) and ligaments (*sïmanta*) in the muscular order. It is evident from close comparative study that the Suśruta school of anatomy had tolerably sound knowledge of the human muscular system for all practical purposes.

Suśruta mentions 14 joints of more than 2 bones (*saṃghāta*) which are held together by a band or sheet of fibrous tissue, which he calls '*sïmanta*' that is ligament. He enumerated them in the following junctions :—"Three are in each foot at the ankle (a joint of *tibia, fibula* and *astragalus*, held together by,—*anterior tibio-fibular ligament, posterior tibio-fibular lig., talo-fibulare anterius, calcaneo-fibulare, talo-fibulare posterius* and *ligamentnm deltoideum*), at the knee (a joint of the *femur, tibia*, capped by the *patella*, held together by *ligamentum patellae, lig. Posticum Winslowii, lig. collaterale tibiale, lig. collaterale fibulare* and *ligamenta cruciata genu*), at the hip-joint (of the *femur, ilium* and *pubis*, held together by *lig. Transversum acetabuli, lig. ilio-femorale, lig. pubo-femorale, lig. ischio-capsulare*, and *lig. teres femoris*) : so in the arns at the wrist (a *radiocarpal articulation* between the *radius* and the *scaphoid, semilunar and cuneiform bones,* held together by the *external lateral ligament, internal lateral ligament, anterior* and *posterior ligaments*), at the elbow (a joint of *humerus, radius* and *ulna,* held together by the *anterior* and *posterior ligaments, lig. collaterale ulnar* and *lig. collaterale radiale*), and at the arm-pit (the shoulder-joint of the head of the *humerus, glenoid fossa* of *scapula* and the *coracoid process,* held together by *labrum glenoidale, capsula articularis* and *ligamentum coraco-humerale*). Accoding to others, there are 18 (ligaments). The above-mentioned 14, one at the pelvis (*sacro-iliac joint* of *sacrum, ilium* and *pubis,* held together by *lig. sacro-iliacum anterus, lig. sacro-iliacum posterus breve, lig. sacro-iliacum posterus longum, lig. ilio-lumbale, lig. sacro-tuberosum, lig. sacro-spinosum, lig. pubicum posterius, anterius, superius* and *inferius*), at the upper-breast (*sterno-clavicular* joint of the *sternum* and *clavicles* held together by *lig. sterno-claviculäris* and *lig. rhomboidale*) and the lower-breast (*sterno-costal* joints of the sternum and the seven costal cartilages held together by *lig. costo-sternalium radiatum. ligg. sterno-costalia interarticularia*) and at the neck (*scapulo-clavicular* joint held together by *lig. coraco-claviculare, lig conoideum* and *lig. trapezoideum*) *Suśruta* III. 5. 15-16[5]

It is very likely that Suśruta by *'sïmanta'* means only the synovial capsule and the membrane which are usually found at the joint of more than two bones and which he calls *'saṃghāta'*. By the general term *'sandhi'* he has designated the articular joint and which he has enumerated as 210 and the fibrous band which binds the bones at the joints together (*ligament*) and the muscles to the bones (*tendons,*) whether it is ligamentous or tendonous, he calls by the common designation *'snāyu'*-'to bind' and which he describes to be nine hundred (*III. 5. 30.*) And the large and strong tough fibrous longitudinal bands and chords are called *'kaṇḍara'*.

"*Kaṇḍaras* are 16 : 4 in feet (*tendo achilis* in the leg and *semimarbransus tendon* in the thigh), 4 in the arms (*supinator longus tendon* in the forearm, and the *semilunar* or *biceptial fascia tendon* in the arm,) 4 in the neck (*sterno-cleido-mastoid tendon, membrana tectora, membrana atlanto-occipitalis posterior, lig.cruciatam atlantis*

5. चतुर्दशास्थ्नां सङ्घाताः। तेषां त्रयो गुल्फजानुवङ्क्षणेषु। एतेनेतरसक्थि बाहू च व्याख्यातौ। त्रिकशिरसोरेकैकः ॥१५

चतुर्दशैव सीमन्ताः। ते चास्थिसंघातवद्गणनीयाः, यतस्तैर्युक्ता अस्थिसङ्घाताः। ये ह्युक्ताः सङ्घातास्तु खल्वष्टादशैकेषाम् ॥१६

with *crus superius* and *inferius*), 4 in the spinal column (*lig. longitudinale anterius, lig. longitudinale posterius, lig.flavum*, and *lig. supraspinale*). The terminals of the '*kaṇḍaras*' of the hand and feet are in the nails; those of the neck passing through the heart terminate in the sexual organ (*meḍhra*) and those of the spinal column passing through the pelvis terminate in the pubis." *Suśruta* III. 5. 10.[5a]

	Suśruta	Ligaments Tendons	
		1. The Extremities.	
Toe	5 × 6 = 30	27 + 5 = 32	Palmar band lig collateralia and synovial membrane at each interphalangeal joint, 2 in each toe and 1 in the large toe(*2 × 4 + 1 = 9*)and 5 dorsal extensor tendons.
Ankle }		5	Four ligaments and one synovial membrane
Heel }	30	5	Five tendons.
Sole }	28	18	intratarsal ligg. and 10 s. membrane.
Leg	30	28	
Thigh	40	34 .	
Hip-joint	10	8 + 1 = 9	
Knee-joint	10	7 + 3 = 10	
	150 × 4 = 600		

5a. षोड़श कण्डराः ; तासां चतस्रः पादयोस्तावत्यो हस्तग्रोवापृष्ठेषु । तत्र हस्तपाद-गतानां कण्डराणां नखाः प्ररोहाः । ग्रीवाहृदयनिबन्धिनीनामधोभागगतानां मेढ्रम् । श्रोणिपृष्ठनिबन्धिनीनामधोभागगतानां विम्बः । मूर्द्धोरुवक्षोऽंसपिण्डादीनाञ्च ॥१०

II. The Trunk.

Loin.	60	18	
Back-bone	80	71	Lig. interspinalia, lig. supra-spinalia, lig. flava—vel subflava and synovial membrane for each of the 12 thoracic and 5 lumbar vertebrae and 3 common ligaments for all.
Sides (24 ribs)	60	72	Lig. capituli costae radiatum, lig. capituli costae interarticulare and synovial membrane for each of the 24 costo-vertebral articulations.
	30	56	Lig. costo-sternalium radiatum, lig. costo-xiphoidea, lig. sterno-costalia interarticularia and the posterior costo-sternal ligament for each of the 14 ribs (7 *pairs*)
	230		

III. The Neck and the Head.

Neck	36	52	4 Ligaments for each of the 7 cervical vertebrae, sterno-clavicular 12 and acromo-clavicular ligaments 12.
Head	34	31	Occipito-atloid joints 2 and each is provided with 8 ligaments, membrana atlanto occipitalis anterior, membrana occipitalis posterior, membrana tectora, lig. cruciatum atlantis, lig. alaria, lig. apicis dentis, capsular ligament and synovial membrane; atlo-axoid joints are three, each supplied with 5 ligaments, lig. transversum atlantis, capsular, anterior and posterior atlo-axoid ligaments and synovial membrane.
	70		
Total	900[6]		*Suśruta* III. 5, 30—32[6]

6. नव स्नायुशतानि। तासां शाखासु षट् शतानि। द्वे शते त्रिंशच्च कोष्ठे। ग्रीवां प्रत्यूर्द्ध्वं सप्ततिः ॥३०

एकैकस्यान्तु पादाङ्गुल्यां षट् निचितास्तास्त्रिंशत्। तावत्य एव तलकूर्चगुल्फेषु। तावत्य एव जङ्घायाम्। दश जानुनि। चत्वारिंशदूरौ। दश वङ्क्षणे। शतमध्यर्द्धमेवमेकस्मिन् सक्थनि भवन्ति। एतेनेतरसक्थिबाहू च व्याख्यातौ ॥३१

षष्टिः कट्याम्। अशीतिः पृष्ठे। पार्श्वयोः षष्टिः। उरसि त्रिंशत् ॥३२

It will be noticed that there is a marked discrepancy between the two figures. And it may be due to the different methods of calculation and classification, or it is possible that by *'snāyu,'* Charaka and Suśruta meant something entirely different from the ligament and the tendon. The general tendency of the Sanskrit scholars is to regard *'snāyu'* as nerve. But this is contradicted by its etymological derivation from *'snā'*. or *'si'*, to bind and the Suśruta mentions 210 joints, but does not say anything anywhere else of the binding material that holds them together excepting of 14 *'sīmanta'* at the junction of more than two bones (*saṃghāta*).* He could not possibly omit to mention the binding material of the rest of the joints, when he has been minute in every other detail. And moreover the internal evidence tends to prove that he meant by *'snāyu'*, ligaments and tendons as he says :—"*Snāyus* are of four kinds—branching (*pratānavatī*), globular (*vṛtta*), extensive (*pṛthu*) and perforated (*śuṣira.*) The *'snāyus'* in the four branches and joints are branching ; *'kaṇḍaras'* (the large *snāyus*) are globular; the *'snāyus'* of the anterior parts of the stomach, intestine and the bladder are perforated ; the *'snāyus'* of the sides, breast, back-bone and the head are extensive.

"As a boat of wooden planks well tied by many knots, can bear the weight of animals and goods in water, so a man can carry weight as his joints are knotted together by '*snāyus*'. The body does not suffer as much by the destruction of the bones, muscles or joints as by the destruction of '*snāyus*'. The physician that knows well the internal and superficial '*snāyus*' can only extract from the body, the deeply impregnated missiles". "*Suśruta* III. 5. 34-36."[7]

"The flesh (of the body) being tied to the bones by vascular system and '*snāyus*', do not tear out and fall down". *Suśruta* III. 5. 22.[8]

---

7. स्नायुश्चतुर्व्विधा विद्यात् तास्तु सर्ब्बा निबोध मे ।
प्रतानवत्यो वृत्ताश्च पृथ्वयश्च शुषिरास्तथा ॥३४
प्रतानवत्यः शाखासु सर्व्वसन्धिषु चाप्यथ ।
वृत्तास्तु कण्डराः सर्ब्बा विज्ञेयाः कुशलैरिह ॥
आमपक्वाशयान्तेषु वस्तौ च शुषिराः खलु ।
पार्श्वोरसि तथा पृष्ठे पृथुलाश्च शिरस्यथ ॥३५
नौर्यथा फलकास्तीर्णा बन्धनैर्बहुभिर्युता ।
भारक्षमा भवेदप्सु नृयुक्ता सुसमाहिता ॥
एवमेव शरीरेऽस्मिन् यावन्तः सन्धयः स्मृताः ।
स्नायुभिर्बहुभिर्बद्धास्तेन भारसहा नराः ॥
न ह्यस्थीनि न वा पेश्यो न शिरा न च सन्धयः ।
व्यापादितास्तथा हन्युर्यथा स्नायुः शरीरिणाम् ॥
यः स्नायूः प्रविजानाति वाह्याश्चाभ्यन्तरास्तथा ।
स गूढ़ं शल्यमाहर्त्तुं देहाच्छक्नोति देहिनाम् ॥३६

8. मांसान्यत्र निबद्धानि शिराभिः स्नायुभिस्तथा ।
अस्थीन्यालम्बनं कृत्वा न शीर्य्यन्ते पतन्ति वा ॥२२

IV.—The Vascular System.

The *vascular system* (*Śira* = tubular vessel) is no less difficult, rather more so, as it defies all human ingenuity to describe it in tabulated figures. For the arteries bifurcate into branches and twigs, and spread out all over the body in infinite shape and size; the veins commence at the terminations of the capillaries and as they converge towards the heart, they form larger and still larger vessels, uniting with one another until finally seven large trunks empty their contents into the auricles of the heart; likewise the lymphatic and the nervous networks. Hardly two vessels are of equal length, size, shape and dimension in two different parts of the body. Therefore any comparison is necessarily to be more or less of guess-work. In the following table only the large and distinctive longitudinal vessels have been counted from the '*Atlas of Applied Topographical Anatomy*' of Karl von Bardeleben and Heinrich Haeckel and the '*Regional Anatomy*' of George Mc Clellan. It seems that Suśruta includes the nervous net-work in the vascular system which he divides into four classes, nervous (*Vāta*—air), venous (*pitta*-bile), lymphatic (*kapha*-phlegm) and arterial (*raktavaha-śira*-blood-carrying vessel). The identification of the '*vāta, pitta, kapha* and *raktavahā śiras*' with the nervous, venous, lymphatic and arterial systems is not far-feched and fanciful. For Suśruta says :—"The '*vāta*'-carrying vessels are of tawny or light-golden-brown (*aruṇa*) colour, and are filled with air; '*pitta*'-carrying vessels are all warm and of blue (*nīla*) colour ; '*kapha*' bearing vessels are cool and of white (*śveta*) colour; the blood-carrying vessels are of red (*lohita*) colour and are neither warm nor cold." III. 7. 13[8a].

"There are seven hundred tubular vessels : as gardens by water-conduits and fields by canals are irrigated and nourished, so by the irrigating and draining action of the '*śiras*,' the body is nourished and sustained. As the midrib of a plant-leaf gives off laterally countless veins, so from the main (*śiras*) small and smaller branches spread out." *Suśruta* III. 7. 2[9].

8a. तत्रारुणा वातवहाः पूर्य्यन्ते वायुना शिराः।
पित्तादुष्णाश्च नीलाश्च शीता गौर्य्यः स्थिराः कफात्।
असृग्वहास्तु रोहिण्यः शिरा नात्युष्णशीतलाः॥ १३

9. सप्त शिराशतानि भवन्ति ; याभिरिदं शरीरमाराम इव जलहारिणीभिः केदार इव च कुल्याभिरुपस्निह्यतेऽनुगृह्यते चाकुञ्चनप्रसारणादिभिर्विशेषैः। द्रुमपत्रसेवनीनामिव च तासां प्रतानाः। तासां नाभिर्मूलं, ततश्च प्रसरन्त्यूर्द्ध्वमधस्तिर्य्यक् च ॥२

	Suśruta	Nerve-trunks	Veins	Arteries	Lymph vessels	Lymph
I. The Four Branches						
Foot (Lower extremity)	25	30	22	19	16	
Arm (Upper extremity)	25	26	33	21	23	
II. The Trunk						
Pelvic region	8	7	8	10	12	19
Sides	2p	9p	9p	9p	9p	* (p = pair)
Back-bone	6	17				
Breast	10	15	7	10	10	12
Stomach	6	9	6	7	6	11
III. Neck and Head.						
Neck	14	15	14	15	16	10
Ear	2p	2	1	1		Nerves : ramus vestibularis and cochlearis ; auditory artery dividing into 3 branches ; internal auditory vein.
Nose	6	7	6	5	3	
Tongue	9	5	4	5	4	
Eye	4p	4	5	5		Nerves : frontal, oculo-motor, optic,

trochlear ; Veins : vena vorticosa, retinal, conjunctival, choroid and ciliary ; arteries ; arteria centralis retinae, suprascleral, ciliary, choroid & conjunctival.

"The nervous (*vāta*), the venous (*pitta*), lymphatic (*kapha*) vessels are 175 each as well as the arterial (blood-carrying *śiras*) passing the liver and the spleen. Thus seven hundred '*śiras*' spread out all over the body. In one foot, there are 25 nerve-vessels; likewise in the other foot and each of the arms. There are 34 nerve-vessels in the trunk of the body: in the pelvic region 8, in the sides 2 each, in the back 6, and in the breast 10, above the shoulder, there are 45: in the neck 14, in the two ears 4, in the tongue 9 and both the eyes 8. Thus 175 nerve-vessels are described. And this description also corresponds to that of the venous, lymphatic and the arterial (blood-carrying) vessels, with this exception that instead of 8 nerve-vessels in the eyes and 4 in the ears, there are 10 (in the eyes) and 2 (in the ears) of the venous, lymphatic and blood-carrying (arterial) vessels." *Suśruta* III. 5. 7. 5-7[10].

---

10. तासां मूलशिराश्चत्वारिंशत्—तासां वातवाहिन्यो दश, पित्तवाहिन्यो दश, कफवाहिन्यो दश, दश रक्तवाहिन्यः। तासान्तु वातवाहिनीनां वातस्थानगतानां पञ्चसप्ततिशतं भवात, तावत्य एव पित्तवाहिन्यः पत्तस्थाने, कफवाहिन्यश्च कफस्थाने, रक्तवाहिन्यश्च यकृत्प्लीह्नोः—एवमेतानि सप्त शिराशतानि ॥५

तत्र वातवाहिन्यः शिरा एकस्मिन् सक्थ्नि पञ्चविंशतिः। एतेनेतरसक्थिबाहू च व्याख्यातौ। विशेषतस्तु कोष्ठे चतुस्त्रिंशत्;—तासां गुदमेढ्राश्रिताः श्रोण्यामष्टौ,

That the heart was the centre of the circulatory system, of the blood, was well understood by *Suśruta* (1. 14. 3-6) and according to Charaka it has 10 out-going (*arterial*) and in-coming (*venous*) trunk-vessels (1. 30. 1).

"Though chyle [*rasa*] circulates all throughout the body, its principal centre is the heart (*hṛdaya*). That chyle in 24 tubular vessels, 10 upwards, 10 downwards and 4 sideways, enters into every part of the body, irrigates and maintains its growth, vitalizes and supports life...... . Though chyle is aquatic in nature but in its passage through the liver and the spleen, it becomes blood. *Suśruta* 1. 14. 3-5.[11]

द्वे द्वे पार्श्वयोः, षट् पृष्ठे, तावत्य एव चोदरे, दश वक्षसि। एकचत्वारिंशज्जत्रुण ऊर्द्ध ;—तासां चतुर्द्दश ग्रीवायां, कर्णयोश्चतस्रः, नव जिह्वायां, षट् नासिकायाम्, अष्टौ नेत्रयोः। एवमेतत् पञ्चसप्तत्यधिकशतं वातवहानां शिराणां व्याख्यातम् ॥६

एष एव विभागः शेषाणामपि। विशेषतस्तु पित्तवाहिन्यो नेत्रयोर्दश, कर्णयोर्द्वे। एवं रक्तवहाः कफवहाश्च। एवमेतानि सप्त शिराशतानि सविभागानि व्याख्यातानि ॥७

11. तस्य हृदयं स्थानं, स हृदयाच्चतुर्व्विंशतिं धमनीरनुप्रविश्योर्द्धगा दश दश चाधोगामिन्यश्चतस्रस्तिर्य्यग्गाः कृत्स्नं शरीरमहरहस्तर्पयति वर्द्धयति धारयति यापयति जीवयति चादृष्टहेतुकेन कर्म्मणा ॥३

तस्य शरीरमनुधावतोऽनुमानाद्गतिरुपलक्षयितव्या क्षयवृद्धिवैकृतैः। तस्मिन् सर्व्वशरीरावयवदोषधातुमलाशयानुसारिणि रसे जिज्ञासा, किमयं सौम्यस्तैजस इति। अत्रोच्यते स खलु द्रवानुसारी स्नेहनजीवनतर्पणधारणादिभिर्विशेषैः सौम्य इत्यवगम्यते ॥४

"In the heart there are ten great out-going [*mahāmulā*] and in-coming [*mahāphalā*] tubular vesseles [*dhamanī*]." Charaka 1. 30. 1[11a]. The ten great vessels are the seven main trunk veins and three arteries as follows: (1) superior vena cava, [2] interior vena cava, [3] coronary sinus, [4-7] vena pulmonalis ; [8] left pulmonary artery, [9] aorta, [10] right pulmonary artery.

"Below the heart, on the left side the liver and the lung, and on the right side, the spleen and the lung, are situated." *Suśruta* III. 4. 30[12].

According to Charaka the skin consists of six strata (IV. 7. 2)[13] but Suśruta more accurately describes them to be seven. III. 4. 3[14].

11a. अर्थे दश महामूलाः सिराः सक्ता महाफलाः।
महच्चार्थश्च हृदयं पर्य्यायैरुच्यते बुधैः॥

12. शोणितकफप्रसादजं हृदयं, यदाश्रया हि धमन्यः प्राणवहाः। तस्याधो वामतः प्लीहा फुस्फुसश्च, दक्षिणतो यकृत् क्लोम च ॥३०

13. सर्व्वं शरीरमभिसंचक्षाणाद् यथाप्रश्नमेकमनाः। यथावच्छरीरे षट् त्वचस्तद्-यथा—उदकधरा त्वग् बाह्या, द्वितीया त्वग्रसृग्धरा, तृतीया सिध्मकिलाससम्भवाधिष्ठाना, चतुर्थी कुष्ठसम्भवाधिष्ठाना, पञ्चमी अलजीविद्रधीसम्भवाधिष्ठाना, षष्ठी तु सा यस्यां छिन्नायां ताम्यत्यन्ध इव च तमः प्रविशति यां चाप्यधिष्ठायारूंषि जायन्ते पर्व्वसन्धिषु कृष्णरक्तानि स्थूलमूलानि दुश्चिकित्स्यतमानि चेति, षट् त्वच एताः षडङ्गं शरीरमवतत्य तिष्ठन्ति।

14. तस्य खल्वेवंप्रवृत्तस्य शुक्रशोणितस्याभिपच्यमानस्य क्षीरस्येव सन्तानिकाः सप्त त्वचो भवन्ति। तासां प्रथमावभासिनी नाम, या सर्व्वं वर्णानवभासयति पञ्चविधाञ्च च्छायां प्रकाशयति ; सा व्रीहेरष्टादशभागप्रमाणा, सिध्मपद्मकण्टकाधिष्ठाना द्वितीया लोहिता नाम, षोड़शभागप्रमाणा तिलकालकन्यच्छव्यङ्गाधिष्ठाना। तृतीया

Suśruta		Strata of the skin according to Modern anatomy	
Avbhāsinî	Epidermis	Stratum corneum	
Lohitā		Stratum intermedium	Stratum lucidum
Śvetā		Stratum disjunctum	
Tāmrā		Stratum granulosum	
Vedinî		Stratum mucosum	
Rohiṇî		Stratum germinativum	
Māṃsadharā		Corium	

From the foregoing comparative charts, it will be seen, that though the ancient Hindu anatomical school erred in some details, but in fundamentals, their knowledge was remarkably accurate, minute and thorough, especially when we take into consideration the dim and distant age, in which these medical treatises were composed. The study of anatomy was regarded essential in the medical education and practice. Charaka says :—"In the medical science, knowledge of anatomy is necessary ; one can only understand principles of hygiene, when he has

श्वेता नाम, द्वादशभागप्रमाणा चर्म्मदलाजगल्लीमशकाधिष्ठाना। चतुर्थी ताम्रा नामाष्टभागप्रमाणा विविधकिलासकुष्ठाधिष्ठाना। पञ्चमी वेदिनी नाम, ब्रीहिपञ्चभागप्रमाणा कुष्ठविसर्पाधिष्ठाना। षष्ठी रोहिणी नाम, ब्रीहिप्रमाणा ग्रन्थ्यपच्यर्व्वुदश्लीपदगलगण्डाधिष्ठाना। सप्तमी मांसधरा नाम, ब्रीहिद्वयप्रमाणा भगन्दरविद्रध्यर्शोऽधिष्ठाना। यदेतत् प्रमाणं निर्द्दिष्टं तन्मांसलेष्ववकाशेषु; न ललाटे सूक्ष्माङ्गुल्यादिषु। यतो वक्ष्यत्युदरेषु ब्रीहिमुखेणाङ्गुष्ठोदरप्रमाणमवगाढं विध्येदिति ॥२

studied bodily sciences (anatomy and physiology) IV. 6. 1[15].

Suśruta recommends dissection. He says: "The parts and the parcels (of the body) that have been mentioned up to the skin, can not at all be described without dissection. So if a surgeon wants to aquire positive (doubtless) knowledge, he should analyse thoroughly all the parts and organs of a body, after disinfecting it. Occular observation easily supplements studies and adds to knowledge. (The way a corpse should be taken for observation is described thus). The corpse should possess all the organs and not be deceased of any long illness or of poisoning, nor should it be of a man of a hundred years of age. The contents of its viscera (urine and feces) should be removed and it should be kept in a stream without current to rot. A platform should be made in the water to lay the corpse on it and cover the whole body with hay, grasses and leaves, so that fish can not eat it, and it is not put out of its place. In seven days, it will decompose sufficiently and then rub it gently from the skin to the interior with

---

15. शरीरविचयः शरीरोपकारार्थमिष्यते भिषग्विद्यायाम। ज्ञात्वा हि शरीरतत्त्वं शरीरोपकारकरेषु भावेषु ज्ञानमुत्पद्यते तस्मात् शरीरविचयं प्रशंसन्ति कुशलाः।

grass, hair or bamboo-skin and observe minutely every organ and every part of the body. *Suśruta*, III. 5. 49-50[16].

In the Hippocratic collection of writings, though there is no systematic presentation of muscles, ligaments, blood-vessels and glands, yet their knowledge and position are clearly indicated in the books '*peri arthron*' (articulations) '*peri osteon physios*' (the nature of bones), '*peri adenon*' (glands), '*peri sarkon*' (flesh) and '*mochaikos*'. However their description is very vague and meagre, as being mentioned indirectly in connection with the treatment for dislocation and fracture of bones.

Galen was undoubtedly, par excellence, the greatest of ancient anatomists. The manner

16. त्वक्पर्य्यन्तस्य देहस्य योऽयमङ्गविनिश्चयः ।
शल्यज्ञानादृते नैष वर्ण्यते ऽङ्गेषु केषुचित् ॥
तस्मान्निःसंशयं ज्ञानं हर्त्रा शल्यस्य वाञ्छता ।
शोधयित्वा मृतं सम्यग्द्रष्टव्योऽङ्गविनिश्चयः ॥
प्रत्यक्षतो हि यद्दृष्टं शास्त्रदृष्टञ्च यद्भवेत् ।
समासतस्तदुभयं भूयो ज्ञानविवर्द्धनम् ॥४९

तस्मात् समस्तगात्रमविषोपहतमदीर्घव्याधिपीड़ितमवर्षशतिकं निःसृष्टान्त्रपुरीषं-पुरुषमवहन्त्यामापगायां निवद्धं पञ्जरस्थं मुञ्जवल्कलकुशशणादीनामन्यतमेनावेष्टिताङ्गम प्रकाशे देशे कोथयेत्। सम्यक् प्रकुथितञ्चोद्धृत्य ततो देहं सप्तरात्रादुशीरवालवेणु वल्कलकूर्चीनामन्यतमेन शनैः शनैरवघर्षयंस्त्वगादीन् सर्व्वानेव वाह्याभ्यन्तराङ्गप्रत्यङ्ग-विशेषान् यथोक्तान् लक्षयेच्चक्षुषा ॥५०

and methods of his narration, the style of his language, the accuracy of his description, make the anatomical study, not only instructive, but captivating and refreshing. He divides his monumental work, "*The Utilities of the Human Body*" which became the classic and the standard authority in human anatomy in Europe and the Saracen empire for more than fourteen centuries, into 17 books or chapters as follows: —I. Hand; II. Hand, fore-arm and the arm; III. Abdomen; IV. Alimentary organs and their auxiliaries; V. Alimentary organs and their auxiliaries; VI. Respiratory organs; VII. Vocal organs; VIII. The head, brain and the senses; IX. The cranium, the brain and the cranial nerves; X. The eyes and their auxiliaries; XI. The face, especially the jaw-bones; XII. The neck and the rest of the spine; XIII. The pelvic structure; XIV. Genital organs; XV. Genital organs; XVI. Nerves, arteries and veins; XVII. Epilogue—Difference between function and utility. On every organ and every part of the body, Galen gives a comparative review of the similar structure of other animals and philosophic generalisations as to the origin and development of organs, which he ascribes to functional utility and adaptation as a means of self-preservation and reproduction and thereby anticipating Lamarck (1744-1829) by nearly seventeen centuries. Below is given a short translation of his introductory general remarks on the 'genital organs', as a sample, believing that it will interest more readers than any other part of the body.

"Nature has three objects in view in the structural formation of the animal; she has created them really, either for preservation of life as the brain, heart and the liver, or for the convenience of life as the eyes, ears, nose and hands, or for the perpetuation of the race as the external genital parts as the testicles and the matrix; now we have previously demonstrated in detail, that any of the parts, either created for (preservation of) life, or for its embellishment, could not be better devised than what they are actually. It still remains for us to explain in this book, the parts, destined for the perpetuation of race among us.

"First of all, nature would have desired, if it were possible, to create her work immortal. Nature not permitting it, she has invented the expedient she could to obtain immortality for it (her creation), as a clever founder of a city, who not only cares that his city is actually peopled, but takes all precautions that it lasts for ever, at least as long as possible. However it does not appear that any city has been fortunate on that point, to have lasted so long that time has completely effaced the memory of its founder. But works of nature have lasted for thousands of years and shall live still, by the admirable means, she has invented to substitute always a new animal for a dead animal.

"What is then the means adopted among animals and man, so that no race perishes, on the contrary each race remains intact and immortal? That is what I propose to explain in this book, in commencing with my exposition. Nature has given to all animals organs of conception and she has associated with those organs a special impulse of pleasure of generation and filled the soul with such an irrestable desire, quite unexplainable with their functional uses, that the animals erotically excited and impassioned, especially the adolescent, though deprived of reason and understanding, attend to the perpetuation of the race, as if they were completely reasonable. One should think that nature really knowing that the objects she has created, being not susceptible of perfect wisdom, has given the animals, as a substitute for that wisdom, the allurement of intense pleasure, associated with the usage of those organs to assure the salvation and conservation of the race.

"It is just to admire, first, the ingenious device of nature and then the structure of the organs which naturally correspond for each animal to its bodily form. You would learn from us one day, concerning other animals when we fill the gap, left by Aristotle. For the human species, all the world knows and understands, to what degree of utility, the external genitals by their convenient situation, their dimension, their figure and their entire conformation, have attained. When you will know the utility of each organ, profoundly hidden, organs which are revealed by dissection, you will admire, I am sure, the art that has created them.

"In fact, nature has placed the matrix beneath the stomach, the region she has recognized as the most favourable for copulation, reception of the sperm and especially for the growth of the embryo so that the fetus can attain to a perfect state. You could not find, in fact, in any part of the animal, another region more suitable, for any of the purposes above-mentioned ; this is the best (place)for copulation, being far removed from the facial organs; most favourable for the growth of the fetus, being capable of considerable distension without difficulty and finally, the most convenient for the child-birth, as it is the easiest for the baby to slip off downwards to the inferior parts and the legs. In fact, the mouth of the matrix, which nature has formed as a passage for the entrance of the sperm and the departure of the embryo when it has reached its complete development, opens in the vagina. When the animal has conceived, the mouth(of the matrix)closes so firmly, it will not permit the least thing either to escape or to penetrate; during copulation, it dilates and extends in such a way that the sperm has an easy and large passage to the matrix."

II. PHYSIOLOGY

"*'Anna'* (food) supplies the body with *'dhātu'* (elements) for its up-building and preservation." *Suśruta* 1. 14. 11 [17]. Food is converted in the alimentary tract into *'rasa'* (chyle) by *'antaragni'* (internal fire or combustion, that is oxidation). Oxidation takes place by the natural warmth of the *'pitta'* (bile = sanguinary principle) of the body. "As fire in a hearth converts rice and water of a cooking pot into food and foam, so the digestive-fire (*pachatyagni*) converts the ingested food and drink into chyle and *'mala'* (excreta = feces and urine)." Charaka VI. 15. 6 [18]. The bile-duct being situated above the alimentary receptacle, digestion is facilitated by the favourable situation as that of the sun and the moon. (The idea being that as cooking easily takes place when the cooking-pot is placed upon the fire and not below it or sideways, so the stomach being situated above the bile-duct, which was regarded as the fire-principle, easy

---

17. अन्नात् पानाच्च मतिमानाचाराच्चाप्यतन्द्रितः ।
तत्र रस गतौ धातुरहरहर्गच्छतीत्यतो रसः ॥११

18. एवं रसमलायान्नमाशयस्थमधःस्थितः ।
पचत्यग्निर्यथा स्थाल्यामोदनायाम्बु तण्डुलम् ॥

digestion was the natural consequence). Due to the rich aquatic content of the place, ingested food and drink are easily softened, favouring digestion. *Suśruta* 1. 21. 16.[19]

"Now the question is whether the (digestive) fire is a different thing from '*pitta*' (the bile) or the bile is the fire ? The answer is that due to its caloric quality, '*pitta*' acts as fire in its action of cooking (*pachana*) and oxidation (*dahana*) and therefore, the bile is called the 'internal fire' (*oxidase*). *Suśruta* 1. 21. 9[20].

"The chyle (*rasa*) though aquatic, becomes red during its passage through the liver and the spleen. In the radiant heat of the body, the qualified chyle becomes red, and is called the '*rakta*' (blood)." *Suśruta* 1. 14. 5-6.[21]

---

19. श्लेष्मस्थानान्यत ऊर्द्ध्वं वक्ष्यामः। तत्रामाशयः पित्ताशयस्योपरिष्टात् तत्प्रत्यनीकत्वादूर्द्ध्वगतित्वात् तेजसश्चन्द्र इवादित्यस्य ; स चतुर्व्विधस्याहारस्याधारः। स च तत्रौदकैर्गुणैराहारः प्रक्लिन्नो भिन्नसङ्घातः सुखजरो भवति ॥१६

20. तत्र जिज्ञास्यं, किं पित्तव्यतिरेकादन्योऽग्निः, आहोस्वित् पित्तमेवाग्निः इति। अत्रोच्यते,—न खलु पित्तव्यतिरेकादन्योऽग्निरुपलभ्यते, आग्नेयत्वात् पित्ते दहनपचनादिष्वभिवर्त्तमानेऽग्निवदुपचारः क्रियतेऽन्तरग्निरिति। क्षीणे ह्यग्निगुणे तत्समानद्रव्योपयोगादतिप्रवृद्धे शीतक्रियोपयोगादागमाच्च पश्यामो न खलु पित्तव्यतिरेकादन्योऽग्निरिति ॥९

21. स खल्वाप्यो रसो यकृत्प्लीहानौ प्राप्य रागमुपैति ॥५

भवतश्चात्र

रञ्जितास्तेजसा त्वापः शरीरस्थेन देहिनाम्।
अव्यापन्नाः प्रसन्नेन रक्तमित्यभिधीयते ॥६

"Chyle is transformed into blood, blood into flesh, flesh into fat, fat into bone, bone into marrow and marrow into semen." *Suśruta* 1. 14. 10.[22]

"Because the chyle is transformed into '*dhātu*' (elements or bodily substances), and it constantly circulates in the body, it is called the '*rasa*'.

"This '*rasa*' remains in each '*dhātu*' 3500 moments (that is, the chyle is formed the same day, but it takes five days for the chyle to be transformed into blood and blood into flesh etc.) and thus in one month it is converted into the semen of man and '*ārttava*' (the rupture of the Graafian vesicles with the ripeness of the ova, or the menstrual blood which is associated with the occurrence) of woman." *Suśruta* 1. 14.11-12[23].

Semen "circulates in every part of the body of all living beings ; as fat in the milk, sugar in the sugar-cane juice, so is the semen (*śukra*)

---

22. रसाद्रक्तं ततो मांसं मांसान्मेदः प्रजायते ।
मेदसोऽस्थि ततो मज्जा मज्ज्ञः शुक्रस्य सम्भवः ॥१०

23. तत्र रस गतौ धातुरहरहर्गच्छतीत्यतो रसः ॥११
स खलु त्रीणि त्रीणि कलासहस्राणि पञ्चदश च कला एकैकस्मिन् धाताववतिष्ठते ।
एवं मासेन रसः शुक्रीभवति स्त्रीणाञ्चार्त्तवमिति ॥१२

present in the human body." *Suśruta* III. 4. 20-21[24]. It is not manifest in the children for it is present in a small quantity as the sweet aroma and delicate fragrance of a flower is not perceived in a young bud before time develops and ripens it, though its presence can not be doubted in an elementary state. *Suśruta* I. 14. 15[24a].

"In the living body, there are as many circulations as are present in the body like the chyle and the blood etc. for in the living body without circulation, they can not be produced or reduced." *Charaka* III. 5. 1[25].

"The centre of the vitalizing (*prāṇavaha*) circulation is the heart and the great trunks (*mahāsrota*) of arteries and veins). *Charaka* III. 5. 3[26].

---

24. सप्तमी शुक्रधरा नाम, या सर्व्वप्राणिनां सर्व्वशरीरव्यापिनी ॥२०

भवन्ति चात्र

यथा पयसि सर्पिस्तु गुड़श्चेचो रसे यथा ।
शरीरेषु तथा शुक्रं नृणां विद्याद्भिषग्वर: ॥२१

24(a). यथा हि पुष्पमुकुलस्थो गन्धो न शक्यमिहास्तीति वक्तुं नैव नास्तीत्यथवास्ति, सतां भावानामभिव्यक्तिरिति ज्ञात्वा केवलं सौक्ष्म्यान्नाभिव्यज्यते स एव गन्धो विवृतपत्रकेशरे कुसुमे कालान्तरेणाभिव्यक्तिं गच्छति ; एवं बालानामपि वय:परिणामात् शुक्रस्य प्रादुर्भावो भवति । रोमराज्यादयोऽथार्त्तवादयश्च विशेषा नारीणां रजसि चोपचीयमाने शनै: शनै: स्तनगर्भाशययोन्यभिवृद्धिर्भवति ॥१५

25. यावन्त: पुरुषे मूर्त्तिमन्तो भावविशेषास्तावन्त एवास्मिन् स्रोतसां प्रकारविशेषा: । सर्व्वे भावा हि पुरुषे नान्तरेण स्रोतांस्यभिनिर्व्वर्त्तन्ते चाप्यधिगच्छन्ति ।

26. तत्र प्राणवहानां स्रोतसां हृदयं मूलं महास्रोतश्च ।

"As the fibres of the water-lily and lotus stalks are naturally perforated, so in the tubular vessels, there are minute pores in the tubular vessels (*dhamanï*) throuch whigh the *'rasa'* circulates." *Suśruta* IV. 9. 9;.

I. Digestion.

From the above quotations, it can be seen that the ancient Hindu school of medicine grasped the essential fundamentals of digestion and circulation, though the intricate and complex process of their mechanism was not and could not be understood by them. Physiological chemistry is of but very recent development and growth. A few years ago, it was not even suspected that the digestion and absorption were due to the fermentative action of the glandular secretions. The digestive ferments or enzymes reduce the ingested food particles by cleavage into their elemental compounds by creating molecular instability through their electro-chemical action and in proportion as the food-stuffs are altered thus in the alimentary canal and transformed from insoluble into soluble substances, from such as are not diffusible into such

---

27. यथा स्वभावतः खानि मृणालेषु विसेषु च ।
धमनीनां तथा खानि रसो यैरुपचीयते ॥९

as are easily diffused, and they are absorbed by the epithelium of the gastro-intestinal mucous membrane and are synthetized into chyle during the passage through the restitutive secretion of the cells. The reaction of the enzymic activity upon the ingested food-particles, is the reduction and cleavage into their component elements, which is the same thing as oxidation The Hindus understood that digestion was concommitant with oxidation (*antaragni*), but did not know that the oxidation was caused by the digestive ferments.

'*Rasa*' has been translated as the chyle, for it is the most appropriate available term. But '*rasa*' is more than chyle. '*Rasa*' is the whole of the soluble and diffusible solution of the digested food which being partially regenerated and synthetized during its passage through the mucous membrane by the anabolic restitutive secretions of the living cells, either enters into the lymph sinuses of the mucosa, or are absorbed by the solitary and agminated follicles and by the lymph-glands interposed along the lacteals or are taken up by the blood capillaries of the mucous coat, especially in the villi of the small intestine. Whether the '*rasa*' forced into the lymph torrent is carried along the thoracic duct which pours its contents (lymph and chyle) into the left subclavian vein or absorbed in the blood capillaries of the villi, travel by the venous portal system, it has to pass through the hepatic cells for further synthetic transformation, before it is driven to the heart for general circulation.

The blood is red in color, for it is caused by the mass of red-corpuscles (*erythrocytes*) held in suspension in the plasma. The blood is composed of a liquid part, the 'plasma', in which float a vast number of microscopical bodies, the red corpuscles (*erythrocytes*), the white corpuscles (*leucocytes*) and the blood plates or platelets (*hematoblast*). The red corpuscle has the shape of a biconcave disk with bevelled edges with a diameter of 0.0075 millimeter in man and for each cubic millimeter of blood, there are red corpuscles in man from 4 to 5 millions, in goat 9 to 10 millions, in sheep 13 to 14 millions, in birds 1 to 4 millions and in fish quarter million to two millions. The chief function of the red corpuscle is to carry oxygen, which it owes to its principal ingredient—haemoglobin and which possesses the special quality of chemically combining with oxygen and yielding up the same oxygen, whenever there is decrease in the concentration of oxygen in the solvent. In performance of this important function, the red corpuscles soon lose their vitality, deteriorate and are disintegrated in the liver. The liver eliminates the wastes and the pigments as an excretory product, which thus receives the golden brownish tinge. The bile is essentially the excretory product of the metabolic wastes which are formed in the hepatic cells as a result of their detoxicating and metabolic activities, but the bile has adapted in the economy of the system, to the functional utility of zymo-exciters, particularly of the lipolytic enzymes. The red corpuscles are newly formed again in the red bone marrow and the spleen, where special cells are provided for their reproduction. But it is probable that the spleen plays a more important role in the integration and synthesis of the haemoglobin molecules, for iron is its important component element, having special chemical affinity for oxygen, and iron is principally metabolized in the spleen.

It is therefore a delightful surprise to read in Charaka and Suśruta that they attributed to the liver and the spleen of transforming '*rasa*' into blood, and heart was the centre and medium of the blood circulation to irrigate, feed, nourish and sustain tissues and life. Of course it was a fanciful speculation that the blood is transformed in five days into flesh and in a month into semen. But the blood supplies the nutrient materials for the cellular sustenance, growth and upbuilding. And it is a fact, though 'spermin', the special substance of the semen, is found in concentrated form in the testes and prostate, it is found in a considerable quantity in the thymus, milt, ovaries and the blood and plays an important role in the general oxidation of the tissues and in the metabolic reduction of the intermediate regressive albuminous substances as leucomines into harmless products as urea. *

'*Rasa*' contributes to health, pleasant countenance and nourishes the blood ; the blood contributes to the brightness of the skin, nourishment of the flesh and keeps one alive ; fat contributes to the adipose tissues, perspiration, hardihood and health of the bone ; the bone keeps the bodily frame and nourishes the bone-marrow ; the bone-marrow contributes to the pleasant countenance, adipose tissues, strength (of the body), increase of the semen and fills the bone ; the semen contributes to the personal bravery, resistance to disease (*chyavana*),

---

* (A. Poehl : *Einwirkung des Spermins aufden Staffumsats*. Züit für klin. Med., 1894, p. 135)

inclination to pleasure, physical strength and reproductive power. *Suśruta* I. 15. 6 [28].

"'*Śleṣma*' (lymph) is produced in the intestine, sweet and cool; from the sweetness, viscosity, and humidity from the digested food." *Suśruta* I. 21. 17[29].

"'*Śleṣma*' is white (chyle in the lacteal, especially after the heavy ingestien of fat), heavy and cool; when it is unoxidized (*avidagdha* in the lacteal and in the thoracic duct, still in the condition of chyle), it is sweet, but when oxidized, it is alkaline." *Suśruta* I. 21. 19[30].

Śleṣma "lubricates joints (*snovia*), is fattening, healing, flesh-giving, causes growth, refreshing through moistening, strengthening, adds to the thickness of the subcutaneous fat, and thus '*śleṣma*' doing five functions according to the position, benefits the body." *Suśruta* I. 15. 5[31].

---

28. रसस्तुष्टिं प्रीणनं रक्तपुष्टिञ्च करोति। रक्तं वर्णप्रसादं मांसपुष्टिं जीवयति च। मांसं शरीरपुष्टिं मेदसश्च। मेदः स्नेहस्वेदौ दृढत्वं पुष्टिमस्थ्नाञ्च। अस्थि देहधारणं मज्ज्ञः पुष्टिञ्च। मज्जा प्रीतिं स्नेहं बलं शुक्रपुष्टिं पूरणमस्थ्नाञ्च करोति। शुक्रं धैर्य्यं च्यवनं प्रीतिं देहबलं हर्षं बीजार्थञ्च ॥६

29. माधुर्य्यात् पिच्छिलत्वाच्च प्रक्लेदित्वात् तथैव च।
आमाशये सम्भवति श्लेष्मा मधुरशीतलः ॥१७

30. श्लेष्मा श्वेतो गुरुः स्निग्धः पिच्छिलः शीत एव च।
मधुरस्त्वविदग्धः स्याद्विदग्धो लवणः स्मृतः ॥१९

31. सन्धिसंश्लेषणस्नेहनरोपणपूरणबृंहणतर्पणबलस्थैर्य्यकृत् श्लेष्मा पञ्चधा प्रविभक्त उदककर्म्मणानुग्रहं करोति ॥५

That by '*śleṣma*' or '*kapha,*' lymph was understood, is proven by the fact that Suśruta describes in the vascular system (III. 7. 1-13) the tubular lymph-vessels with arteries, veins and nerves and that his '*śleṣma*' corresponds to the synovial lymph, is corroborated by this passage :—"As it works well, if oil or fat is applied to the axle of a carriage wheel, so the '*śleṣma*' acts in the joints of the living beings." III. 4. 15[32].

II. Circulation

The lymph is a colorless liquid found in the lymph vessels as well as the extravascular parts of the body, having almost the same constituents as the blood-plasma. The lymph is at least in part the mediator in the exchange of constituents between the blood and the tissues. Throughout the entire body, there is a rich supply of blood vessels penetrating every tissue with the exception of the epidermis and epidermal structures as the nails and hair. In the ground-work of the tissue, there is space and this interstitial space is filled with lymph and thus all the tissue elements, in fact, may be regarded as being bathed

32. स्नेहाभ्यक्ते यथा तूचे चक्रं साधु प्रवर्त्तते ।
सन्धय: साधु वर्त्तन्ते संश्लिष्टा: श्लेष्मणा तथा ॥१५

in lymph. From this fluid the cell takes the necessary nutrients dissolved in it, and into it the cell discharges its waste products. In the interstitial space, the lymph freely intercommunicates, finally connecting with a number of fine tubes—the lymphatics, through which excess of fluid, tissue wastes, pathogenic germs and their products are drained off. The lymphatics like the blood-vessels freely anastomose, thus forming large trunks which finally empty their contents in the main venous trunks at both the junctions of the jugular and subclavian veins. In the course of the lymphatics, there are numerous adenoid structures (lymph-glands) which act as a filter as the fluid passes through them, retaining all the pathogenic germs, their deleterious products as well as various excretory products, which the lymph-glands either destroy or make them comparatively harmless.

The flow of the blood-plasma into interstitial space, where it is known as the lymph, is governed by the principles of pressure, filtration, diffusion, osmosis and the relative permeability of the capillary walls. The intracapillary pressure tends to filter the plasma through the endothelial cells composing the walls of the capillaries ; the force of diffusion arises from the inequality of the chemical composition of the blood-plasma and the interstitial fluid; osmosis from different molecular concentration and relative permeability according to the regional capillary structure.

Though lymph lacks any central heart system as the blood vessels, the flow of its circulation is perhaps regulated by the relative pressure-level from the higher tension in the capillaries to lower in the lymphatic space and in the minute vessels considerably much greater than in the larger ones as in the veins, and as this difference of pressure is the cause of the flow of venous blood from the capillaries to the heart. This flow may be accelerated by other factors. The lymphatics are provided with muscular wall of automatically oscillating tanus under the influence of special vascular nerves and as with each systolic efflux, there is an increased pressure of the arterial flow, muscular and nervous dilation which make the perivascular lymphatic valves act like tiny pumps, accentuating the momentum of the centripetal evacuation of the contents. Perhaps inspiration also exerts a sucking action by positively lowering the pressure at the subclavian vein in which the thoracic duct empties its contents.

The lymph fluid is not uniform in composition in every part of the body. The lymph originates from three sources : (a) by filtering from the blood through the capillary wall; (b) from exudation of the tissues with their anabolic and catabolic wastes ; (c) the digested nutrient solution which is absorbed by the lymphatic roots of the intestinal villi and which is known as the chyle.

The composition of the lymph, therefore, is variable. In the lacteals, the lymph mixed with the chyle has often after the ingestion of heavy fat and protein, a milky white appearance and contains a good deal of sugar. The lymph which flows from the fistula of the thoracic duct, is a watery, slightly opalescent fluid. In the capillary lymph-space and in the large serous cavities as the peritoneum, pleura, pericardium, tunica vaginalis of testicles, where there is always a sufficient quantity of the lymph to keep the walls lubricated and moistened, it is a colorless liquid, almost like water, but decidedly alkaline.

The lymph does not coagulate as easily as the blood. But it contains fibronogen and in case there is any rupture of the lymphatic, it readily clots so that no serious damage be done to the tissues. But unlike the blood, the lymph contains a very few corpuscles. Platelets and functions (*thrombocytes*) are always absent ; the red-corpuscles (*erythrocytes*) are met with on very rare occasions ; but the *leucocytes*—the wandering cells, are always found, though smaller in size and fewer in number. Perhaps the leucocyte through its ameboid movement traverses through the capillary membrane and enters into the lymph-stream and acts as useful scavenger and devourer of any pathogenic germ that might have gained access in the tissues ; or the leucocyte may be produced in the lymphatic glands and enter into the arterial circulation when the lymph trunks empty their contents at the junctions of the jugular and subclavian veins and are carried to the heart. In the blood the leucocytes are seen larger and with developed phagocytic power for the reason that the blood contains opsonin and alexin which sensitize the pathogenic micro-organisms, thus facilitating phagocytosis. The destroyed germs are dissolved in the blood, increasing thus the protein content, which is a nourishing food to the leucocytes.

So lymph glands not only filter and purify the lymph stream, they are ever watchful sentinels to catch and retain any dangerous marauder that may be in the lymph torrent, but also are active synthetic laboratories for the origin and development of the leucocytes. In this vital work with the lymph-glands in the lymphatics, all the lymphoid adenoid bodies as the spleen, bone-marrow and the thymus have their important share. In malarial fever, it is a well known fact that the spleen is enlarged. This only means that the spleen is hyperactive, destroying the minute protozoa that are attacking the red-blood corpuscles and producing an excessive number of leucocytes for the bodily defence. This also explains that with the ablation or total extirpation of the spleen, there is no serious consequence or there is any marked reduction of the leucocytes in the blood. The task of the spleen is supplemented and functioned by the bone-marrow and the numerous lymph-glands which are numerous and are scattered either single or in cluster all throughout the lymphatics.

On the whole the flow of the lymph is very sluggish and much slower not only than the arterial, but also than the venous blood.

Suśruta also mentions twenty-four '*dhamanī*' and passage of some other liquids in the body. But he does not confound '*dhamanī*' with *'śira'* (vascular system) like Charaka (I. 30. 10). He says : "There are some who say that *dhamanī* and *srota* are not different from the *śira* (vascular system). But this is not just; *dhamanī* and *srota* are different from the *'śira'*. For the characteristics of the *'srota'* and *'dhamanī*, differ from those of *'śira.'* How ? For the *'śiras'* have main central trunks and their action is also otherwise. In the medical science, they are mentioned separately. Only because they are situated close to each other, they are minute and there is some similarity in their action, therefore in spite of their dissimilar activities, they are often confounded with each other. *Suśruta* III. 9. 2[33].

"There are two vital streams—*srota* : their main bearers (*mūlasthāna*) are the heart and chyle-carrying tubes (lacteals and thoracic duct); if they are penetrated (by any wound), involuntary cries, syncope, hallucination, illusion and trembling appear and death might even take

---

33. चतुर्विंशतिर्धमन्यो नाभिप्रभवा अभिहिताः। तत् केचिदाहुः शिराधमनीस्रोतसामविभागः, शिराविकारा एव धमन्यः स्रोतांसि चेति। तत् तु न सम्यक्। अन्यथा एव हि धमन्यः स्रोतांसि च शिराभ्यः। कस्मात्? व्यञ्जनान्यत्वान्मूलसन्नियमात् कर्म्मवैशेष्यादागमाच्च। केवलन्तु परस्परसन्निकर्षात् सदृशागमकर्म्मत्वात् सौक्ष्म्याच्च विभक्तकर्म्मणामप्यविभाग इव कर्म्मसु भवति ॥२

place. Alimentary canals are two and their bearers are the intestine and the lacteals : if they are penetrated, pain, loss of appetite, vomiting, thirst, blindness or immediate death take place. Serous (*udaka*) tubes are two and their bearers are '*tālu*' (between the meningeal membranes surrounding the central nervous system) and the '*kloma*' (*pleura*) ; if they are penetrated, thirst and immediate death take place. Chyle-carrying tubes are two and their main bearers are the heart and the chyle-carrying vessels (the lacteals and the thoracic duct) ; if they are penetrated, there is edema or immediate death with symptoms the same as if the heart and the main arteries are wounded. The blood-vessels are two (the hepatic artery and the portal vein) and their main bearers are the liver and the spleen, and the blood-vessels ; if the sources of the two vessels (the liver and the spleen) are penetrated, there are paleness of the skin or jaundice, fever, burning sensation, bleeding and redness of the nose. Streams of circulating protein (*māṃsavaha*) are two and their main sources are ligaments, skin and the blood-vessels; if their main sources are penetrated, edema, emaciation, vascular obstruction and even death might take place. The urine-bearing tubes are two, the bladder and the penis ; if their main sources are penetrated, there are suppression of the urine in the bladder, anuria and paralysis (insensibility) of the penis. The feces-carrying tubes are two ; their sources are the intestine and the anus ; if they are penetrated, there are constipation, offensive odor, and the tying down of the entrails (*antra*-the bowel). The seminal tubes are two : their sources are the mamma and the testicles ; if they are penetrated impotence, difficulty in seminal discharge take place. The ovarian (*ārttava-vaha*) tubes are two : their sources are the matrix and the ova-carrying tubes (the *ovi-ducts*—Fallopian tubes) ; if they are penetrated, sterility, pain in copulation and amenorrhea take place." *Suśruta* III. 9. 12[34].

---

34. तानि तु प्राणान्नोदकरसरक्तमांसमेदोमूत्रपुरीषशुक्रार्त्तववहानि. येष्वधिकार एकेषां बहूनि। एतेषां विशेषा बहवः। तत्र प्राणवहे द्वे, तयोर्मूलं हृदयं रसवाहिन्यश्च धमन्यः; तत्र विद्धस्य क्रोशनविनमनमोहनभ्रमणवेपनानि मरणं वा भवति। अन्नवहे द्वे, तयोर्मूलमामाशयोऽन्नवाहिन्यश्च धमन्यः; तत्र विद्धस्याध्मानं शूलान्नद्वेषौ छर्द्दिः पिपासान्ध्यं मरणं वा। उदकवहे द्वे, तयोर्मूलं तालु क्लोम च; तत्र विद्धस्य पिपासा सद्यो मरणञ्च। रसवहे द्वे, तयोर्मूलं हृदयं रसवाहिन्यश्च धमन्यः; तत्र विद्धस्य शोषः प्राणवहविद्धवच्च मरणं तल्लिङ्गानि च। रक्तवहे द्वे, तयोर्मूलं यकृत्प्लीहानौ रक्तवाहिन्यश्च धमन्यः; तत्र विद्धस्य श्यावाङ्गता ज्वरो दाहः पाण्डुता शोणितातिगमनं रक्तनेत्रता चेति। मांसवहे द्वे, तयोर्मूलं स्नायुत्वचं रक्तवहाश्च धमन्यः; तत्र विद्धस्य श्वयथुर्मांसशोषः शिराग्रन्थयोर्मरणं वा। मेदो-

Here of course Suśruta has used *'srota'* in the generic sense of what are described in modern anatomy as tubes, ducts, canals and cavities.

III.—The Nervous System

"The normal *'vāyu'* (nervous system) is the regulator of the physical mechanism. The nerves are of five kinds, *'Prāṇa, apāna, samāna, udāna* and *vyāna.'* It carries out the physical attempts (muscular contractions), reveals the senses and is the carrier of the sense-perceptions as the impression, taste, smell, touch and hearing. It is the strengthener of the bodily elements (*dhātu*) and the co-ordinator of the bodily organs. It activates speech, bases of sound and hearing and is the main cause of the consciousness

---

वहे द्वे, तयोर्मूलं कटीवृक्कौ च ; तत्र विद्धस्य स्वेदागमनं स्निग्धाङ्गता तालुशोषः
स्थूलशोफता पिपासा च। मूत्रवहे द्वे, तयोर्मूलं वस्तिर्मेढ्रं च ; तत्र विद्धस्यानद्ध-
वस्तिता मूत्रनिरोधः स्तब्धमेढ्रता च। पुरीषवहे द्वे, तयोर्मूलं पक्वाशयो गुदश्च ;
तत्र विद्धस्यानाहो दुर्गन्धता ग्रथितान्त्रता च। शुक्रवहे द्वे, तयोर्मूलं स्तनौ वृषणौ
च ; तत्र विद्धस्य क्लीवता चिरात् प्रसेको रक्तशुक्रता च। आर्त्तववहे द्वे, तयो-
र्मूलं गर्भाशय आर्त्तववाहिन्यश्च धमन्यः। तत्र विद्धायां वन्ध्यात्वं मैथुनासहिष्णुत्व-
मार्त्तवनाशश्च। सेवनीच्छेदाद्रुजाप्रादुर्भावः। वस्तिगुदविद्धलक्षणं प्रागुक्तमिति। स्रोतो-
विद्धन्तु प्रत्याख्यायोपचरेदुद्धृतशल्यन्तु क्षतविधानेनोपाचरेत् ॥१२

of sound and touch. It is the source of pleasure and cheerfulness. It increases the digestive fire and eliminates from the body all the waste-products." *Charaka* 1. 12. 7[35].

"The '*prāṇa*' nerves (*cerebrospinal*) are located in the brain, thorax, ears, tongue, face and nose. Spitting, sneezing, vomiting, respiration and digestion are the functions of the '*prāṇa-vāyu*'. '*Udāna*' nerves (cervical, thoracic and brachial plexus) are located in the umbilicus, thorax and in the neck ; speaking, exertions, heat, strength and complexion are its activities. '*Samāna*' nerves (*vasodilator*) are located in the sudoriferous glands and ducts, and in the lymphatics (*amvu.*) It being situated by the side of the digestive fire (bileduct ?), it increases digestive fire. '*Vyāna*' (motor) nerves are spread over the entire body. Their conduction is very rapid. By '*vyāna*' nerves, walking, extension, movements of the hands and feet, contraction

---

35. वायुस्तन्त्रयन्त्रधरः, प्राणोदानसमानव्यानात्मा, प्रवर्त्तकश्चेष्टानामुच्चावचानां, नियन्ता प्रणेता च मनसः। सर्व्वेन्द्रियाणामुद्योतकः, सर्व्वेन्द्रियार्थानामभिवोढ़ा, सर्व्वशरीरधातुव्यूहकरः, सन्धानकरः शरीरस्य, प्रवर्त्तको वाचः, प्रकृतिः स्पर्शशब्दयोः श्रोत्रस्पर्शनयोर्मूलम् हर्षोत्साहयोर्योनिः। समीरणोऽग्नेर्दोषसंशोषणः ; क्षेप्ता बहिर्मलानां ; स्थूलाणुस्रोतसां भेत्ता ; कर्त्ता गर्भाकृतीनाम् आयुषोऽनुवृत्तिप्रत्ययभूतो भवत्यकुपितः ॥

(of muscles), the twinkling of the eyes and other activities are accomplished. *Apāna* (automatic or sympathetic) nerves are located in the testicles, bladder, reproductive organs, umbilicus (abdomen), knee, hip and the anus. The *apāna* nerves residing in the bowels, cause the elimination of semen, urine and feces and the expulsion of the ova and the fetus." *Charaka* VI. 28. 4-9[36].

"The brain is the centre of the senses." *Suśruta* III. 3. 18[37].

"The ten nerves (*dhamanī*) of the upper

---

36. स्थानं प्राणस्य शीर्षोरःकर्णजिह्वास्यनासिकाः ।
ष्ठीवनक्षवथूद्गारश्वासाहारादि कर्म्म च ॥
उदानस्य पुनः स्थानं नाभ्युरः कण्ठ एव च ॥
वाक्प्रवृत्तिः प्रयत्नोर्ज्जोबलवर्णादि कर्म्म च ॥
स्वेददोषाम्बुवाहीनि स्रोतांसि समधिष्ठितः ।
अन्तरग्नेश्च पार्श्वस्थः समानोऽग्निबलप्रदः ॥
देहं व्याप्नोति सर्व्वन्तु व्यानः शीघ्रगतिर्नृणाम् ।
गतिप्रसरणाक्षेपनिमेषादिक्रियः सदा ॥
वृषणौ वस्तिमेढ्रञ्च नाभ्यूरू वङ्क्षणौ गुदम् ।
अपानस्थानमन्त्रस्थः शुक्रमूत्रशकृत्क्रियः ।
सृजत्यार्त्तवगर्भौ च युक्ताः स्थानस्थिताश्च ते ॥
स्वकर्म्म कुर्व्वते देहो धार्य्यते तैरनामयः ।
विमार्गस्था ह्ययुक्ता वा रोगैः स्वस्थानकर्म्मजैः ॥
शरीरं पीड़यन्तीते प्राणानाशु हरन्ति वा ॥

37. शिरोमूलत्वाद्धीन्द्रियाणाम् ।

extremities, by activating sound, touch, impressions, taste, smell, respiration, sighing, yawning, hunger, laughing, speech, and crying, maintain the body. ···Two (auditory) carry sound; two (optic) carry impressions; two (lingual) carry taste and two (olfactory) carry smell. By two man speaks, by two makes (vocal) sound, by two he is asleep and by two he is awakened." *Suśruta* III. 9. 4[38].

"Man sleeps when sense-organs cease to operate, being tired by the fatigue of the mind." *Charaka* 1. 21. 35[39].

"Memory is caused by the following eight causes :—From the cause of impressions, (their) similarities and dissimilarities, co-ordination of the mind, practice, consciousness, concentration (of attention), what is remembered from repeti-

---

38. ऊर्द्ध्वगाः शब्दस्पर्शरूपरसगन्धप्रश्वासोच्छ्वासजृम्भितक्षुद्धसितकथितरुदितादीन् विशेषानभिवहन्त्यः शरीरं धारयन्ति। तास्तु हृदयमभिप्रपन्नास्त्रिधा जायन्ते—तास्त्रिंशत्। तासान्तु वातपित्तकफशोणितरसान् द्वे द्वे वहतः—ता दश। शब्दरूपरसगन्धानष्टाभिर्गृह्णीते। द्वाभ्याञ्च भाषते, द्वाभ्यां घोषं करोति, द्वाभ्यां स्वपिति, द्वाभ्यां प्रतिबुध्यते। द्वे चाश्रुवाहिण्यौ। द्वे स्तन्यं स्त्रिया वहतः स्तनसंश्रिते; ते एव शुक्रं नरस्य स्तनाभ्यामभिवहतः। तास्त्वेतास्त्रिंशत् सविभागा व्याख्याताः। एताभिरूर्द्ध्वं नाभेरुदरपार्श्वपृष्ठोरःस्कन्धग्रीवाबाहवो धार्य्यन्ते याप्यन्ते च ॥४

39. यदातु मनसि क्लान्ते कर्म्मात्मानः क्लमान्विताः।
विषयेभ्यो निवर्त्तन्ते तदा स्वपिति मानवः॥

tion of sight, hearing or perception (as tasting or smelling), is called the memory." *Charaka* IV. 1. 117-118[40].

"The side-way four (cutaneous) nerves, branching into hundreds and thousands, they have become countless. They open in the hair follicles by which they carry the sweat (*sveda*) and sebaceous secretion (*rasa*). By these secretions the internal and external body is moistened and refreshed...By them the pleasure and pain of touch are felt." *Suśruta* III. 9. 8[41].

---

40 वक्ष्यन्ते कारणान्यष्टौ स्मृतिर्यैरुपजायते ।
निमित्तरूपग्रहणात् सादृश्यात् सविपर्य्ययात् ॥
सत्त्वानुबन्धादभ्यासाज्ज्ञानयोगात् पुनः श्रुतात् ।
दृष्टश्रुतानुभूतानां स्मरणात् स्मृतिरुच्यते ॥
एतत्तदेकमयनं मुक्तैर्मोक्षस्य दर्शितम् ।
तत्त्वस्मृतिबलं येन गता न पुनरागताः ॥
अयनं पुनराख्यातमेतद्योगस्य योगिभिः ।
संख्यातधर्म्मैः सांख्यैश्च मुक्तैर्मोक्षस्य चायनम् ॥

41. तिर्य्यग्गाणान्तु चतसृणां धमनीनामेकैका शतधा सहस्रधा चोत्तरोत्तरं विभज्यन्ते, तास्त्वसङ्ख्याः । ताभिरिदं शरीरं गवाक्षितं विबद्धमाततञ्च । तासां मुखानि रोमकूपप्रतिबद्धानि ; यैः स्वेदमभिवहन्ति रसञ्चापि सन्तर्पयन्त्यन्तर्व्वहिश्च, तैरेव चाभ्यङ्गपरिषेकावगाहालेपनवीर्याण्यन्तःशरीरमभिप्रतिपद्यते त्वचि विपक्वानि तैरेव स्पर्शसुखमसुखं वा गृह्णाति । तास्त्वेतास्तिस्रो धमन्यः सर्व्वाङ्गगताः सविभागा व्याख्याताः ॥८

"The waste-products (*mala*) of digested aliment, are the feces and the urine......,of lymph mucous exudation, of blood, the bile, of flesh, as the wax in the ear-tube (sebaceous secretions), of fat the sweat, of bones the nails and hair, of bone-marrow wax in the eye-pits, and of the skin oil (sebaceous fatty secretion). *Suśruta* 1.46.550[42].

Kapha (lymph), *pitta* (bile = oxidation) and *vāyu* (air = nerves) maintain the body as the moon, the sun and the air vitalize the earth by their activities of humidity (of the moon), heat (of the sun) and the conduction of heat and cold (by the air current). *Suśruta* 1.21. 8[43].

The above quotations tend to prove that the ancient Hindu schools of medicine believed that the body was nourished by the lymph and the blood formed out of the chyle during its passage within the liver and the spleen, was the medium of circulation and the neryes acted as the conductor of sense-perceptions of which the brain was the centre.

In the Hippocratic writings we find almost

---

42. कफ: पित्तं मल: खेषु स्वेद: स्यान्नखरोम च ।
नेत्रविट् त्वचु च स्नेहो धातूनां क्रमशो मला: ॥५५०

43. विसर्गादानविक्षेपै: सोमसूर्य्यानिला यथा ।
धारयन्ति जगद्देहं कफपित्तानिलास्तथा ॥८

similar views, though with less clearness and positive assertions. In *'peri physios anthropoy'* 4-5(=the nature of man), there are four ground principles—the blood (*aima*), phlegm (*phlegma*), yellow bile (*cholen xanthen*) and black bile (*cholen melainan*), which are described to be mixed and to circulate in the body. In the *'peri noison to tetarton*= the fourth book of the Maladies 33), only bile is mentioned without any qualification and for the other bile, water (*udrops*) is substituted. "The sources for the blood are the heart, for the phlegm the brain, for the water the spleen, for the bile a section of the liver." 33. They are introduced into the system with the ingested food and drink, containing these principles (*peri noison* IV. 35-38). Many glands (*peri adenon*= glands 1-10) as the tonsil, mamma, lymphatic ganglions in the neck, arm-pit and groin as well as the brain, have been mentioned but not the pancreas, testicles or ovaries. The function of the glands is to absorb the superfluous liquid in the body and thus to preserve the bodily equilibrium. The largest and the most important gland par excellence was supposed to be the brain and its function was to pump and distribute the liquid in all parts of the body according to the organic needs.

Galen distinguished between the arteries and the veins. According to him the blood was formed in the liver and it was sent to the heart for the distribution in all parts of the body after the volatilized '*pneuma*' (air = the spirit = the soul) has been separated. The '*pneuma*' mixed with the air brought from the lungs, becomes the vital essence of life (animal spirit) and from the brain, circulates to all parts of the body with the nerves. Before Galen it was believed that the vital spirit (*pneuma* = air) circulated in the arteries, for arteries are always found empty after death.

According to Charaka (IV. 7. 8) there are eight handfuls (*añjali*) of blood and six of lymph in a normal healthy human body. (Because the body fluid constantly increases, or decreases, any calculation by the '*añjali*' measure can be but conjectural). There are ten handfuls of water, according to each individual's own measure—the water that after absorption, becomes mixed with feces, urine, blood and other materials of the body ; which circulating in the system, nourishes the outer skin ; which entering into the abscess under the skin, is known as '*lasīkā*'; which being evaporated by the heat of the body, is eliminated as perspiration ; that water (*udaka* = serous fluid) is ten handfuls. The material that is first formed out of the digested food and which is known as the chyle, is nine handfuls. The blood is eight handful, feces seven, lymph six, bile five (or the venous blood), urine four, *'vasā'* (serum of the flesh) three, fat two, bone-marrow one, brain (or brain-serum) half handful, semen half handful and *'ojas'* (prostate gland secretion) half handful." *Charaka* IV. 7. 10[44].

According to Foster (*Physiology*, p. 49), "the total quantity of blood in the human body is about one thirteenth of the body weight." Howell (*Physiology*, p. 458) says: "The ratio of weight of blood to weight of body is in the dog 7. 7 per cent; rabbit and cat 5 p. c.; birds 10 p c.; in man we have upon record two determinations on guillotined criminals made by Bischoff, which

44. यत् त्वञ्जलिसङ्ख्येयं तदुपदेक्ष्यामः, तत्परं प्रमाणमभिज्ञेयं तच्च वृद्धिह्रासयोगि तर्क्यमेव। तद्यथा दशोदकस्याञ्जलयः शरीरे स्वेनाञ्जलिप्रमाणेन यत् तु प्रच्यवमानं पुरीषमनुवध्नात्यतियोगेन तथा मूत्रं रुधिरमन्यांश्च शरीरधातून्, यत् तु सर्व्वशरीरचरं बाह्यत्वग् विभर्त्ति यत् त्वगन्तरे व्रणगतं लसीकाशब्दं लभते यच्चोष्मणानुबन्धलोमकूपेभ्यो निष्पतत् स्वेदशब्दमवाप्नोति तदुदकं दशाञ्जलिप्रमाणम्। नवाञ्जलयः पूर्व्वस्याहारपरिणामधातोर्यं रसमित्याचक्षते। अष्टौ शोणितस्य, सप्त पुरीषस्य, षट् श्लेष्मणः, पञ्च पित्तस्य, चत्वारो मूत्रस्य, त्रयो वसायाः द्वौ मेदस, एको मज्ज्ञः, मस्तिष्कस्य अर्द्धाञ्जलिः, शुक्रस्य तावदेव प्रमाणं, तावदेव श्लैष्मिकस्यौजस इत्येतच्छरीरतत्त्वमुक्तम्।

gave 7. 7 and 7. 2 per cent. Haldane and Smith however have devised a modification of Grehant's carbon monoxide method, which they have applied to living men. The results of some 74 experiments gave them an average value of only 5 per cent per man. The distribution of this blood in the tissues of the body at any time has been estimated by Ranke from experiments on freshly killed rabbits, as follows: spleen, 0. 23 p. c.; brain and cord, 1. 24 p. c.; kidneys, 1. 63 p. c.; skin, 2. 10 p. c.; intestines, 6. 30 p.c.; bones, 8. 24 p. c.; heart, lungs and great blood-vessels, 22. 76 p. c.; resting muscles, 29. 20 p. c.; liver, 29. 30 p. c."

The blood circulates in the tubular closed vessels, for thereby the pressure is increased and the time for completing the circulation is reduced. "If we take 180 grams, as the quantity in man, ejected at each stroke at a pressure of 250 mm. of mercury, which is equivalent to 3. 21 meters of blood, this means that the left ventricle is capable at its systole of lifting 180 grams 3. 21 m. high, i. e. it does 578 gram-meters of work at each beat. Supposing the heart to beat 72 times a minute, this would give for the day's work of the left ventricle nearly 60,000 kilogram-meters. Calculating the work of the right ventricle at one-fourth of the left, the work of the whole heart during the day would amount to 75,000 kilogram-meters." Foster's *Physiology*, p. 218.

The blood is the medium through which every cell of the body is supplied with its nutritive needs. In blood circulate the synthetized elements of the ingested food. In the capillaries, the blood-plasma filters through and fills the interstitial space, bathing every tissue in the lymph-fluid, from which the cells extract the nutritive materials they need for their sustenance and growth and to which they discharge their waste products. Without blood-circulation there can be no supply of the lymph fluid for the preservation of the tissues. This is easily seen in the occlusion of the main artery of the extremity when putrefactive fermentation takes place of an animal tissue still attached to the body, known as the 'gangrene' with the production of gases as sulphuretted hydrogen and volatilized fat, which gives the bad odor and the iron-content of the hemoglobin is precipitated into sulphide of iron which imparts to the limb a range of colors commencing in green and terminating in black.

In addition to supply the nutritive fluid to the cells, the chief function of the blood is to carry oxygen with hemoglobin, hormones and glandular secretions for tissue respiration, oxidation, and stimulation and in the intercellular oxidation, heat of the body is generated. When the oxygen of the blood is reduced and it comes back to the heart through the veins to be sent to the lungs, to be charged with oxygen, it is of purple color, but when it is loaded with oxygen, it is sparkle bright-red. The venous blood contains many waste products of the cells, dissolved in it as the amonium carbonate, urea, urates, xanthin bases, carbonic acid as carbonates, cholesterin and other substances.

Charaka and Suśruta formed right conception of the function of the blood and the lymph in broad general outlines. Of course it was not possible for them to know their complex functional utilities in detail. Nor do we yet know. But they thought that the nerves were also tuberal vessels, through which flowed the vital force of life, something too fine for the eyes to see and which brought the sensory impressions to the central nervous system for co-ordination and carried the motor impulses to the periphery. It was invisible but mighty like the air which brings heat and cold waves, storms and tempests (*Charaka* 1. 12. 6) or like blowing with bellows which intensifies the fire of the furnace and which it was compared to and identified with. But the exact nature of the nerve impulse and the mode of its conduction, is not yet completely understood. It is usually compared with the electric current. But the sensory and the motor nerves are different, the sensory fibres only bring impressions to the nerve-centre, while the motor only carry them from the centre to the periphery. Yet histological or chemical examination hardly reveals any structural differentiation. Moreover the propagation and the velocity of the nerve-force depends on the nature and locality of the nerve fibre, the temperature and the pressure. The nerve-fibre is one of the units of a nerve-trunk : it is the axis-cylinder process of a neuron and is either medullated, that is, surrounded by a white substance called myelin, or non-medullated ; either the medullated or the non-medullated may or may not be surrounded by the primitive sheath or neurilemma, so that there are four forms of nerve-fibres. The neuron is the cell unit of the nerve-fibre and the neurons propagate their impulse by contact of the dendrites, the terminal arborization round the axon. The neurons also differ greatly in size, shape and internal structure and they are generally classified as the bipolar and multipolar cells.

This structural variation explains the difference in speed of nerve impulstion. Helmholtz found that the motor nerve of a frog travels with the velocity of 28 to 30 meters per second and the researches of Piper indicated that the motor nerve of a man travels at the velocity of 117 to 125 meter per second. There does not seem to be any structural difference between two afferent or efferent nerves, as for an example, between auditory and olfactory, and in their mode of conduction and speed, and if they carry different impressions and impulses, it is because their terminal endings have been developed to catch particular impressions and the lobe in the brain has been specialized as an economy to the system to receive, co-ordinate and react only to special impulses. It is just like two electric wires one of which has been connected to ring the bell and the other to make light.

By the specially adapted peculiar structure of the retina, the vibrations of light (color-images = *rūpa*) can be focussed upon it, setting up nerve-impulses that are transmitted by the fibres of the optic nerve and optic track to the visual centre in the cortex in the brain, which is situated in the occipital lobes, for co-ordination, color-consciousness and response to the stimuli. Total blindness follows the removal of both occipital lobes. But if only one lobe is ablated or injured, there is a partial blindness, affecting the symmetrical halves of both eyes known as '*hemipia*'; the right one influencing the two right halves of the eyes, and the left one, the two left halves of the retinas.

The *outer ear* is so constituted that when the vibrations of matter, the rapidly alternating variations of pressure, what is commonly known as the 'waves of sound', forced through the accoustic apparatus, strike against the auditory epithelium, richly supplied with the nerve-fibres of the cochlear branch, and the sensory impulse thus generated is carried over the auditory nerve (eighth cranial nerve) and track to the auditory centre in the first convolution of the 'temporal auditory lobe,' where auditory consciousness is developed.

The *taste* (*rasa*) nerve fibres are distributed to parts of the buccal cavity and especially the tongue, of which the most sensitive parts are the tip, the borders, and the posterior portion of the dorsum in the circumvallate papillae. The anterior two-thirds of the tongue are supplied with sensory fibres from the lingual nerve (a branch of the fifth nerve) and the posterior third from the glossopharyngeal. The nerve track has not yet been definitely known, but it is supposed to terminate in the hippocampal convolution, posterior to the olfactory lobe. The gustatory sensation is possibly complex. There are but four fundamental taste sensations, —namely, sweet, bitter, acid, and salty and the rest are but the combinations of these primary tastes, for the experience of which we are dependent on the terminal organs which are chiefly present in the fungiform and circumvallate papillæ. And there are so many complex and multiple junctions between the fifth nerve, the seventh nerve and the glossopharyngyal nerve, by way of the Vidian nerve, petrosal nerves, tymphanic plexus, the otic and the splenopalatine ganglia, that it is hard to determine, how the taste sensation travels, but perhaps through the chorda tympani nerve.

In the *nasal septum* and a portion of the upper turbinate bone, the area corresponding to about 250 square millimeters in each nostril, there is a profuse distribution of the fibres of the olfactory (*gandha*) nerve, in the shape of elongated, epithelial like cells, each of which bears on its end a tuft of six to eight hair-like processes. And there are tiny glands which keep the mucous always humid and moist.

Particles of odoriferous matters, carried in a gaseous medium, namely the air, to the olfactory epithelium, become dissolved in the thin layer of fluid that keeps the nasal membrance moistened and this percolates through and stimulates the nerve-endings. But if the membrane be too dry or the secretion be too abundant or altered in quality, the power of smelling is diminished and even may be wholly suspended. The olfactory nerve terminates in the cortex of the brain in the '*cornu Ammonis and hippocampus.*' The animals with highly developed sense of smell possess a large '*limbic lobe.*' Some of the substances retain their odoriferous quality even in minute dilution as camphor 1 : 400,000 ; musk 1 : 8,000,000 ; vanilin 1 : 10,000,000 parts.

The touch (*sparśa*) is a compound sensation of pressure, warmth, cold and pain, through four distinct kinds of nerve-fibres which are not only richly distributed over the general cutaneous surface, but also in the buccal and rectal membranes. But the alimentary membranes, or the superfaciæ in the interior of the body are supplied with nerve-fibres of pain and devoid of those of touch and temperature sensations. Application of cocaine on the eye or throat paralyzes the feeling of pain and pressure, but the sensations of heat and cold are not influenced, which proves that their nerve-fibres are different and mediate through different channels. It has been clinically observed that the compression of the cords of the brachial plexus, resulted in the insensiblity of the arm to pressure and temperature, but not of pain. And it is supposed the nerve-endings of pain lie deeper than the tactile senses, which are superficial ; the former mediating through the spinal cord and the latter through the posterior funiculi, together with some of the fibres of the muscle sense and they do not cross until after they reach the medulla and perhaps they are represented in the rolandic area.

The vocal sound or voiçe (*ghoṣa*) is distinct from speech, which is an articulate sound to express definite ideas. The animals are endowed with vocal power, but not with speech. And there may be speech without voice as in whispering and voice without speech as in singing a musical tone. The vocal organ, the larynx, resembles to a great extent the siren in the production of tone. The larynx is a framework of cartilages, connected with elastic ligaments, which are vocal cords, and it opens above into the cavity of the pharynx and below into the trachea or windpipe. With respiration, the lung acts as bellows, pressing a blast of air through the thin tube of the windpipe and the escaped air is modulated by the movable ligaments into various tones. The voice has three characteristics, (1) '*loudness*,' which depends on the force of the expiratory blast; (2) '*pitch*,' which depends on the rapidity of vibrations and (3) the '*quality*' which depends on the capacity of the resonance chamber and the muscular strength and pliability of the laryngeal ligaments (vocal cords). The alternate expansion and contraction of the ligaments and muscles of the larynx (*glottis*) are made by the bulbar and recurrent laryngeal nerves. If any of these nerves is destroyed, the rythmic widening and narrowing automatically cease and the glottis remains immobile and no voice (vocal sound) can be produced.

There are four *speech* (*bhāṣā*) *centers*, situated along the Sylvian fissure, in the left hemisphere for the right-handed and in the right hemisphere for left-handed individuals. The motor center for pronouncing and articulating words, occupies the foot of the third frontal convolution (left), immediately in front of the centers of phonation, utilized in speech. The destruction of this center produces motor aphasia (*aphemia*). In aphemia one is able to hear and to understand when spoken to, and is able to emit sound, to move the tongue and the lips, but he has lost his vocabulary, in other words, the faculty to articulate words. But if the injury is not complete; that is, in partial aphemia, the patient can utter a few incoherent words and syllables according to the nature of the lesion. The center for auditory images, that is, for comprehending spoken words, occupies the posterior fourth of the first temporal convolution (left). The destruction of this center causes sensory *aphasia* (word-deafness). In sensory aphasia, one can hear the voice, as the faculty of hearing is not affected, but he can not understand the spoken words, and the words are to him mere sounds and do not express any idea. The center for visual graphic images, that is, for distinguishing written or printed words, occupies the left angular gyrus(posterior inferior part of the left parietal lobe). The destruction of this center causes *alexia* (word-blindness). In alexia, one can not read even his own writing, although his vision and intelligence are not affected and he can see the form of the letters, but has lost the faculty of comprehending ideas, expressed through those words. The center for the faculty of writing, is situated at the foot of the second frontal convolution and the destruction of this center produces the inability to write (*agraphia*). In agraphia, one has lost his faculty of expressing his ideas in writing or any graphic form. Agraphia is usually associated in clinical experience with motor aphasia (*aphemia*).

Sleep (*nidrā*) is evidenced by the cessation of sensory-motor reaction. Various hypotheses have been advanced to explain the causation of sleep. (1) Cerebral anemia was suggested by the old writers; but it is rather the effect than the cause of it. (2) Hyposecretion of the thyroid due to the inhibitive action of the accumulative waste products during waking hours and the hyper-secretion of the pituitary body; but in myxedema, drowsiness is not constant, nor is there any proof that in hypnotic or epileptic somnolence, there is any increased secretion of hypophysis, or diminished secretion of the thyroids. (3) Osmotic theory of Devaux, which tries to explain sleep due to the increased viscocity of blood, through dehydration, is not bsustantiated by observation, as in privation of water—in thirst, the nervous system is rather irritated. (4) Chemico-toxic theory enjoys a better reputation. The accumulated tissue-waste products as lactic acid, cholesterine, leucomaine, exercise an inhibitory action on the cerebral activity, either paralyzing the centre directly, through intoxication or indirectly by reflex vaso-constriction. (5) Accumulation of carbonic acid which has an extreme avidity for oxygen, reduces the minimum ratio of free oxygen, necessary for the central nervous activities. (6) Consumption of the intramolecular oxygen causes cerebral asphyxia, which is expressed as sleep, as during the waking hours, the brain cells use up their store of oxygen more rapidly than it can be replenished by absorption from blood ; the consequence is that for lack of respiration, the brain-cells can not react to the sensory stimuli and gradually losing consciousness, store up sufficient oxygen through the anabolic process to be awakened up again. (7) The neuron theory tries to explain sleep on the histological principle that the nerve track is not continuous like the electric wire, but composed of the cell-units (neuron) which transmit their impulse from one to the other by their contact through the interlacings of dendrided and terminal arborizations, and when there is sufficient accumulation of fatigue products, the dendrides contract and retract, so that the nerve-path being broken and the brain being automatically relieved from sensory stimulation, sleep is mechanically produced. But it has not yet been proved that the dendride processes are contractile enough as to lose all connections with the neighborly cells. (8) A central nervous mechanism produces sleep, not as a result of asphyxiation, toxins or neuro-toxins (*Bouchard*), but to prevent them and to protect the brain-cells from the evil effect of their further accumulation, so that during enforced involuntary rest, the obnoxious products can be eliminated and the brain-cells can be refreshed and revitalized through the anabolic process (the income of energy being more than its expenditure)—as an economic accommodation to self-preservation. If the sleep is deep, profound and undisturbed, it will take less time than otherwise to oxygenate, tonicize, recuperate and vitalize the brain-cells for the resumption of their activities of sensory-motor co-ordination and reaction.

Hunger and thirst (*kṣut-pipāsā*) sensations are mediated, probably through the nerve endings in the stomach and pharynx. Normal hunger is known as the appetite and it is not yet definitely determined whether this impression is conveyed by sensory fibres, distributed to the mucous membrane of the stomach or of the muscular coat. When the stomach is empty, these peripheral nerve-endings are excited. That it has nothing to do with nutritive needs of the organism, is evidenced by the fact that when water or indigestible substances are taken in to fill the stomach, the hunger sense is allayed. From this, it can be concluded that hunger is a gastric sense. Of course, when there is a general tissue hunger for lack of nutrition, a general nervousness and discomfort are experienced, due to the resultant nervous excitation. The water needs of the body are experienced through the fibres of the glosso-pharyngeal nerve as an end organ of thirst, for we know, that if the pharynx is dried up either by salty or saccharine food, dried air or dust, at once there is a sensation of thirst, though there may be no bodily need for it and it can be appeased by removing the irritant substances and moistening the spot. It is possible that when the tissues give up their storage of reserve-water to compensate the loss of the blood, it constantly incurs through respiration, perspiration and urination, there is a general call for supply of water, and it first expresses the demand through the excitability of the glossopharyngeal nerve, and if it is extreme through general nerve excitation and irritation, as in tissue hunger.

Sweat (*sveda*) is the secretion of the sudoripareous glands, of which, there are nearly two millions (*Krause*), distributed all over the cutaneous surface, except the glans penis, prepauce and the deeper portion of the external auditory meatus. It is known that with vaso-dilation, their secretion is increased. But it can be also produced independently, directly through the excitation of the nervous mechanism, as is seen in strong emotion, cold-sweat of phthisis and other diseases, when the skin is in anemic state. The stimulation of the sciatic nerve in cat, has been demonstrated to produce profuse sweating on the hairless balls of the feet. But when an animal with sciatic nerve divided on one side, is made dyspenic, no sweat appears on the hind limb of that side, though there is abundance in the other, thus clearly proving a central nervous mechanism, regulating sweat-glands as vaso-dilation. It seems that picrotoxin and strychnia induce sweating action by influencing the central nervous system while nicotin induces perspiration by acting both centrally and peripherally. As histologically and anatomically the nerve-fibers of the sweat glands and the vaso-constrictors resemble very closely, it is reasonable to presume, that like the latter, the central nervous regulator of the sweat glands is in the medulla.

Sebum (*rasa*) a semiliquid oily material, that is secreted by the sebaceous glands, distributed all over the cutaneous surface, chiefly associated with the hair follicle, but also without it as in the glans penis, lips and the deeper portions of the external auditory meatus, is meant possibly to protect the skin from bacterial invasion, and to prevent the hair from being brittle. Sebum on exposure to air forms a waxy cheesy mass as is seen in the comedones from the occlusion of the ducts, or in the glans penis (*Smegma preputti*) or in the auditory meatus (*cerumen*= ear-wax) and it contains fats, soaps, cholesterin, albuminous material (casein like), remnants of epithelial cells and inorganic salts. As the sebaceous secretive activites are associated with vaso-dilation, it is presumed that their nervous mechanism is the same, although sebum by its oil coating over the skin prevents the undue loss of heat as well as prevents the undue absorption of moisture. Vaso-dilation and vaso-constriction are regulated by the nerve-fibres belonging to the sympathetic or automatic nervous system.

Heat (*uṣmā*) is produced as a reaction of the intracellular oxidation or vital process and absorbed in the blood, it is conveyed to every part of the body to preserve the temperature equilibrium of the hot-blooded animal. For heat is being constantly lost from the body through radiation (conduction), evaporation (perspiration from the skin), respiration (vaporization of water through lungs), and with urine and feces. If there is excess of heat, it is conducted to the periphery and is radiated with sweat by vaso-dilation. If on the other hand, the surrounding air is cold and the body needs to conserve its heat, there is vaso-constriction so that the escape of heat is reduced, as well as the production of heat is stimulated by increased oxidation. In cold-blooded creatures as fish, amphibia, reptiles or in the hibernating animals (*poikilothermos*), either the oxidizing process is not yet intense as in the former, or the heat-regulating mechanism is absent or poorly developed as in the latter, and the consequence is that their body temperature fluctuates with that of the surroundings. While the hot blooded animal (*homoiothermous*) keeps relatively a constant temperature independent of the surroundings. There:is every reason to believe that the heat-regulating mechanism (tissue-oxidation for the prduction of heat, conservation of heat through vaso-constriction, and radiation of heat through vaso-dilation) is controlled by a nervous center, which perhaps is situated either in the pons or medulla.

III. PATHOLOGY

"Whatever causes pain, is a disease (*vyādhi*). Diseases are of four kinds: accidental or mechanical (*āgantu*), physical (*śārira*), mental (*mānasa*), and natural (*svābhāvika*). Diseases caused by injuries are *'āgantu'* ; of alimentary origin and by the derangement of the nervous, venous, lymphatic and arterial systems, *'śārira'* ; through anger, sorrow, fear, joyousness, sadness, jealousy, concentration of mind, misery, haughtiness, greed, envy, desires and longings, *'mânasa'* ; hunger, thirst. senility, sleep and death, are 'natural' diseases". *Suśruta* I.I. 20[44a] .

"Again, the diseases originate from seven sources as follows: hereditary (*ādivala*), maternal (*janmavala*), alimentrry (*doṣavala*), mechanical (*saṃghātavala*), physical (*kālavala* = seasonal),

---

44(a). तद्दुःखसंयोगा व्याधय इत्युच्यन्ते । ते चतुर्व्विधा आगन्तवः शारीरा मानसा स्वाभाविकाश्चेति । तेषामागन्तवोऽभिघातनिमित्ताः । शारीरास्त्वन्नपानमूला वात-पित्त-कफ-शोणित-सन्निपातवैषम्यनिमित्ताः । मानसास्तु क्रोध-शोक-भय-हर्ष-विषादेर्ष्याभ्यसूया-दैन्य-मात्सर्य्य-लोभ-काम-प्रभृतय इच्छाद्वेषभेदैर्भवन्ति । स्वाभाविकाः क्षुत्पिपासाजरामृत्युनिद्राप्रभृतयः । सुश्रुत, सूत्रस्थानम्, १, २० ।

contagious (*daivavala*), and natural (*svabhāvavala*) *Suśruta* I, 24. 4[45].

"The diseases that are transmitted through the lesion in the sperm or the ovum of the parents, are hereditary, as '*kuṣṭha*' (leprosy—there is every reason to belive that the syphilic eruption of the skin and ulceration were regarded as varieties of leprosy) and '*arśa*' (hemorrhoids). The hereditary diseases are of two kinds and might come either from father or mother's side.

"The diseases that are produced through the improper regimen (*apachara* = wrong food and injurious exercise) of the mother (during the intra-uterine life of the fetus) are called maternal as born—lame, blind, deaf, mute, '*minmina*' (one who speaks with a hissing nasal accent, due to overgrowth of adenoid tissue in the rhino-pharynx) and the dwarf. These diseases (acquired during the intra-uterine life) are caused by either) mother's (defective) circulation (*rasakṛta*) or miserable living.

"The diseases that are produced through improper food and living, or (reacting through

---

45. तत् तु सप्तविधे व्याधावुपनिपतति । ते पुनः सप्तविधा व्याधयस्तद्यथा—आदिवलप्रवृत्ता जन्मवलप्रवृत्ता दोषवलप्रवृत्ताः संघातवलप्रवृत्ताः कालवलप्रवृत्ता दैववलप्रवृत्ताः स्वभाववलप्रवृत्ता इति । सुश्रुतसंहिता, सूत्रस्थानम्, २४, ४ ।

digestion) anxiety, are '*alimentary*'. Alimentary diseases are of two kinds—gastric and intestinal occasioned by physical causes (as improper food and living) or mental causes (as anxiety, fear or nervous excitement).

"(The diseases occasioned by) the injuries struck with force on the weak, are '*mechanical*' whether by instruments or by ferocious animals.

"The diseases that are producd by cold, heat, wind and rain, are '*physical*', whether (they) are natural or unnatural.

"The diseases that are produced by the tyranny of the gods (through thunder and lightning), through curses (*phobia*), sorceries of the *Atharva-veda* (infectious diseases), and through contagion (syphilis) are *daiva-vala* (god-sent, i. e. beyond human control). These diseases are of two kinds as occasioned by thunder-lightning or by demons (infectious diseases as cholera or small-pox). And again they are of two kinds—through accident (as thunder-lightning) or through contact (as syphilis).

"Hunger, thirst, senility (old-age), sleep and death etc. are natural diseases. They are of two kinds—timely or untimely. They can be cured when they are untimely (i. e. if there is hunger, thirst or premature senility, when there is no reason for it, they are proper subjects for treatment), but not so when they are timely."

Suśruta 1, 24. 5-7[46].

"In addition to (parasitic) animalcules (that cause disease), there are twenty kinds of microbes (*krimi*) divided into four classes." *Charaka* III. 7. 6[47].

"The origin of the microbes of the blood-vessels (veins), is like that of leprosy. Their

---

46. तत्रादिबलप्रवृत्ता ये शुक्रशोणितदोषान्वयाः कुष्ठार्शःप्रभृतयः ; तेऽपि द्विविधा मातृजाः पितृजाश्च। जन्मबलप्रवृत्ता ये मातुरपचारात् पङ्गुजात्यन्धबधिरमूकमिन्मिन-वामनप्रभृतयो जायन्ते ; तेऽपि द्विविधा रसकृता दौहृदापचारकृताश्च। दोषबलप्रवृत्ता य आतङ्कसमुत्पन्ना मिथ्याहाराचारंभवाश्च ; तेऽपि द्विविधा आमाशयसमुत्थाः पक्वाशय-समुत्थाश्च, पुनश्च द्विविधाः शारीरा मानसाश्च। एत आध्यात्मिकाः ॥५

संघातबलप्रवृत्ता य आगन्तवो दुर्ब्बलस्य बलवद्विग्रहात् ; तेऽपि द्विविधाः शस्त्रकृता व्यालादिकृताश्च। एत आधिभौतिकाः ॥६

कालबलप्रवृत्ता ये शीतोष्णवातवर्षाप्रभृतिनिमित्ताः। तेऽपि द्विविधा व्यापन्नर्त्तुकृता अव्यापन्नर्त्तुकृताश्च। दैवबलप्रवृत्ता ये देवद्रोहादभिशप्तका अथर्व्वकृता उपसर्गकृताश्च, तेऽपि द्विविधा विद्युदशनिकृताः पिशाचादिकृताश्च, पुनश्च द्विविधाः संसर्गजा आकस्मिकाश्च। स्वभावबलप्रवृत्ताः क्षुत्पिपासाजरामृत्युनिद्राप्रभृतयः ; तेऽपि द्विविधाः कालकृता अकाल-कृताश्च। तत्र परिरक्षणकृताः कालकृता अपरिरक्षणकृता अकालकृताः। एत आधिदैविकाः। तत्र सर्व्वव्याध्यवरोधः ॥७॥ सुश्रुतसंहिता, सूत्रस्थानम्, १४, ५-७।

47. विंशतिविधाः क्रिमयः पूर्व्वमुद्दिष्टा नानाविधेन प्रविभागेनान्यत्र सहजेभ्यः। ते पुनः प्रकृतिभिर्विभज्यमानाश्चतुर्व्विधा भवन्ति। चरकसंहिता, विमानस्थानम्, ७, ६।

habitat is the blood-vessels. They are very minute, globular and without feet. Many of them are so minute that they are invisible." *Charaka* III. 7. 7[48].

Pathology or the science of disease, has up to the last century, been rather vague owing to the complexity of reaction of the pathogenic agents upon the living matter. Bacteriology is entirely a modern science. A few years ago it was not even suspected that infectious diseases are due to the intervention of morbific microbic agents. Their very existence was not even known. Microscopy and chemical reagents have but recently revealed the most interesting teeming world of animalcules, which though invisible to the naked eye, are no less potent adversaries of the living beings, and there is a constant struggle between life and these invisible foes, to which it ultimately succumbs, and in spite of the relentless war of science for the last generation, it has not been able, but partially, to conquer and to control them. Even the diseases that we call organic, as the cardiac

---

48. शोणितजानान्तु कुष्ठैः समानं समुत्थानम्। स्थानं रक्तवाहिन्यो धमन्यः संस्थानमणवो वृत्ताश्चापादाश्च। सूक्ष्मत्वाच्च एके भवन्त्यदृश्याः। चरकसंहिता, विमानस्थानम्, ७, ७।

affection, or metabolical as gout, may be the manifestations of the accumulated reactions of pathogenic germs, which have disappeard long ago, as pneumococci and gonococci respectively. This is clearly seen in tabes dorsalis, as a sequel of syphilis, after twenty or thirty years of infection.

The ancient conception of disease was based more or less on humoral pathology, i. e. disease originated from the derangement of the humors and it was the function of the diet and medicine and proper living, to bring them back to their normalcy and equilibrium. According to the Hindu schools of medicine, there were three fundamental humors (*vāyu*, *pitta*, *kapha*), according to the Greek, four (blood, phlegm, bile and water by some, yellow and black biles by others) in the human body. '*Vāyu*' is the active principle like the wind, which brings hot and cold waves ; '*pitta*' is the heat principle like the sun ; and the '*kapha*' is the cold principle like the moon, whose beams were reputed to exercise a very soothing and beneficial influence on plant life, in contradistinction of the sun's rays which were supposed to have a scorching effect, as it usually happens in an arid tropical climate. (*Suśruta* 1. 21. 8). As for the luxuriant vegetable life and growth, all these three elements in their right proportion are necessary, and excess of either, heat, cold or wind, is injurious to the plant, as in the animal kingdom.

However fanciful and grotesque this appears at the first glance to the moderner, it is not really so when it is seen with clear perspective and sharp analysis. It is true that concrete facts and statements appeal more to reason than vague generalization and abstract philosophy. But by close observation it will be easily observed that their *'vāyu, pitta, kapha'* correspond, to what is expressed in vulgar terminology, as *'nervous, sanguine and phlegmatic temperaments* and which can be translated into medical nomenclature as *'hypermetabolism, normal metabolism and hypometabolism.'* The following citations tend to lead to the aforesaid conclusion :—

"The bodily oxidation (*agni*) is classified into four kinds according to its activities as follows :— hyper-(*tīkṣṇa*), hypo-(*manda*), normal (*sama*) and abnormal (*viṣama*). Of them (one of) hypermetabolism is able to bear all abuses (i. e possesses a great resisting power against infection) ; hypometabolism has its opposite qualities ; normal metabolism becomes (easily) upset by abuse, but without abuse, remains natural ; abnormal metabolism has the opposite qualities of the normal,." *Charaka* III. 6. 6[49].

"These four kinds of oxidation pertain to man. Those who have *vāyu, pitta, kapha,* in propotion (equal), enjoy normal oxidation. In the case of those who have predominance of *vāta* (nervous temperament), oxidation beomes abnormal by association with *vāyu.* In those who have predominance of *pitta* (sanguine temperament), oxidation becomes accentuated by its association (hyper-oxidation). In those who have predominance of '*śleṣma*' (phlegmatic temperament), their oxidation becomes lowered by its association (hypo-oxidation)." *Charaka* III. 6. 7[50].

"The dominant qualities at the time of union of

---

49. अग्निषु तु शारीरेषु चतुर्व्विधो विशेषो बलभेदेन भवति। तद्यथा तीक्ष्णो मन्दः समो विषमश्चेति। तत्र तीक्ष्णोऽग्निः सर्व्वापचारसहः, तद्विपरीतलक्षणस्तु मन्दः, समस्तु खल्वपचारतो विकृतिमापद्यते, अनपचारतस्तु प्रकृतावेवावतिष्ठते। समलक्षण-विपरीतलक्षणस्तु विषमः। चरकसंहिता, विमानस्थानम्, ६, ६।

50. इत्येते चतुर्व्विधा भवन्त्यग्नयश्चतुर्व्विधानामेव पुरुषाणाम्। तत्र समवातपित्तश्लेष्मणाम् प्रकृतिस्थानां समा भवन्त्यग्नयो वातलानान्तु वाताभिभूतेऽग्न्यधिष्ठाने विषमा भवन्त्यग्नयः। पित्तलानान्तु पित्ताभिभूते ह्यग्न्यधिष्ठाने तीक्ष्णा भवन्त्यग्नयः। श्लेष्मलानान्तु श्लेष्माभिभूते ह्यग्न्यधिष्ठाने मन्दा भवन्त्यग्नयः। चरकसंहिता, विमानस्थानम्, ६, ६।

the sperm with ovum, are inborn (with the baby), as temperament (*prakṛti*). *Suśruta* III. 4. 48[51].

"The man of nervous (*vāta*) temperament, is sleepless (*jāgaruka*), sensitive to cold, ill-tempered, exclusive (*stena*=thievish), haughty, unmannerly (*anārya*=un-arian), fond of music, songs, dance and arts (*gandharvachitta*), whose hands and feet are long, whose beard, hair and nails are very dry, who is excitable (*krodhālu*= angry) and strike people with handand nails. That person is impatient, whose friendship is unstable, (who is) ungrateful, thin, violent, whose veins show out throughout his body, (who is) garrulous, who walks fast, is fond of walking and is fickle-minded." *Suśruta* III 4. 59[52].

"The man of sanguine temperament (*pitta*) perspires freely, smells come from his body (from volatile oil), his body has the yellowish color

---

51. शुक्रशोणितसंयोगे यो भवेद्दोष उत्कटः।
प्रकृतिर्जायते तेन तस्या मे लक्षणं शृणु॥ सुश्रुतसंहिता, शारीर-
स्थानम्, ४, ५८।

52. तत्र जागरूकः शीतद्वेषी दुर्भगः स्तेनो मत्सर्य्यनार्य्यो गान्धर्व्वचित्तः स्फुटित-
करचरणोऽतिरूक्षश्मश्रुनखकेशः क्रोधी दन्तनखखादी च भवति॥
अधृतिरदृढसौहृदः कृतघ्नः कृशपरुषो धमनीततः प्रलापी।
द्रुतगतिरटनोऽनवस्थितात्मा वियदपि गच्छति संभ्रमेण सुप्तः॥ सुश्रुतसंहिता,
शारीरस्थानम्, ४, ५९।

and is relaxed; and his nails, eyes, forehead, tongue, cheeks, and palms of hands and soles of feet are copper-colored (indications of good circulation of blood); he becomes repugnant when he gets wrinkled (*vali*), gray-haired (*palita*) and bald-headed (*khālitya*): he is a voracious eater, sensitive to heat and he becomes easily angry and easily satisfied; his strength and longevity are medium. A man of sanguinary temperament is brainy (*medhāvī*), clever and is an authoritative speaker; in combat he is brave and irresistible." *Suśruta* III. 4. 61[53].

"The complexion of a man of phlegmatic (*śleṣma*) temperament, is like the grass, blue lotus blossom or wet *ariṣṭa* (soap-tree), sharpened sword or the shaft of an arrow (i. e. fat and bright.) He is pleasant to look at, fond of eating sweet things (it is well-known that in myxedema or cretinism there is a great fondness

---

53. स्वेदनो दुर्गन्धः पीतशिथिलाङ्गस्ताम्रनखनयनतालुजिह्वौष्ठपाणिपादतलो दुर्भगो वलीपलितखालित्यजुष्टो बहुभुगुष्णद्वेषी क्षिप्रकोपप्रसादो मध्यमबलो मध्यमायुश्च भवति ॥६१

मेधावी निपुणमत्तिर्विगृह्य वक्ता
तेजस्वी समितिषु दुर्निवारवीर्य्यः। सुश्रुतसंहिता, शारीर-
स्थानम्, ४, ६१।

for sugar and high tolerance for carbohydrates), obliging, lazy, patient, without desires, heavy, indifferent and thick-bodied." *Suśruta* III. 4. 65[54].

One can see here almost the true clinical picture of hyper-thyroidism in an advanced state, in the primary stage and hypo-thyroidism. Thyroid influences metabolism. With metabolsim is inter-locked the automatic bodily mechanism of self-defence against infection. It is well-known that our integuments and mucous membranes swarm with innumerable pathogenic germs which almost live a harmless, vegetative parasitic life, but if the organism is devitalized by overwork or malnutrition, if its immunizing resisting power is lowered, in other words, if its defensive mechanism has been weakened, then infection takes place. We inhale almost with every inspiration plenty of *bacillus tuberculosis* and they lodge in our nostrils and lungs, we harbour in our intestine enough of *coli-group*, but they can not do any harm as long as our metabolic activities have not been lowered

54. दूर्व्वेन्दीवरनिस्त्रिंशार्द्रारिष्टशरकाण्डानामन्यतमवर्ण: सुभग: प्रियदर्शनो मधुरप्रिय: कृतज्ञो धृतिमान् सहिष्णुरलोलुपो बलवांश्चिरग्राही दृढ़वैरश्च भवति ॥ सुश्रुत-संहिता, शारीरस्थानम्, ४, ६५ ।

beyond the danger point. So far pathogenesis, vitality of the organism, is the important factor. This vitality classification, coefficient with metabolism and oxidation, is practically synonymous with *vāyu* (= air) as a conductor of hot and cold waves, *pitta*(= heat principle), *kapha* (= cold principle), which we are justified to translate as the nervous (*hypermetabolism*), sanguine (*normal metabolism*) and phlegmatic (*hypometabolism*) temperaments, and on which the whole system of the Hindu medicine is based. If there are points in which the picture drawn by Charaka varies from modern clinical observation (as bad smell and premature senility in sanguine temperament, and strength in phlegmatic type), it should not be forgotten that, there have been evolutive changes with time both in the pathogenic agents and our system, from the time of the ancients and consequently reactions have been partially modified. Moreover, it is good to remember that for the age in which Charaka and Suśruta lived, their studies strike our admiration from the comparative historical point of view, but for modern practical needs, they are nothing but crude and vague generalizations.

I. Constitutional Pathogenesis

We can quite agree with Suśruta (I. 120) that 'whatever causes pain, is a disease'. But the definition will be more logical and correct if we say, "Disease is the state of body and mind, produced in the organism, by a morbific agent and the organism reacting against it."

It is yet controversial whether infections are transmitted by heredity (*ādivala*). According to Weissman (*gemules* of Darwin and *plastidules* of Haeckel are now practically discarded as bearers of heredity) the germplasm is a bridge between the past and the present, linking man to the first-developed unicellular existence. The germplasm or the germinative cell assures the continuity of life and progress. In the lowest step of the ladder in animal life, among protozoa, reproduction takes place by fission, budding or both combined when the mother cell, through excess of nutrition divides into two as a relief of cellular tension. With the growth of organic life and specialization of cells as an economy for functional utilities, special cells (*gamets*) have been developed for reproduction. In further evolution, gamets have been differentiated into female gamet (*ovum*) and male gamet (*spermatozoon*). Their amphimixis tends to cause variation, while the germ-plasm tries to conserve the type. Hence inspite of infinite variety, never two beings being the same, there is a fundamental unity of the species, as modifications are very slow.

The germplasm—the bearer of heredity, is the "*chromatin*' substance of the reproductive cell-nucleus. The chromatin divides into chromosomes (*idants*) and when they break up again, the smaller units are called chromomeres (*ids*) and each chromomere or '*id*' contains all the dynamic potentialities—generic, specific, individual, which under appropriate nutrition and temperature, forms the organism. Each '*id*' is surrounded by hypothetical units, called the '*determinants*' and determinants by '*biphores*' which are supposed to exercise the directing influence in the development of phylogenic evolutive transformations. Though immortality of the germ-plasm can be maintained without amphimixis, as in parthenogenetic eggs or by artificial parthogenesis in normal ova as demonstrated by J. Loeb, in higher plants and animals however, sexual conjugation is the normal process. Conjugation or fertilization means the reducing division of the chromosomes and the restoration of the normal bulk in the fertilized ovum by equal contribution from both the parent cells. The stimulus which activates the fertilization is a chemotactic substance liberated by both the cells, but it seems that if the ovum is stronger as in the final stage, there is a protoplasmic outgrowth towards the spermatozoon. The protoplasm contains nutritive materials for the embryo.

Inheritance of heredity is complicated by two factors. Somatic characteristics are not transmitted—but only germinal. Yet the germinal materials are influenced by somatic behaviour or functional uses. One might lose his limbs and his children would not be born without them. The Jews have been practising circumcision for the last four thousand years, yet the Jewish male babies are born with prepuce. But according to the experiments of Brown Sequard, if the sciatic nerve of a guinea pig be cut, the animal becomes epileptic and if mated, brings forth offsprings that are epileptic, though the sciatic nerve is there and has not been severed, but its functional disturbance has been fixed by heredity.

Somatic cells undergo the evolutionary modifications of the functional exercise of an organ, by which its development is regulated. Therfore the hereditary transmissions are of two kinds, germinal and epigenetic, i. e. the germplasmic material becomes influenced and modified by the somatic behaviour, that is, by external conditions. And though the amphimixis takes place, the characteristics of both the parents are not equally blend d in the offspring. It might receive the prepotent characteristics of one as in a cross between a Negro with a White, pigment and hair etc., or the recessive charcteristics of the other. The sex of the offspring, according to some, depends on the maturity of the ovum, and if the fertilisation takes place in the beginning, it is male and if at the terminating period of the catamenia, it is female. If the twins are not of the same sex, it is because two ova have been fecundated at two different periods. Consanguineous marriages produce evil effects, for heredity fixes and accentuates the weak characteristics of both the parents. If a blind man marries a blind woman, there is a possibility that the offsprings of the mating would have defective eye-sight, if they are not born totally blind, but if a blind man marries a woman with good eye-sight, the negative characteristic of one would be counterbalanced by the other and children born of that marriage would not be affected probably in their eye-sight. Of course, the laws of heredity are not so simple. According to some biologists, one does not inherit more than

50 p. c. from the parents, i. e. half from the father and the mother, each one of the parents cotributing about one-fourth, and each one of the grand-parents one-eighth and so on according to the geometric regressive proportion. But there may be also sudden reversion to the ancestral type and what is known as '*atavism.*' So no fixed rules of heredity can be determined. But it is certain that the parents transmit to their offspring their psychic and bodily impressions. For germ-plasms must be certainly very sensitive to the somatic impressions and transformations.

We have no definite proof that the pathogenic germs are directly transmitted with the germ-plasms. For if really the ovum or the spermatozoon be infected, then they would be incapable of fertilization, growth and development, lacking impulsive momentum, vitality and nutrition, necessary for amphimixis and embryonic formation. The frequent abortion that takes place in the primary state of syphilis, is not probably due to the presence of *treponema pallidum* in the germplasms, but due to their low vitality and exhausted condition of nutrition or the invasion of the embryo by the pathogenic germs through the placenta. Of course, there are cases known in medical history where the offspring has been born with all the stigmata of syphilis, acquired from the father, while the mother has acquired immunity from its infection from the fetus through gradual elaboration of the antibodies, as a reaction of the organism. But it does not necessarily imply that the spermatozoon that fertilized the ovum and caused conception, had living syphilic germ in it, or it might have been simply saturated with attenuated syphilic virus—mild enough not to interfere with embryonic and fetal growth, yet a sufficient cause to bring forth immunizing reactions in the maternal organism, without infecting her. In the matter of hereditary transmission of infectious diseases, the question is whether the germplasms can be carriers of infective microbes? In this the father is concerned only at the time of conception. Of course at the time of copulation and conception, the father's state of health and condition, are reflected in the offspring. If the father is youthfnl, healthy and in happy mood, the offspring acquires a gay and cheerful disposition of mind. If on the contrary, the father is aged, or suffers from dyspepsia, malaria or liver troubles, which naturally create a melancholy frame of mind, the children inherit the appearance of premature senility. The children of youthful parents usually inherit a mobile and agile nervous system, as in youth nerves are very sensitive and responsive to impressions. The children of gouty, tubercular or hemophiliac parentage aquire a diathetic predisposition to these diseases. In an arthritic family often are seen manifestations in different members of the family of gout, eczema, nervous affections, hepatic and renal lithiasis, diabetes and Bright's disease. But there is no conclusive evidence that the germ-plasm is a carrier of infectious germ.

But the mother's influence is much more preponderant. The fetus lives and grows in the mother's womb as a parasite for eight to ten months. For its nutrition it is dependent on the maternal circulatory system. Spermatozoon practically acts simply as a stimulant and gives the momentum to the ovum to start its anabolic evolutionary course. The child is really formed of the mother's nutrition. So her psychical and physical life vitally reflects in the formation and growth of the fetus, during the long period of gestation. If she has any infectious disease, it is very unusual, if she does not transmit it to the fetus through the placenta.

Nutritional (*doṣavala*) disturbances are many and varied, and are known as metabolic diseases. Nutrition is the function of every living cell, consisting in the taking in and assimilation through fermentative changes, whereby tissue is nourished and built and energy is liberated : its successive stages are known as digestion, absorption, assimilation, disassimilation and excretion.

Anabolism is the assimilative synthetic process, while catabolism is the retrograde disassimilative metabolism. For both these functions a liquid medium is necessary in which the nutritive substances can be in a soluble state, so that by osmotic pressure, it can percolate through the capillary wall and enter into interstitial space, from which the cells extract their food needs by endosmosis, and by exosmosis, throw out the metabolic waste products formed in the organic synthesis into the lymph stream. If any of the waste products be allowed to accumulate, the organism would die out of auto-intoxication.

So nutrition comprises various functions. (1) Transmission and transformation of food in the alimentary canal by the digestive enzymes, from insoluble into soluble products so that they become dialyzable: starches are saccharified, albumines are peptonised and fats are partly emulsified and partly split up into fatty acids and glycerine. (2) Absorption of the digested soluble nutrients. (3) Detoxication, synthesis and fixation of the nutrients in the liver, especially the glucose, which is converted into glycogen. (4) Transportation of the nutrients with the blood-circulation to every tissue of the body for the food-supply of the cells, the extraction of the food-material from the plasma by the cells, and ejection into it of the waste-production of catabolism. (5) Regressive metamorphosis and reduction of harmful disassimilative products into harmless substances, chiefly in the liver as the conversion of the nitrogenous end-products into urea. (6) Elimination of the metabolic wastes through the kidneys, lungs and the skin. It has been estimated that an adult voids daily 250 grams of iarbon and 18 grams of nitrogen. This must be replaced to preserve the equilibrium between the cncome and the expenditure of the bodily energy, or it will slowly starve to death.

Death takes place through starvation, when the body has lost nearly 45 per cent of its weight. When food is withdrawn, the orgainism performs its multifarious functional activities, as the pulsation of the heart, metabolism, respiration, maintenance of the body temperature, muscular contraction and excretion of waste products, by consumption of the body fat and protein, sacrificing the less useful to the more useful in the economy. Death is postponed if plenty of water is taken, for it maintains the integrity of the circulatory system and aids in the transportation of the metabolic wastes for expulsion from the body. Without sufficient consumption of water, the increased viscosity of blood and the retention of the toxic excretory substances hasten death. However, death through absolute starvation is very rare. But death through malnutrition—insufficiency or bad quality of food, especially during famine—is very common, indirectly or directly. Malnutrition weakens the vital resisting power of the organism and clears the way for the invasion of epidemics, which is usually the case, or death is slowly preceded by gradual emaciation, anemia, dropsy, cardiac and cerebral disturbances, especially delirium.

If the aliments are too abundant or of bad quality, the undigested food falls an easy prey to microbes that swarm in the alimentary canal, provoking fermentation and putrefaction, thus causing dyspepsia, lientery auto-intox icationn dlatation and catarrh of the digestive tube. In the children, it is manifest by gradual emaciation, nervous irritability and erethema of the buttocks, vulva and thighs. But even if it be digested and absorbed, overnutrition is liable, with excess of carbohydrate consumption to engender glycosuria, if it be coupled with hepatic and pancreatic insufficiency, with excess of protein consumption into peptonuria and albuminuria with heptal insufficiency under certain pathological conditions. The evil effects of over-nutrition did not escape Charaka. For he says: "If any one accustomed to day-sleep and the comforts of bed (i. e. does not take sufficient exercise) indulge in excess of oily, sweet and slimy substances, new rice, new wine, meat, fish, milk, butter, and cakes, he becomes subject to many diseases. If he does not reduce (the excessive consumption) of restorative dishes, he will suffer from diabetes (*prameha* = glycosuria and albuminuria), cutaneous irritation (*kaṇḍu*), pain (*gouty*), eczema (*koṭha*), jaundice, fever, leprosy, alimentary diseases, strangury (*mūtra-kṛchchhra*), loss of appetite, lassitude (*tandrā*), impotence, emaciation, lethargy, heaviness of the body, burdening the circulatory system with waste products, dullness of sense-impressions, mental cloudiness, drowsiness (*pramīlaka*), edema (*śotha*), and other diseases." *Charaka* I. 23. 1-5[55]

II. MECHANICAL PATHOGENESIS.

Mechanical (*ādhibhautika*) *agents* can be the means of causing bodily suffering and death in various ways under different circumstances. If a man falls from a tree, the injury would depend on the pressure of contact, based on force (weight, height of the position and the gravitation of the earth, as well as the nature of the ground). Even one can suffer fatal injury, especially to the nervous system, by the rapid vibration of air, as near the passage of a high-speed projectile, of which there have been numerous victims in the recent war and it is known as *'shell-shocks'*. Whatever may be the injury, it is due to the conflict of power and resistance. When one falls from a tree, he is the body in motion : when a sword or a bullet strikes him, he is the resistance. The injury on the wound depends on their mutual relation. One might strike another with a sword, lacking force without causing more than a bruise, but the same

55. प्रकृतिमिह नराणां भौतिकीं केचिदाहुः
पवनदहनतोयैः कीर्त्तितास्तास्तु तिस्रः । चरकसंहिता, सूत्रस्थान, २३, १—५ ।

sword can cut him in twain, if struck with vigor. The nature of a wound depends on the instrument and the force with which it is struck. With sharp-pointed intruments as the needle, pin, cannula of hypodermic syringe, sting of certain insects and scorpions, any wound is called the '*puncture*' and puncture is usually harmless. Even the heart can be punctured without any serious consequence. Neither is the puncture of the nerve serious, unless the vital centres are penetrated which might cause sudden death. A bruise in the soft parts without a break in the skin is called '*contused wound*' which heals very quickly. A clean cut with a sharp instrument is called the '*incised wound*' and though there is profuse bleeding as long as the incised parts are not tightened together, it heals rapidly usually without infection. Lacerated wounds are those which are inflicted with a blunt instrument or by biting of animals. They generally take a longer time to heal, as it is very hard to keep the torn out tissues in aseptic condition. The seriousness of a gun-shot wound depends on three factors, namely, the point of entrance, the tract and the point of exit. When the bullet has lodged in the tissues of the body, the tract is known as '*blind*'. The wound at the point of entrance is always smaller, due to the contractibility of the tissue than the aperture of the exit, as it is more subjected to pressure and distension and is consequently more or less lacerated whether the tract of the bullet is direct or tortuous. When a bullet lacks a great velocity, it slunts by, if it meets a bone and becomes tortuous, but if it be driven with a great force, it might drill clear through a bone or cause a fracture and impart to the fragments sufficient momentum to act as glancing missiles and aggravate the lesion. The wounds caused by explosives are more serious, as aside from the mechanical effect, the tremendous sudden increase of pressure and temperature, as well as the liberation of toxic gases cause a very severe nerve shock. In any gun-shot or explosive wound, it is the nerve-shock, that is the serious matter. Otherwise in a simple wound not affecting any vital part in the economy, if there is no introduction of any septic matter, and bleeding can be arrested and suppuration prevented, there need not be any fatal consequence.

The physical (*kāla-vala*) agents are many as heat, cold, air-pressure, sudden seasonal changes, dazzling light, the sun (sun-stoke), sound and electricity. It seems that the human organism can stand cold much easier than heat. Of course with the rising temperature, metabolism is slowed up and the consequence is less oxidation, which means in other words, less production of heat. And there is vaso-dilatation, and the blood rushing to the periphery loses part of its heat by radiation in the surrounding atmosphere, and with the evaporation of perspiration, there is not only further loss of heat, but also a noticeably cooling sensation. However, when the evaporation from the skin is not rapid as in humid heat, it is more unpleasant. The dog or the cat whose body is covered with hairy coating and can not perspire freely, put out their tongue, execute rapid respiratory movements and thus facilitate evaporation through their gustatory organ. But when due to excessive consumption of alcohol, the vaso-motor mechanism does not react, or due to burn, perspiration is interfered with, or in the close overheated chamber near a furnace or boiler, prostration comes with high fever, rapid pulse, stertorous respiration, hot and dry skin and delirium. Perhaps this symptoms-complex is due to the chemical change in the nerves, brought about by excessive heat and not to the coagulation of myosin as it was supposed before. Exposure to the strong sun for a long time, principally the unprotected head, affects the nervous mechanism directly, especially in one who has not been gradually accustomed to it, by the penetrating actinic rays, creating perhaps molecular changes in the nerve-cells. The prostration is extreme, rapid and sudden, but often the high temperature is missing, though in other ways, the symptoms are those of heat-stroke. Though cold can be better borne than heat, yet after heavy consumption of alcohol, which causes vaso-dilatation and consequently loss of heat, one can be easily frozen to death. The action of cold is intensified by humidity which absorbs a good deal of heat and wind which drives away the warm layer of air surrounding the body. Even a healthy person with prolonged exposure to cold and sudden fall of temperature, might get a frost-bite. The frost-bite is manifest in the first stage by erythema and rubefaction, in the second stage by ulceration and finally by eschars, entailing the loss of the organ. Even when it does not directly cause any lesion, indirectly in a weak, debilitated or undernourished organism, it causes the development of various germs as pneumococci; or there is an irresistible tendency to sleep from which one hardly wakes; or the physical and mental apathy may be interrupted by cerebral derangement and delirium, and one dies of heart-failure. The influence of the variations of the atmospheric pressure is not very negligible. At the sea level, the air exerts a pressure of 1.03 kilogramme per square centimeter, that is, about 18,000 kilogrammes for the human body. When a man makes an abrupt ascent to a high altitude in an aeroplane or makes a descent as a sea-diver, the sudden pressure variation is apt to cause various disturbances. At the sea level, at zero altitude, there is a barometric pressure of 76 centimeter of mercury; in Cashmere at the altitude of 7,000 feet, 56; at Mt. Everest at the altitude of 29,000 feet, 24.8. If a deep-sea fish is brought to the surface, it bursts from the expansion of the gas contained in the fish, so a man by a sudden high ascent not only finds it hard to breathe owing to the rarefaction of the air and consequent diminution of oxygen, but also the intestinal gases expand and cause tympanites and the blood rushing towards the periphery provoke diverse disorders from the results of anemia of the internal organs. At the altitude of 2000 meters, the oxygen diminishes 13 per cent; at 3000,21 per cent; at 6500,43 per cent and at 8500,50 per cent. To counteract this influcnce, the aeronauts are supplied with oxygen tanks, and the deep sea divers with compressed air to two or three atmospheres. The benefit of a mountain resort is in the purity of air and its higher ozone content. But above 11,000 feet, one who is not accustomed to high-mountain climbing, mountaineering may provoke '*mountain sickness*' with a symptom-complex of giddiness, nausea, dyspnea, headache, thirst, malaise and a slight rise of temperature, almost like the sea-sickness, and with weakness of heart may prove fatal. But when a deep-sea diver comes to the surface, he feels a buzzing sensation in the ears, due to the difference of pressure between the two surfaces on the tympanum, and this difference may be sufficiently great to cause rupture of the membrane, and there is a complaint of great fatigue and tendency to fainting. If the reduction of pressure is rapid, there is hemorrhage from the nose, ears and lungs and on the skin in puntiform shape, which the divers designate as '*flea bites.*'

Light is visible between 497,000,000,000 and 728,000,000,000 vibrations per second. Below or above this figure, there is no sensory impression. Yet within this narrow limit of our visibility, we can see that light plays an important part in stimulating our nervous system and general metabolism and killing many of the microbes exposed to it. It is well known how the sun light activates plant growth. Under its influence, carbonic acid—a waste product of the cellular metabolism, is made to unite with water—and thus reconstituting a hydrate of carbon—which is the principal mainstay of energizing food supply of human beings and herbivorous animals. And though light is used very effectively as a valuable therapeutic agent in dermatosis, a strong light might cause erythema and reflected light, either from sand as in the desert or snow, might provoke opthalmia and blepharitis. The harmfnl effects of light can be avoided by using blue or black glasses over the eyes, and covering the body, especially the head with black or blue cloth through which the ultra-violet rays can not penetrate and to which the irritation is due.

Sound is only audible within the close range of 30 and 30,000 vibrations per second. Prolonged harsh sounds may cause mechanical lesion, even perforation of the timpanum and reflexibly nervous irritation. The soothing and restorative effect of the mountains and country places is often in the freedom from noise. And music which is nothing but the harmyon of sound, is now well recognised as an important therapeutic agent for calming and soothing nervous irritation and in various other nervous derangements.

The nature of electricity is not fully understood. Life itself possibly is an electro-chemical reaction, brought about and maintained by the interchange of the intercellular fermentative activities. And the human body is a complicated electrical apparatus : the lungs are the battery and the nerves are the wires insulated with sheaths of medulated and lipoid coatings. If the nerve current propagates at the rate of 120 meters per second only, while electricity at 3000 miles, it is because the nerve is not a homogenous wire, but interrupted by thousands of sympathetic junctions. It is now recognised that the insignificant quantity of minerals in the diet plays a vital role in the economy. It is very likely that they are intimately connected with the generation of electric current. And like vibrations of light and sound waves, the human organism can only adjust within a limited range. Beyond that, it provokes death by molecular change in the nervous system as in electricution. The alternative current of 200 voltage kills a dog within 30 seconds, 700 a horse and about 2000 a human being. This also proves that the human body is a better electrical machinery, withstanding the shocks of 2000 voltage, while the horse though superior to man in body weight and muscular strength, succumbs to shocks of 700 voltage.

Infectious (*daiva-vala*) *agents* are of various kinds as a sporozoid in malaria (*plasmodium malaria*), a high fungus akin to streptothrix actinomyces in tuberculosis (*bacillus tuberculosis*) or a bacterium like gonococcus in gonorrhea. It seems that the pathogenic microbic agents are almost ubiquitous. They are in the soil, water and the air. They find themselves upon our skin from all sources. But they usually live there a harmless saprophytic life, as the horny epidermis underlined by a layer of fat offers resistance to their penetration. With each inspiration countless bacteria get admission in the respiratory passage, but they are retained by the hair in the nasal orifices and by the vibratile cilia of the mucous membrane. Those who penetrate farther, are either expelled with the mucous secretions, or by the germicidal mucus they are disinfected and pasted on the walls of the nasal orifices. The microorganism invade in large colonies the alimen tary canal with the ingestion of food and drink, but the hydrochloric acid content of the gastric juice possesses a considerable germicidal power. The intestine unquestionably is a fovorable place for their growth, as sufficient humidity, warmth and nutrition from the residue of the food are found ideally combined, and there is hardly any antiseptic secretion there to arrest their development. In the gastric cavity are found nearly 50,000 microbes, in the mouth of duodenum 30,000, in the cecum 25,000 and in the lower intestine about 100,000 per cubic millimeter. On the whole, on the same basis of computation there are about 412,000,000,000 microbes in the whole of the alimentary canal and every day with the feces from 12 to 15 billions are evacuated. That they do not increase usually more than that, is due to the fact that the fermentative bacterial colony counteracts the luxuriant growth of the putrefying germs which cannot flourish in the acid medium and thus they preserve a mutual balance against each other so that they can not easily become obnoxious to the economy. But in case the vegetative microbic flora become active and virulent, they reach the lymphatic glands and the liver, where tney are destroyed. Of course the toxins liberated by the pathogenic micro-organism can be absorbed, but they are more or less attenuated, modified and made innocuous in the hepatic cells and other mechanisms of the body. Though the vulva and vagina swarm with pathogenic germs, infection through the genito-urinary passages is very rare except in venereal diseases as gonorrhea, soft chancre and syphilis, where even an abrasion, wound or cut is necessary which generally takes place through the sexual congress by the sharp edges of the hair, so that the venereal disease-producing germs can find a safe lodging place to develop in vitality and virulence, as they are partly disinfected by the germicidal mucous secretion and washed away by the force of urination. When the morbific agents as streptococcus are introduced in the vaginal canal, they are all destroyed within forty-eight hours (*Menge*) by the abundant vaginal secretions.

But even when the pathogenic germs force through and invade the economy, the body is not defenceless. When their morbific action is not very virulent, the leucocytes rush up to the locality and destroy them ; if complete destruction is not possible for the phagocytes, the lesion is circumscribed by the leucocytes and the exudation. However, if the morbific invading micro-organisms are very virulent, then of course the leucocytes are repelled by the negative chemotoxic action of their secretory toxins. And then they invade the economy by the lymphatic or venous path. For blood has a considerable germicidal power due to its opsonic content. But even in case the microbes enter by way of the stomach or the intestine and reach the portal vein, they have to pass through the formidable fortresses of the bodily defensive mechanism—the liver and the lungs which exercise a tremendous germicidal action, before they can enter into the left heart to be thrown into the general circulation. And whether the microbes enter into the circulatory system by the portal vein or penetrating through the capillaries, any way in blood they have but short-lived existence, for either they are destroyed or driven into the capillaries, within less than ten to fifteen minutes.

Life is indeed a continuous struggle with the micro-organisms to preserve its integrity. Even when there is a general invasion, the body does not give up the task of self-preservation hopelessly. The body enjoys more or less various immunities—racial, ancestral, seasonal, inoculationary acquired and passive as a natural reaction of the organism to counteract the toxic products of the disease germs. We know that the Negro races possess a remarkable immunity against *yellow fever* while they are very susceptible to tetanus and tuberculosis. The Mongolian race is very predisposed to small-pox, but not to tuberculosis. It is well known that the offsprings of a gouty family are almost immune against tuberculosis. And syphilis runs in Europe a benign form, which when introduced among savages, rages like an epidemic and exterminates the population. Seasonal preference for diseases is also well marked as the typhoid and the gastro-intestinal diseases in the summer, malaria in the autumn, thoracic disorders in the winter and pneumonia in the spring. It is the Chinese who first noticed about four thousand years ago that certain diseases like the small-pox gave an immunity to its victim against its recurrence. On this principle, vaccination has driven away small-pox practically from all civilized countries. As a prophylaxis against infectious diseases, *serum therapy* is being built up on the same basis, inoculating an animal with the virus and thus gradually attenuating the virus through a few successive animals, a serum can be obtained which contains enough of antibodies, but not strong enough to cause any malaise, in the human system. The inoculation of the attenuated serum is not only a prophylaxis against the disease, but even when the infection takes place, it stimulates the resisting power of the organism by its bacteriolytic (*lysogenic*), agglutinative and opsonic action. Various sera have been made and tried as that of typhoid, pneumonia, cholera, but yet only the vaccine of small-pox has given completely satisfactory result. But undoutedly with the improvement of technique and with better knowledge of bio-chemistry and bacteriology, modified bacterial sera promise great results in therapeutics in no distant future.

Incubation Period of the Infectious Diseases.

Disease	Microbe	Average	Minimum	Maximum
Anthrax	Bacillus anthracis	2 days	1 day	3 days
Cholera	Spirillum cholera Asiatic	2 to 4 ,,	1 ”	6 ,,
Diphtheria	Klebs-Loeffler bacillus	2 ,,	2 ”	15 ,,
Erysipelas	Streptococcus erysipelatos	4 to 6 ,,	7 hours	22 ,,
Gonorrhea	Gonococcus	3 to 5 ,,	1 to 2 ”	7 to 28 ”
Influenza	Pfeiffer's bacillus	3 to 4 ,,	1 ”	5 ,,
Malaria	Plasmodium malariae	6 to 10 ,,	4 ”	Several months
Measles	...	8 to 12 ,,	4 ”	14 days
Plague	Bacillus pestis	1 to 3 ,,	8 hours	10 ,,
Small-pox	...	12 ,,	7 ”	15 ,,
Chicken Pox	...	15 ,,	14 ”	17 ,,
Syphilis	Treponema pallidum	20 to 30 ,,	10 ”	50 ,,
Tetanus	Bacillus tetani	2 to 3 ,,	7 hours	30 ,,
Typhoid	Bacilius typhosus	14 ,,	3 ”	21 ,,
Whooping cough	...	8 ,,	2 ”	10 ,,

All infectious diseases are now ascribed to microbic agents and they have been all identified except in some eruptive fevers as the scarlatina, measles, small-pox, varcella (*chicken pox*) and ere long, it is expected they will be isolated. The parasytic diseases can be classified this way.

Diseases due to pyogenetic micrococci :—Suppuration, septicemia, erysipelas and gonorrhea.

Acute diseases due to specific bacilli :—Cholera, diphtheria, influenza, meningitis, plague, pneumonia, tetanus, typhoid, yellow-fever.

Chronic diseases due to tissue bacilli :—Glanders, leprosy, tüberculosis, mycetoma (*Madura foot*).

Diseases due to protozoa :—Dysentery, filariasis, kala-azar, malaria, sleeping sickness, syphilis.

But the same morbific agent may cause local or general pathogenesis as for example, when pyogenic streptococcus is inoculated subcutaneously, only a local lesion—erysipelas is produced, but when it is injected into the veins, it causes general infection—septicema.

The microbes (*krimi*) in the feces originate in the same way as those in the lymphatics. Their habitat is the intestine. If some of them (*krimi*) travel towards the stomach, then in the breath and in the vomiting, there is bad odor. They are minute, globular (*micrococci*), white-complexioned, long (rod-like bacteria as that of the anthrax), and like the lamb-hair (*leptothrix*)." *Charaka* III. 7. 9[56].

Dental caries : "In this disease the microbes (*krimi*), orginating from corrupt blood, blacken, perforate and loosen the teeth." *Suśruta* II. 16, 27[57].

The disease-producing germs are introduced into the system either through the air as tuberculosis, food and drink as in cholera, through soil as in tetanus, personal contact as in gonorrhea, or through an intermediatory as in malaria (*anopheles*). As long as the microbes remain in vegetative state, they simply live as parasites, but sparing the host and doing the least harm to the economy, as they take only the minimum food for their maintenance. It is only when the organism is devitalized due to over-work, fatigue,

---

56. पुरीषजास्तुल्यसमुत्थानाः श्लेष्मजैः। तेषां पक्वाशय एव स्थानम्। प्रवर्द्धमानास्त्वधो ते विसर्पन्ति, यस्य पुनरामाशयोन्मुखाश्च स्युः, तदनन्तरं तस्योद्गारनिश्वासाः पुरीषगन्धिनः स्युः। संस्थानवर्णविशेषास्तु सूक्ष्मवृत्तपरीणाहाः श्वेता दीर्घोर्णांशुसङ्काशाः केचित्। चरकसंहिता, विमानस्थानम्, ७, ९।

57. कृष्णश्छिद्री चलः स्रावी ससंरम्भो महारुजः। अनिमित्तरुजो वाताद्विज्ञेयः कृमिदन्तकः॥ सुश्रुतसंहिता, निदानस्थानम्, १६, २७।

malnutrition, or undernutrition that they become virulent and by their toxic secretion cause functional disturbances and reactions.

Flies deposit microbes in the ulcer and when the ulcer is eaten up by those microbes, (local) edema is produced. *Suśruta* IV. I. 103[58].

Chemical (biṣa) agents are many, but they can be divided into two classes as endogenous and exogenous. The endogenous toxins are those that are produced autogenously in the cells as metabolic wastes or engendered by the microbes that live on the body as parasites. The exogenous toxins may be introduced with rotten, poisonous, indigestive or disharmonious combination of food and drink, bites of venomous snakes and insects, occupations in lead, copper, corrosive chemicals, sulphur, arsenic, quick-silver mines or ovens, especially of coke-coals where in addition carbon monoxide may be absorbed

"Toxins are of two kinds : stable (*vegetable and metallic*) and mobile (of animal origin).

---

58 मक्षिका व्रणजातस्य निक्षिपन्ति यदा क्रिमीन् ।
श्वयथुर्भक्षिते तैस्तु जायते भृशदारुणः ॥

सुश्रुतसंहिता, चिकित्सितस्थानम, १, १०३ ।

Stable toxins are divided into ten classes and the mobile toxins into sixteen classes. Root, leaf, fruit, flower, skin, exudation, juice, extract, '*dhātu*' (*chemical principle or metal*) and bulb are the sources of *sthāvara* (*stable*) poisons." *Suśruta* V. 2. 2-3[59].

"Retention of feces and urine (through absorption of their poisonous contents), day-sleep, keeping vigil at night, drinking of liquor, exposure to cold and wind, sexual excess, exposure to foul odor, dust, smoke, wind and the sun, ingestion of (excessive quantity of) foods that are hard to digest, acid or vegetables (*śāka*= leaves of plants), drinking of very cold water, receiving a wound in the head, acidity due to indigestion, weeping, retention of tear, cloudy weather, extreme depression, some misfortune to the country and untimely season, derange the nerve, venous and lymphatic systems and vitiate the blood of the brain and

---

59. स्थावरं जङ्गमञ्चैव द्विविधं विषमुच्यते ।
दशाधिष्ठानमाद्यन्तु द्वितीयं षोड़शाश्रयम् ॥
मूलं पत्रं फलं पुष्पं त्वक् चीरं सार एव च ।
निर्य्यासो धातवश्चैव कन्दश्च दशमः स्मृतः ॥२

सुश्रुतसंहिता, कल्पस्थान, २, २-३ ।

thus cause headache with varied symptoms." *Charaka* 1. 17. 4[60].

"Foods that are turned into poison by (disharmonious) combination, are being mentioned...... Do not eat meat or fish with the grains of sprouting rice, fat, honey, milk, molasses or with bean (*māṣa-paseolus radiatus*). Do not take clarified butter, if it has been kept more than ten days in a brass vessel." *Suśruta* 1. 20. 12-13[61].

---

60. सन्धारणाद्दिवास्वप्नाद्रात्रौ जागरणान्मदात् ।
उच्चैर्भाष्यादवश्यायात् प्राग्वातादतिमैथुनात् ॥
गन्धादसात्म्यादाघ्रातादजोधूमानिलातपात् ।
गुर्व्वम्लहरितादानादतिशीताम्बुसेवनात् ॥
शिरोभिघाताद्दुष्टामाद्रोदनाद्बाष्पनिग्रहात् ।
मेघागमान्मनस्तापाद्देशकालविपर्य्ययात् ॥
वातादयः प्रकुप्यन्ति शिरस्यस्रञ्च दुष्यति ।
ततः शिरसि जायन्ते रोगा विविधलक्षणाः ॥

चरकसंहिता, सूत्रस्थानम, १७, ४ ।

61. अतोऽन्यान्यपि संयोगादहितानि वक्ष्यामः । न च विरूढ़धान्यैर्वसामधुपयोगुड़माषैर्वा ग्राम्यानूपौदकपिशितादीन्यभ्यवहरेत् । न पयोमधुभ्यां रोहिणीशाकं जातुशाकं वाश्नीयात । बलाकां वारुणीकुल्माषाभ्याम्, काकमाचीं पिप्पलीमरिचाभ्यां, नाड़ीभङ्गाशाककुक्कटदधीनि च नैकध्यम् । मधु चोष्णोदकानुपानं पित्तेन वा मांसानि । सुराकृशरापायसांश्च नैकध्यम् । सौवीरकेण सह तिलशष्कुलीम् । मत्स्यैः सहेक्षुविकारान् । गुड़ेन काकमाचीम् । मधुना मूलकम । गुड़ेन वाराहं मधुना सह विरुद्धम् । क्षीरेण मूलकम् । आम्रजाम्बवश्वाविच्छूकरगोधाश्च सर्व्वांश्च मत्स्यान्

"Poison is not the only toxin; unpurified copper (that has not been incinerated and calcinated) is a terrible poison." *Rasendra-Sāra-saṃgraha* 1. 136[62].

"Unpurified sulphur (that has not been incinerated and calcinated) produces fever, eczema, delirium and bilious disorders." *Rasendra-sāra-saṃgraha* 1. 50[63].

Purified mercury (that has been incinerated and calcinated) is like real ambrosia, but faulty (i. e. incompletely purified or unpurified) is harmful like venom." *Rasendra-sāra-saṃgraha* 1. 7[64].

विशेषेण चिलिचिमं पयसा। कदलीफलं तालफलेन पयसा दध्ना तक्रेण वा। लकुचफलं पयसा दध्ना माषसूपेन वा मधुना घृतेन च, प्राक पयसः पयसोऽन्ते वा ॥१२

अतः कर्म्मविरुद्धान् वक्ष्यामः। कपोतान् सर्षपतैलभृष्टान् नाद्यात्। कपिञ्जलमयूरलावतित्तिरिगोधाश्च एरण्डदार्व्वग्निसिद्धा एरण्डतैलसिद्धा वा नाद्यात्। कांस्यभाजने दशरात्रपर्युषितं सर्पिः। मधु चोष्णं उष्णे वा। मत्स्यपरिपचने शृङ्गवेरपरिपचने वा सिद्धां काकमाचीम्। तिलकल्कसिद्धमुपोदिकाशाकम्। नारिकेलेन वराहवसापरिभृष्टां बलाकाम्। भासमङ्गारशूल्यं नाश्नीयादिति ॥

सुश्रुतसंहिता, सूत्रस्थानम्, २०, १२-१३।

62. न विषं विषमित्याहुस्ताम्रञ्च विषमुच्यते। रसेन्द्रसारसंग्रह, १, १३६।

63. अशुद्धगन्धः कुरुते तु तापं कुष्ठं भ्रमं पित्तरुजां करोति।

रसेन्द्रसारसंग्रह, १, ५०।

64. शुद्धोऽयममृतः साक्षात दोषयुक्तो रसो विषम् ॥ रसेन्द्रसारसंग्रह, १, ७।

Poisoning might also take place from the ingestion of some fish-eggs at the breeding season, some fish and molluscs which live on putrefied matter, from the cooking earthen vessels that are varnished with substances containing lead, arsenic or vermillion, foods that are colored and flavored with aniline products or preserved with an excessive dose of salicylic acid.

All the snakes are not poisonous however, for though they are provided with a venom gland, all of them do not possess an excretory duct, so that the venom can not be poured out.

But all poisons do not act immediately on the organism. Some poisons especially the metallic ones as arsenic, mercury, lead, sulphur have cumulative effect. Though they may be taken in small doses, they may be accumulated in the liver and the osseous system and after months or even years, they might express in violent reaction of their cumulated effect. But in other poisons as that of morphine, alcohol and tobacco, the harmful reaction ceases more or less after a while when the organism aquires the habit of neutralising the noxious substances of those poisonings. Tobacco not only harms the organism by the partial absorption of nicotine, but also by the inhalation of carbonic acid, carbonic oxide, sulphuretted hydrogen, hydrocyanic acid and pyridic bases, which the tobacco smoking produces.

According to Charaka (III. 6. 4), the diseases are innumerable, but Suśruta (VI. 66. 6.) calculates them as eleven hundred.

IV. DISEASES AND THEIR DIAGNOSIS.

"The physician in order to make a prognosis, must examine by *direct* (*pratyakṣa*), *indirect* (*anumāna* = inference) and *differential diagnosis*, the *color* [of the skin : lemon yellow tint in pernicious anemia, waxy pallor in nephritis, bronzing in Addison's disease, greenish hue in chlorosis, blue skin (*cyanosis*) in conjenital heart disease, brownish-yellow coloration in jaundice, grayish tinge in the long-continued therapeutic ingestion of silver nitrate, yellow tint in cancer and a permanent pallor in malarial cachexia, tuberculosis, leucemia, syphilis, chronic mercurial, lead and arsenic poisoning], *voice* [whispering voice (*aphonia*), coarse or harsh quality of the voice that is generally known as '*hoarseness*' (*dysphonia*) are due to the inflammation of the larynx, or disease, or pressure upon the recurrent laryngeal nerve ; chronic aphonia (hysterical aphonia is only temporary) is said to be prodromal of leprosy and chronic hoarseness that of cancer ; deep, hoarse voice and brassy cough indicate interference with the superior laryngeal nerve and if there is aphonia without cough or dysphonea, it may be due to paralysis of all the laryngeal muscles ; a flat and toneless voice results form one-sided paralysis of a cord and a falsetto voice from paresis of the tensors of the cords ; the open nasal tone is indicative of the paralysis of the soft palate or destruction of the soft palate by ulceration, usually syphilitic or of congenital cleft of the palate, and the closed nasal voice is often suggestive of coryza, hay asthma, hypertrophic rhinitis, nasal polypus, postnasal adenoids, enlarged faucial tonsils, suppurative tonsilitis, acute pharyngitis and retropharyngeal abscess ; the varied forms of aphasia, motor (*aphemia*, *agraphia*), sensory (*visual*, *auditory*), conduction, are the symptomatic expressions of the focal cerebral lesion, occurring in the left hemisphere in the right handed and the right hemisphere in the left-handed, but might also occur in cerebral hemorrhage, thrombosis, embolism, abscess, tumor, gumma, depressed fracture of the skull and more rarely in hysteria, neurasthenia and immediately after epileptic convulsion], *odor*

[an unpleasant odor of breath is usually present in the mouth of those whose teeth are not cleansed and food particles are allowed to accumulate on them and to cause decomposition and fermentation ; a foul odor in stomatitis and glossitis ; a stale and musty odor with the accumulation of sordes upon the teeth as in typhoid ; caries of the teeth, necrosis of the jaw, pharyngeal or tonsillar diphtheria, follicular tonsilitis and locunar concretions also produce bad odor ; but the most fetid odor attends the mercurial and gangrenous stomatitis and less so scurvy ; in uridrosis occurring with diseases in which the action of the kidney has been impaired, the sweat has a urinous odor, and deposits white scales or crystals of urinary solids upon the skin ; there is volatile fatty emanation from the sebaceous secretion and mixed with perspiration, the odor varies in health and sickness, according to age and race : among the Negroes, it is the most pronounced and in the Mongolian race, it is the least], *taste* [a bitter taste is felt in jaundice ; a coppery taste in gastro-duodenal catarrh (biliousness) ; diversified taste sensations as sweetish, sour, foul are felt when the tongue is coated and furred from whatever cause ;

abnormal taste with the long continued use of certain drugs as potassium bromide, iodide or tartar emetic; perversions of taste in hysteria; absence of taste (*ageusia*), if it is unilateral is indicative of the disease of the glosso-pharyngeal nerve, and if it is bilateral, of the diseases of the nose as coryza or polypus; partial impairment of taste (*hemiageusia*) may be due to the facial paralysis, or due to local conditions of the mucous membrane of the tongue, involving the taste buds and end-organs of the gustatory fibers, as in thickly furred or coated tongue, or due to the irritating(as of piperine)or blunting(as of bromides) action of the drugs or condiments), *touch* (*sparśa*) comprises tactile sense (*esthesic*), pain sense (*algesic*), temperature sense (*thermesthesic*), muscle sense (*myesthesic*): the loss of tactile sensibility (*anesthesia*) is indicative of cerebral lesions (*causing hemiplegia*), hysteria, traumatic neuroses, diseases of the spinal cord, especially locomotor ataxia, neuritis and leprosy; hemi-anesthesia, the loss of sensibility confined to one side of the body or to lower extremities or of unequal distribution, are mainly due to hysteria; an excessive sensibility (*hyperesthesia*) is generally met with in hysteria, chiefly in the hysterogenic zones, which are in the breasts and below them in the central part of the chest, in the pelvic region and the back; in neurasthenia there are localized hypersensitive tender spots along the spine, scalp and the chest; in menopause and gouty diathesis, there are also tender points on the scalp; a general hypersensitiveness may be present in influenza, typhoid fever, and in alcoholic intoxication, disturbances in the heat and cold sensation (*thermaesthesic*) are due to syringomyelia and to a less extent to the lesions of the medulla and locomotor ataxia; disturbances of the pain sensation—either hyper—or hypo-sensibility are due to syringomyelia, Morvan's disease, hysteria and syphilic chord disease; loss of muscular sensation is characteristic in locomotor ataxia, paramyoclonus multiplex, myeletic disease, and the lesions in the medulla and the pons; transference of sensation (*allochiria*) so that a touch, on one side of the body is felt on the other, is symptomatic of hysteria, locomotor ataxia, disseminated sclerosis, myeletis; delayed conduction so that a tactile or pain sensation requires 5 seconds or more, instead of one-tenth of a second, is characteristic of locomotor ataxia and peripheral paresis), the *eye* (edema of the eye-lid, particularly the lower one, is usually symptomatic of renal disease; morning puffiness with bloated face is also seen after a night of debauchery or in cases of profound anemia, chlorosis or in neurotic adoloscents; in erysipelas, glanders, severe coryza, hay fever, measles, variola and occasionally in varcella, as well as the prolonged use of arsenic and iodine may induce the swelling of the eye-lids; ptosis—the dropping of the eye-lid—is either congenital or due to the paralysis of the third nerve; lagophthalmos—imperfect closure of the lids follows paralysis of the orbicularis muscle, either due to lesions of the portio dura of the facial nerve or leprosy; blepharospasm—spasmodic closure of the lids is due to the reflex excitability of the fifth nerve in photophobia, in ocular disorders and is symptomatic of meningitis, cerebral tumors, typhus, measles in certain stages of their evolution and may be also present without actual inflammation of the membrane in hysteria and in chorea in children; hordeolum—a sty or minute boil on the palpebral margin, if small and single may be of local origin or indicative of the over-use of defective eyes or more frequently of digestive or genital disorders; blepharitis—inflammation of the margin of the lids which become thick, reddened and crusted with cheesy secretions, is indicative of scrofula or of minute ulceration, resulting from a previous ophthalmia or measles, anemia or in tuberculous diathesis ; verruca—warts upon the eye-lids, are usually found in the old people, indicating the possibility of commencing epithelioma ; syphilic ulceration is generally deeply indurated and accompanies other stigmata of the tertiary stage ; a dusky color of the lids and under the eyes is seen in women during menstruation, in menorrh-agia, long-continued leucorrhea and early in pregnancy : it may also accompany anemia, loss of sleep and in exhausting diseases ; dark circles round the eyes are symptomatic of the abuses of masturbation ; the yellow color of the sclera of the eye is symptomatic of jaundice ; bluish-white or pearly sclerotic is seen in anemia, pthisis and nephritis ; inflamed conjunctiva is usually caused by gonorrheal infection, though it may be present in lesser degree in diphtheria, measles, hay fever, coryza and influenza of the catarrhal type ; the eye may be dry and glazed in collapse or the typhoid status ; an increased secretion of the watery fluid of the eye (*lachry-mation*) accompanies conjunctivitis, irritation of any kind and in alcoholism : inflammation of the cornea (*keratitis*) is mainly of syphilic origin, while the ulceration of the cornea—a reddened, painful, photophobic eye may be in relation with exophthalmic goitre ; protrusion of the eye-ball (*exophthalmos*) is symptomatic of exophthalmic goitre and may be also present in lesser degree in spasmodic asthma or other conditions attended by dyspnoea ; recession of the eye-ball or the sinking of the eye-ball into the orbit (*enophthalmos*)may be provoked by any wasting disease as consumption, malaria, cancerous cachexia, by absorbing the cushion of fat of the orbital cavity ; dimness of vision may be provoked by uremia, diabetes, excessive abuse of tobacco, hysteria and migrane ; light appears yellowish in jaundice, and reddish after nervous irritation, fatigue and in wasting diseases), *ear* (unusally prominent, long or misplaced ears with absence of helix, antihelix, or lobule, are degenerative stigmata ; tophi—small, hard, gritty accretions of chalky masses of sodium urate, seen as nodules in the external ear along the margin or in the depressions, is of gouty diathesis ; a very thin, waxy and bluish ear may indicate general anemia or chlorosis; but a thickened and a deformed ear with the effusion of blood between the cartilages and the perichondrium (*hematoma auris*), is a trophoneurosis of the general paralytic and the insane; the flow of pus (*otorrhea*) from the meatus, which is very common among children and often associated with intense pain, due to inflammation of the tympanum (*otitis media,*) caused by tonsilitis, influenza or measles, is usually without serious consequences, deafness is indicative of the disease of the tympanum, eustacian tube or the auditory nerve: it can be easily found out by placing a watch at a varying distance from the ear and if its ticking sound is not audible by aerial conduction, and then if the same watch is placed upon the mastoid process and the sound becomes audible by bone conduction, then it clearly indicates that there is no nervous lesion and the deafness is due to local hindrances: the auditory nerve and its cortical center may be affected by syphilis, which is usually the case or by tuberculosis by injuring the nerve endings: quinine, salicylic acid or the salicylates may also provoke temporary deafness by causing labyrinthine hyperemia; hypersensitiveness of hearing (oxyacoia) and the buzzing, roaring, hissing sound (*tinnitus aurium*), are due either to nervous irritability or to rhino-pharyngeal catarrh, with involvment of the eustacian tube or the middle ear), *nose* [a coarse and broad nose is symptomatic of myxedema and cretanism ; a depressed and sunken nose is syphilitic unless there is traumatic fracture of the bone ; a pinched and distorted nose may be due to obstruction of polypus, tumor or adenoid growth ; a chronic redness of the nose with dilated capillaries is indicative of alcoholism, otherwise of chronic digestive disorders or amenorrhea ; an intense pain in the nose is symptomatic of syphilic lesion and a burning pain, to catarrhal inflammations ; a sensation of dryness is felt in the preliminary stages of coryza ; sneezing—the spasmodic expiration, is due to the direct (presence of any foreign body or the inhalation of irritant substances as pepper, snuff and in the early stage of coryza, mesales, pertussis, hay fever, asthma) or reflex (as in hysteria) irritation of the sensory nerves of the nose ; nasal stenosis—difficulty of breathing through the nose, if acute, is symptomatic of an acute coryza, diphtheria, hay fever or prodromal of typhus fever, glanders and variola, and if chronic, it is either due to the obstruction to lymphoid growths as in children or to congenital syphilis ; ulceration of the mucous membrane is usually a manifestation of tertiary syphilis or tuberculosis and might be followed by necrosis and caries of the bones: the ulcerated surfaces of syphilic origin is covered with a dry, greenish crust and the stench of the breath is sickening; non-offensive, watery discharge from the nose marks the beginning of acute coryza, hay fever, pertussis, measles, typhus fever, catarrhal form of influenza and iodism; offensive discharge accompanied with greenish-gray crusts and its foul odor imperceptible to the subject, is symptomatic of syphilic necrosis or of atrophic rhinitis; a discharge of blood from the nose (*epistaxis*) may have varied causes as alcoholism which renders the vessels to rupture, adenoid growths, ulceration in the nose, suppressed menstruation, chronic nephritis, cerebral thrombosis, and may be prodromal of typhoid or other eruptive fever infection; loss of sense of smell (*anosmia*) may be due to local obstruction as polipi or adenoid growths, or chronic rhinitis and if it be only temporary, it may be of neurotic origin as hysteria or neurasthenia, and if it be permanent, the olfactory anesthesia may be caused by nasal necrosis of the bone, supporting the tract, or a tumor involving the nerve; hypersensitiveness to smell (*hyperosmia*), hallucinary smell (*parosmia*) and an offensive smell (*kakosmia*) without any physical basis, are all of neurotic origin], *tongue* [the colour of the tongue, the only mucous membrane of the body, except the oral and the faucial, that is open to naked eye inspection, changes according to health, digestion and especially to the gastric condition to which it is closely related : it is pallid in anemia, bluish in cyanosis, reddish in gastric hyper-acidity, bright-red in the first stage of scarlet fever and in the inflammation of the tongue (*glossitis*), and greyish in nigrities ; a great enlargement of the tongue takes place in acromegaly and myxedema, but the tongue also swells considerably in variola, salivary calculus and in angina Ludovici ; the coating of the tongue consists of the accumulated epithelium, micro-organisms and food detritus : a thin-white coated tongue may be normal among the smokers or those who are accustomed to breathe through the mouth, but it usually accompanies mild gastro-intestinal disorder, nasopharyngeal catarrh or light fevers ; a flabby, swollen, indented tongue, covered with a yellow, pasty fur, is symptomatic of catarrhal gastritis, gastro-duodenitis or febrile conditions ; a narrow tongue with a deep median fissure on each side of which there is a rough, thick, brownish fur, or if it be dry, red and glazed, is characteristic in typhoid status in its early and late stages ; a covered tongue with white fur through which project swollen and bright-red fungiform papilla, is indicative of measles and other eruptive fevers ; if one side of the tongue is higher than the other, this is due to the unilateral lingual paralysis and associated with hemiplegia ; if the tongue lies motionless in the floor of the mouth and the subject is unable to protrude it and the functions of speech, mastication and deglutition are seriously impaired, it is due to the total lingual paralysis, caused by thrombosis or syphilic lesion], *skin* [dryness of the skin (*anidrosis*) is observed in cholera, myxedema, diabetes, Bright's disease, dropsy and in the first stage of many acute diseases, attended by high fever ; moist skin and increased perspiration (*hyperidrosis*) occurs in typhoid fever, tuberculosis, trichinosis, tetanus and in rheumatism, but the rheumatic sweat is strong in odor and acid in reaction ; in many acute diseases '*critical sweats*' suddenly break out with the fall of temperature as in pneumonia with the termination of paroxysm as in malaria, or the night sweats of tuberculosis and other wasting diseases ; partial or localized sweating is caused by the deranged innervation of the vaso-motor nerves and by the local vaso-motor paresis : this is particularly marked in rhachitis and in which disease, which usually occurs among children, the sweat is confined to the head and the patient rolls his head at night and the hair on the back of the head is rubbed off ; sweating of the hands and feet are seen in general debility ; unilateral or one-sided sweating of the head and face may arise from destructive pressure on the sympathetic nerves, causing paralysis of the dilator fibers of the ciliospinal branches, as in thoracic aneurism, suppurative parrotities, migrane, neuralgia ; unilateral sweating of the body (*hemodrosis*) occurs in hemoplegia : eccymosis and petechiae—purple patches caused by extravasation of blood into the skin, appear in many diseases and drug poisonings as in acute yellow atrophy of the liver, pernicious anemia, in advanced stage of cancer of the liver and the stomach, cerebrospinal meningitis (epidemic), cyanosis, diphtheria, jaundice (in severe forms), old age (in the extremeties), peliosis rheumatica, pyemia, advanced cirrhosis (hepatic or renal), septicema, tuberculosis (with extreme debility), typhoid fevers, ulcerative (malignant) endocarditis, yellow fever, and the rashes may be caused either by idiosyncrasy or by poisoning with antipyrine, arnica, arsenic, atropine, belladonna, cannabis indica, capsicum, chloral, copper, croton oil, digitalis, iodine, ergot, lead, mercury, morphine, opium, potassium iodide and bromide, quinine, salicylat-es, santonine, silver, sulphur, tar, tartar emetic; inflammatory eruption in cerebro-spinal fever, dengue, glanders (acute), erysipelas, syphilis; exanthematous eruption in measles, rubella, searlatina, varicella, variola], *mind* (dullness of mind is seen in cerebral inflammations, scleroses of the brain, and in brain tumors), *concentration of mind*, *purity* (hygienic conditions), *disposition*, *behavior*, *memory* [memory is impaired (*amnesia*) in paralytic dementia, epilepsy, neurasthenia, the over-use of bromides and in old age], *shape and general configuration of the body* (*ākṛti*--tall, thin subjects with slender ribs, and a long narrow thorax are predisposed to tuberculosis of the lungs; short, stout, thick-boned persons with florid face are predisposed with sumptuous living to obesity and gouty diathesis), *tempera-ment* (irritability of temper is often associa-ted with gout, rheumatism, jaundice and neurasthenia; change of temper is seen in pregnancy, typhoid fever, menopause and at the early stage of the exophthalmic goitre; melancholy mood is marked in hepatic lesions), *perversions* (abnormalities of shape result from the following diseases as rachitis, acromegaly, myxedema, pulmonary osteo-arthopathy, osteitis deformans, osteomalcia), *strength, endurance, intelligence, cheerfulness,* leanness (as in consumption), *obesity, lassitude, beginning of the disease, acuteness* (of the disease), *lightness* (of the disease) *physical characteristics, dietary, habits, quantity of food* (that is consumed), *the prevention of the disease* (prophylaxis), *the cure of the disease, the preliminary symptoms of the disease, pain* (pain is caused by the lesion of the peripheral, or the central nervous system, or indirectly by affecting the general economy; *'acute pain'* is characteristic of acute inflammations of the serous and synovial membranes as in pleurisy or in joint inflammations ; *'dull pain'* is characteristic of the inflammation of the mucous membranes and the parenchymatous viscera ; *'paroxysmal' or remitting pain'* is characteristic of neuralgias and colics ; *'shifting pain'* is charcteristic of rheumatism, hysteria, locomotor ataxia, trichinosis ; *'gnawing or boring pain'* is charcteristic in the diseases of the spinal column, thoracic and abdominal aneurism, periosteal inflammations, gastric carcinoma, and occasionally in gouty and lithemic lesions; '*cramp*'—the sudden painful spasm of certain muscles, aside from the occupation cramps from the over-use of fingers as in writer's cramp, whether it is of the calf, toes or the abdomen is usually characteristic of gastro-intestinal diseases and flatulence by causing an excessive tension to the muscular wall of the stomach and the intestine; diffuse pain as in fever; pain in the vertex—the crown of the head, is characteristic in neurasthenia, diseases of ovaries, uterus, bladder. epilepsy, hysteria, anemia, chlorosis in the frontal and the temporal region of the head, in nephritis, uremia, eye strain, iritis, glaucoma, dyspepsia, constipation, syphilic nodes, lithemia, rheumatism of the scalp; in the occipetal and cervical region: spinal irritation, diseases of the cervical vertebrae, dyspepsia, constipation, syphilis (very frequent), uterine lesions, eye strain, carous teeth, nephritis, uremia, cerebellar tumor, meningitis, adenoids of pharynx, naso-pharyngeal diseases, middle ear diseases, rheumatism; in the parietal region: dysmenorrhea, diseases of ear and bone, cancer of tongue. hysteria, lithemia; in the eye-balls: ophthalmoplegia internaa inflammation of conjunctiva, iris, cornea, coryza, neuralgia of the fifth nerve, asthenopia (eye strain); in the nose: acute rhinitis diphtheria, glanders, primary syphilis; aural region: ottitis media, furuncle of meatus, mastoid abscess, polypus, carous teeth, alveolar abscess, cancer of tongue, aneurism of innominate dentition, temporo-maxillary rheumatism, syphilitic or carous lesion of maxillary or temporal bones; in the front neck: myalgia, cervical caries or abscess, sprains, inflamed lymph glands, aneurism of innominate; nape of neck: rheumatism, neurasthenia, laryngitis, cerebrospinal meningitis, tetanus, cervico-occipital neuralgia; throat: tonsilitis, pharyngitis, scarlatina, diphtheria, cascinoma, laryngitis, irritant poisoning; jaw: dental affections, salivary calculus, neuralgia of maxillary-nerve, parotitis, actinomycosis; shoulder: rheumatism, synovitis, diaphragmatic pleurisy, dilated stomach or colon, duodenitis, colitis, neuritis, gallstone colic, hepatic diseases; sternum: gastric diseases, bronchitis, epidemic influenza, tabes, spinal apoplexy, angina pectoris, mediastinal abscess or tumor; breast: uterine and ovarian lesions, hysteria, menstruation and diseases of mamma; umbilicus: gallstone, hernia, carcinoma of omentum, tumor or ulcer of stomach; chest: pleurisy, acute pneumonia, pericarditis, phthisis, mediastinal tumor; hysteria; flatulence, pericarditis; right hypocondrium gall-stones (particularly) hepatic diseases; carcinoma of stomach, pancreas or duodenum; movable kidney, uremia, pleurisy; left hypochondrium; gastritis, colitis, uremia, peritonitis, enlarged spleen; precordia: functional disorders of heart, endocarditis, thrombosis of pulmonar artery, gout, hysteria, locomotor ataxia, angina pectoris, pyrosis; Interscapular: flatulence, gastric inflammation or ulcer, rheumatism; lumbar: lumbago, fatigue, flatulence, appendicitis, hernia, dysmenorrhea, kidney lesions, prostatis; epigastrum: gastric lesions, appendicitis, gallstones, ulcer of duodenum, carcinoma of pancreas, cholera asiatica; uremia, hepato-optosis, enteroptosis; abdomen: gastralgia, especially hyper-acidity, arsenical, mercurial or lead poisoning, peritonitis, hernia, intestinal tuberculosis, flatulence, tabes, pancreatic lesions, leucemia, dysmenorrhea, diabetes; right iliac: appendicitis, ovaritis, impactedcecum, colitis hernia, varicocele; left iliac: colitis, impacted sigmod, hernia, ovaritis, varicocele; pubic region: cystitis, uterine or ovarian lesions, ectopic pregnancy, pyelitis, carcinoma of the bladder; sacral region: uterine, ovarian, or testicular lesions, excessive venery, ulcer of rectum, sciatica; spine: hysteria, neurasthenia, carcinoma of the liver, rachitis, scurvy, febrile affectations, spinal curvature, mediastinal tumor; anterior thigh: ovarian or uterine diseases, pregnancy or displaced uterus, dysmenorrhea, renal colic, impacted feces; posterior thigh: sciatica, locomotor ataxia, impacted feces; leg: rheumatism, periostitis, leucemia, locomotor ataxia, spinal meningitis; calf: cramp due to nephritis, gout, diabetes, hysteria and over exertion; heel: gout, neurasthenia, ovarian lesion, achilodinia; sole of foot: plantar neuralgia, disease of prostrate, erythromelalgia, ; in the articular joints: rheumatism, gonorrheal arthritis, synovitis, syphilis, tuberculosis, scurvy, neuralgia, pyemia, rachitis; testicle: orchitis, or epididymitis; penis and perinium: vesical calculus, or the passage of the uric acid crystals (gravel), inflammation or ulceration of the bladder, or irritation of the calculus in the ureter or urethra; diffuse pain in the extremities: multiple neuritis, muscular rheumatism, spinal meningitis, influenza, rachitis, trichinosis), *complaints*, *gracefulness* (of the body), *complexion* (a dull, muddy complexion in hepatic lesion, constipation and digestive troubles), *dreams* (dream as a diagnostic aid has not yet been thoroughly evaluated, as the phenomenon of dream is complex and it is hard to analyze it, but it is well known that nightmares are usually caused by indigestion, and it is probable that the dream images are formed by the digestive activity, action of the heart and the peripheral impressions or the indirect pressure of the full bladder or impacted feces during sleep, reacting on the central nervous system, awaking the memory centers which for lack of co-ordination, become distorted and fragmentary), *messenger's countenance, disturbances on the road, the conditions of the sick-room, medicines, the reactions of the medicines* (upon the patient), and *advice about the medical prescriptions.*" Charaka V. I. 1[65].

Predispositions (to diseases) are of six kinds : *racial*, (Negroes are predisposed to tuberculosis, the Mongolian race to small-pox, Whites to yellow-fever, Jews to diabetes and insanity), *ancestral* (congenital syphilis, arthritic diathesis), *geo-*

65. इह खलु वर्णश्च स्वरश्च गन्धश्च स्पर्शश्च चक्षुश्च श्रोत्रञ्च घ्राणञ्च रसनञ्च स्पर्शनञ्च सत्त्वञ्च भक्तिश्च शौचञ्च शीलञ्चाचारश्च स्मृतिश्चाकृतिश्च प्रकृतिश्च विकृतिश्च बलञ्च ग्लानिश्च मेधा च हर्षश्च रौक्ष्यञ्च स्नेहश्च तन्द्रा चारम्भश्च गौरवञ्च लाघवञ्च गुणाश्चाहारश्च विहाराश्चाहारपरिणामश्चोपायश्चापायश्च व्याधिश्च व्याधिपूर्व्वरूपञ्च वेदनाश्चोपद्रवाश्च छाया च प्रतिच्छाया च स्वप्नदर्शनञ्च दूताधिकारश्च पथि चौत्पातिकञ्चातुरकुले भावावस्थान्तराणि च भेषजञ्च भेषजप्रवृत्तिश्च भेषजाधिकारयुक्तिश्चेति परीक्ष्याणि प्रत्यक्षानुमानोपदेशैरायुषः प्रमाणावशेषं जिज्ञासमानेन भिषजा। चरकसंहिता, इन्द्रियस्थानम्, १, ॥

graphical (malaria localized in marshy places, where anopheles—a genus of mosquitos—an intermediatory of its infection can grow and thrive), *periodical* (epidemics—pneumonia is usually prevalent in the spring, influenza in the winter), *according to age* (there are particular diseases of infancy, youth, middle-age and old-age) and *individual* (idiosyncrasy as susceptibility of certain persons to milk, oysters, strawberries etc, producing eczema, diarrhoea etc.) *Charaka* V. I. 3[66].

"So the *respiration* (the respiration rate of the newborn is 44 ; at five years, 26 ; in the adult, 16 to 20 ; in health it is faster standing than lying, during the day than at night, after meals than when fasting, in spring than in autumn, and during exercise, emotional and mental excitement than when at rest ; and there is about four pulse beats for one respiration ; rapid respiration is observed in pulmonary lesions, in lobar pneumonia and also in fever, especially in children by the indirect influence of the heated blood on the medulla ; slow respiration is observed in coma, collapse and poising with

66. तत्र प्रकृतिर्जातिप्रसक्ता कुलप्रसक्ता च देशानुपातिनी च कालानुपातिनी च वयोऽनुपातिनी च प्रत्यात्मनियता चेति । चरकसंहिता, इन्द्रियस्थानम् १, ३ ॥

opium, chloral, chloroform or antimony ; jerking inspiration is indicative of asthma, hystéria, hydrophobia ; jerking expiration in acute pleurisy and fractured rib ; stertorous respiration (snoring) is observed in apoplectic, uremic, diabetic coma, narcotic poisoning and paralysis of the soft palate, aside it is also observed in otherwise healthy individuals, especially children who have adenoids or enlarged tonsils and in grown-ups who are very tired and consequently there is muscular relaxation or are accustomed to mouth breathing, for the snoring sound arises from the vibration from the soft palate when breathing from the mouth and the nose at the same time ; stridulous or harsh respiration is due to some obstruction of the air passage through the larynx, caused through tumor, inflammation or any foreign body; wavy or uneven respiration is symptomatic of pneumonia) ; *neck* (a long, scrawny neck with projecting larynx is indicative of tuberculous diathesis and is usually correlated with the pthisinoid chest, while a short and thick neck with apoplectic predisposition ; rigidity of the neck, if chronic, may arise from the lesion of the, cervical vertebrae, caused by syphilic necrosis, arthritis or the affectation of the cervical muscles by rheumatism and if acute, through the inflammations of cervical glands, tumors or boils interfering with movements of the neck ; nodes upon the clavical bones, resembling the callus, but not caused by trauma, indicate tertiary syphilic lesion ; but tumefaction above the clavicles occur in amphysema and myxedema ; temporary swelling of the thyroid takes place during menstruation, or after sexual union, especially in women after first connubial embrace ; but a chronic enlargement is generally symptomatic of exopthalmic goitre, but may be also due to adenoma, cancer, tuberculosis or gumma of the gland : an atrophied and depressed thyroid is observed in myxedema and cretinism ; tenderness of the neck may be caused by the inflammation of the lymphatic glands of the region from any cause as cervico-occipital neuralgia, cervical myalgia or cervical caries), *teeth* (a baby should have six teeth when one year old, twelve when a year and half old, sixteen when two years old, twenty when two and half years old ; milk teeth : 2 lower central incisors appear between six to nine months ; 4 upper incisors between eight to twelve months ; 2 lower lateral incisors and 4 anterior molars between twelve to fifteen months ; 4 canines between eighteen to twenty-four months ; four posterior molars between twenty-four to thirty months; permanent teeth: 6 first molars appear between six and seven years; 8 incisors between eight to nine years; 8 bicuspids (*premolars*) between 9 to 11 years; 4 canines between 11 to 14 years; 2 second molars between 12 to 15 years; 4 third molars between 17 to 25 years; premature eruption of teeth is indicative of congenital syphilis or tubercular diathesis while delayed dentition that of rachitis or cretinism; if the permanent upper central incisors are dwarfed, narrowed, short, peg-like or somewhat rounded, tapering from gum to edge, with a single, shallow and discolored notch in the edge, it is a sure sign of congenital syphilis, especially if it be associated with keratitis and middle-ear disease; dentated or furrowed teeth originate from malnutrition or an acute illness during infancy, sufficiently severe to interfere with the nutrition; loosening of the teeth in their sockets is associated with the ulcerated, spongy or bleeding gums and therefore it can be ascribed to mercurial or gangrenous stomatitis, pyorrhea alveolaris, scurvy or phosphorus poisoning; a collection of sticky, dark-brown paste (*sordes*) upon the teeth, gums and the lips, sometimes stained with blood oozing from the gums, is very often present in typhoid and other low fevers; gritting or grinding of the teeth among the children is usually associated with gastro-intestinal disorders; erosion of the teeth takes place in gouty subjects, with loss of polish of the labial surface, followed by grooves which extend into the gums, causing inflammation, necrosis, formation of calculi (*tartar*), loosening of the teeth and pyorrhea alveolaris; early, excessive or rapid dental caries may be due to rachitis, but also takes place in pregnancy, diabetes or chronic phosphorus poisoning; dyspepsia, chronic gastritis, constipation, diarrhoea, persistent aural, nasal, opthalmic affections, nervous irritability, neuralgias or migraines may be easily caused by the carous teeth or pus sockets by the absorption of the toxin and the ingestion of microbes with the mastication of food), *liver* and the *spleen* (*pakṣa* = sides : the liver is the largest gland of the body and lies beneath the diaphragm in the right hypocondrium and the upper part of the epigestrum, about the size of 3 by 5 inches and weighing between two and half to three and half pounds; enlargement of the liver which can be felt through palpation, occur in chronic malaria, hypertrophic cirrhosis, leucemia, hydatids, fatty infiltration, abscess, tumor, gummata or cancer; progressive lessening (*atrophy*) of the liver takes place in cirrhosis; displacement of the liver upward may be due to pressure from below by large abdominal tumors, meteorism or ascites, and by downward pressure on the diaphragm by emphysema, spasmodic asthma, large right pleural effusion, large intrathoracic tumor, a dilated heart or a pericardial effusion; abnormal rough, hard and resistant surface is indicative of cirrhosis, carcinoma, amyloid or syphilic lesion: the *spleen* is of oval, flattened shape and lies in the left hypocondriac region between the stomach and the diaphragm, of almost the same size as the liver; the rapid enlargement of the spleen takes place in any acute infection, as in typhoid, malaria and other fevers, tuberculosis, small pox, diphtheria, pneumonia, cerebro-spinal meningitis, puemia or general scepticemia; chronic enlargement of the spleen occurs in pernicious malaria, in splenic anemia, hepatic cirrhosis), *eyes, hairs,* [*keśa*=long hairs as of the head and the beard; *loma*=small and fine hairs of the other parts of the body: the hair is luxuriant, bright, oily and wavy in hyper-secretion of thyroid as in Grave's, Basedow's diseases and the hair is dry, coarse, stiff and sparse in hypo-secretion of the thyroid as in myxedema, cretinism ; early gray hair before forty is usually associated with the premature arterial degeneration (*enderteritis*) but it is said that the sudden loss of pigmentation of the hair may take place at times under the influence of terrible fright, anxiety or deep emotion ; tendency to premature grayness of the hair may be hereditary ; circumscribed grey patches of hair may be due to trophic changes brought about by the lesion of the fifth nerve and its branches ; undue and rapid loss of hair (*alopecia*) is indicative of syphilic lesion, but this must not be confounded with the excessive falling out of hair which takes place during convalescence from acute diseases, as typhoid, malaria, nor with that following an attack of gout or erysipelas, for in syphilis the hair can be easily pulled in large masses without causing pain and the hair does not usually reappear ; in anemia, phthisis pulmonalis, myxedema, hydrocephalis, and the severe neuralgias of the fifth nerve, the hair is usually thinned ; premature loss of hair may be a hereditary family trait], *abdomen* [by inspection, palpation, percussion and auscultation, abdomen can be utilized of a great diagnostic value : smooth, shining and stretched skin (in the abdomen) is observed in abdominal distension ; whitish stricks or striae are indicative of previous long-continued distension as in ascites, fat or pregnancy, and in extreme case, the whitish stricks (*lineae albicantes*) may be observed also on the buttocks and the upper portions of the thigh ; copper-colored, scaly, somewhat circular spots upon the abdomen are indicative of secondary syphilis, as well as the brownish or yellowish macular areas of cloasma, which may be also present; enlarged glands in the groins signify either venerial infection or bubonic plague and their retracted cicatrices of their past lesions ; enlarged superficial abdominal veins, radiating from the umbilicus, appear in portal obstruction, through hepatic cirrhosis or tumor, ascites of long duration or greatly dilated stomach ; the navel (*umbilicus*) is deeply retracted in stout people ; if projecting it may be due to portal obstruction, pregnancy or hernia ; it is flattened or protruding in excessive ascites, or abdominal distentions ; fixation of the umbilicus is significant of hepatic malignant cancer ; the abdominal wall may be thick from the deposit of fat or edema and if it be thin with shrivelled skin, it may be due either to old age, wasting disease, repeated pregnancies or as a reaction of long-standing distension from ascites; the abdomen may be distended by the accumulation of fat in the abdominal wall, or fluid in the perital cavity or gas in the alimentary canal or the presence of a large tumor; swelling in the gastric area may be due to tumor. abscess or cancer on the gastric wall, hepatic cancer or pancreatic cyst or scler-osis or the distension of the gall-bladder either with concretions or pus; swelling in the hepatic area may be due to tumor, cancer, hypertrophic cirrhosis, hydatid cyst or passive congestion of the liver or sympathetically from the distended gall-bladder stuffed with concretions and pus; swelling in the splenic area may be due to mov-able or prolapsed spleen, perinephritic abscess, or congested movable kidney, or cancer of the stomach; the swelling of the appendical area is symptomatic of acute appendicitis; swelling in the pelvic area may be due to distended bladder, or by the distended uterus by tumor or detained menstrual fluid (*imperforate hymen*); swelling in the sigmoid area may be due to the impaction of feces, tuberculous or cancerous peritonitis, ulcer of colon, ovarian tumor or cyst of broad ligament], *nails* (curving of the nails with clubbed fingers, occur only in chronic diseases as phthisis emphysema, aneurism or chronic cardiac diseases; malformation, fragility, dryness or cracking of the nails may be due to injury, syphilis or due to trophic defects, resulting from nerve lesion, neuritis, syringomyelia or pulmonary osteo-arthopathy; arrested growth of nails may be due to hemiplegia from cerebral apoplexy or acute infantile paralysis; enlargement of the nails with thickening and sometimes twisting occurs in the course of syphilis, sclerodactyly and typhoid fevers; the nails in some cases of Raynaud's disease, become dry, scaly and cracked or hypertrophied; ecchymoses and ulcers at the bases of the nails may be due to chloral habit, but in a child (*onychia*) to syphilis or scrofulous diathesis; white marks or transverse grooves on the surface of the nails may indicate, unless due to injury, the period of recovery from a recent acute illness; the growth of the nail from the matrix to the end requires about six months and as the white marks develop at the root of the nail and with the growth of the nail, the transverse goooves also ascend higher and so a rough estimate can be made from their position of the time that has elapsed since the convalescence set in; hard, brittle, and longitudinally striated nails are observed in gouty subjects), *finger* (distorted fingers are due to gout, arthritis deformans and less frequently to chronic rheumatism; hard, white, glissening masses (*tophi*) may be present in the joints or along the tendons, on account of the accumulation of the sodium urate in gout and consequently in gout and rheumatism, the joints of the fingers are enlarged and painful , the tophi is more prominent on the dorsal surface of the joints and it sometimes breaks through the skin, so that the chalk-like concretion exudes; knobby enlargements of the proximal ends of the terminal phalanges (end-joint arthritic nodes) may be due either to gout or arthritis deformans and small crab-eye cysts may be formed over the nodes; the tips of the fingers may be bulbous or club-shaped in chronic lung diseases as phthisis or chronic heart affection; the claw hand occurs in consequence of atrophy and paralysis of the interossei and lumbrical muscles due to neuritis of the median and ulnar nerves; the spade hand with large, coarse, thick fingers and broad nails is observed in myxedema, but in which only the soft parts are affected, while in acromegaly, the bones are enlarged; the hand of the individual of a nervous temperament is firm, fine, delicate and dexterous; of sanguine temperament, broad, heavy, strong and energetic; of phlegmatic temperament soft and clammy; coldness of the hands and feet, with or without tendency to sweating, if persisting for a long time, is due to neurasthenia, anemia, chronic digestive disorders, gout, cardiac or pulmonary diseases, interfering with the circulation) should be observed."

Charaka V. 3. 5[67].

"When he does that (vomits), the physician should examine the expectorated matter from the spittoon with attention." *Charaka* I. 15. 16[68].

Urine was examined for its color, consistence, taste and smell, only in genito-urinary diseases (*Charaka* II. 4; *Suśruta* II. 6) but sputum, feces and semen as a vitality test and as a prognosis in diseases: "According to the sayings of the wise, his life is at an end, whose sputum, feces and semen sink, when thrown into water." *Charaka* V. 9. 14[69]. Suśruta gives elaborate details of the prognostic symptoms :—

---

67. तथास्योच्छ्वासमन्यादन्तपक्ष्मचक्षुःकेशलोमोदरनखाङ्गुलीश्च लक्षयेत् । चरकसंहिता, इन्द्रियस्थानम् ५ ।

68. ततोऽस्य वेगान् प्रतिग्राहगतानवेक्षेत । चरकसंहिता, सूत्रस्थानम्, १५ अः ॥

69. निष्ठ्यूतञ्च पुरीषञ्च रेतश्चाम्भसि मज्जति ।
यस्य तस्यायुषः प्राप्तमन्तमाहुर्मनीषिणः ॥
चरकसंहिता, इन्द्रियस्थानम्, ३ ॥

"He whose *complexion* is changed into pale-brownish (in Addison's disease), reddish (hyperemia; chlorosis rubra), yellowish (jaundice or icterus) or blue-purplish (cyanosis), he is near his death. He who suddenly loses his modesty, beautiful appearance, ability to hold himself upright and personal charms (in apoplexy, a sudden loss of consciousness is followed by paralysis, due to cerebral hemorrhage or blocking of an artery of the brain by an embolus or thrombus), he can be regarded as dead. Whose *lower lip* hangs down (the lips are loose and pendulous in diphtheretic paralysis or chronic bulbar palsy), *upper lip* twitches up (twitching or trembling of the lips is index of general paralysis or bulbar palsy), or both the lips have the colour of ripe plums (the colour of the ripe plum is dark bluish, that is cyanotic : in diseases of the heart or the lungs, especially the chronic forms, owing to dyspnœa, the lips are open, dry and cyanosed), his life is hard to save. He whose *teeth* are reddish (stained with blood—*sordes*—in typhoid prostration), or pale brownish (stained from the deposit of foul matter in jaundice on the tongue), or like polished collyrium (dark black deposit is found on the tongue in Addison's disease or nigritis), or have fallen (loosening of the teeth in their sockets may be due to pyorrhea alveolaris, scurvy, purpura hemorrhagia, and extensive and rapid dental caries is common in diabetes or rachitis), can be regarded as dead. He whose *tongue* is black (in Addison's disease or nigrites) paralyzed (in basal meningitis, syphilic lesion, tumor or cerebral hemorrhage), swollen (glossitis may occur in various diseases as variola, erysipelas or sceptimia), or dry and fissured (in the typhoid status), is near his death." *Suśruta* I. 31. 2-6[70].

He whose hair looks oily (in hyperthyroidism), though not smeared with oil, does not live long,

---

70. श्यावा लोहितिका नीला पीतिका वापि मानवम् ।
अभिद्रवन्ति यं छाया: स परासुरसंशयम् ॥२
छीरपक्रमते यस्य प्रभास्मृतिधृतिश्रिय: ।
अकस्माद्यं भजन्ते वा स परासुरसंशयम् ॥३
यस्याधरौष्ठ: पतित: क्षिप्तश्चोर्ध्वं तथोत्तर: ।
उभौ वा जाम्बवाभासौ दुर्लभं तस्य जीवितम् ॥४
आरक्ता दशना यस्य श्यावा वा स्युः पतन्ति च ।
खञ्जनप्रतिमा वापि तं गतायुषमादिशेत् ॥५
कृष्णा स्तब्धावलिप्ता वा जिह्वा शूना च यस्य वै ।
कर्कशा वा भवेद्यस्य सोऽचिराद्विजहात्यसून् ॥६
सुश्रुतसंहिता, सूत्रस्थानम्, ३१-२-६ ।

and knowing this, the wise (physician) should give him up. *Charaka* V. 8. 7[71].

Susruta says[72]. "Nervous diseases, '*prameha*' (diabetes and gonorrhea), leprosy, hemorrhoids (piles), anal fistula, calculus, '*mūḍhagarbha*' (transverse or scapulo-posterior presentation of the fetus during birth) and abdominal maladies—these eight are naturally hard to cure ; but if these are also complicated with the developments of enervation, emaciation, dyspnea, thirst, '*śoṣa*' (desiccation of the body or pulmonary consumption), vomiting, fever, unconsciousness, diarrhea, hiccup and other complications, then the wise physician, desirous of success, should not untertake their treatment. If

---

71. यस्य केशा निरभ्यङ्गा दृश्यन्तेऽभ्यक्तसन्निभाः ।
उपरुद्धायुषं ज्ञात्वा तं धीरः परिवर्ज्जयेत् ॥
चरकसंहिता, इन्द्रियस्थानम्. ८ ॥

72. व्यातव्याधिः प्रमेहश्च कुष्ठमर्शो भगन्दरः ।
अश्मरी मूढगर्भश्च तथैवोदरमष्टमम् ॥
अष्टावेते प्रकृत्यैव दुश्चिकित्स्या महागदाः ॥३
प्राणमांसक्षयश्वास-तृष्णाशोषवमिज्वरैः ।
मूर्च्छातिसारहिक्काभिः पुनश्चैतैरुपद्रुताः ।
वर्ज्जनीया विशेषेण भिषजा सिद्धिमिच्छता ॥४
शूनं सुप्तत्वचं भग्नं कम्पाध्माननिपीड़ितम् ।
नरं रुजार्त्तिमन्तञ्च वातव्याधिविनाशयेत् ॥५
यथोक्तोपद्रवाविष्टमतिप्रस्रुतमेव वा ।
पिड़कापीड़ितं गाढ़ं प्रमेहो हन्ति मानवम् ॥

in nervous diseases, there are complications of edema, insensibility to touch, paralysis of the body, tremor, tumor and pain in the abdomen, the patient dies. If in urinary diseases these complications develop, and with the urine much substances (*albuminuria*) are discharged and boils appear on the body, that patient dies. In leprosy, if the nodules ulcerate, eyes become red, the voice broken and the five kinds of treatment as vomiting and purgation do not succeed, the death of the patient is near. In hemorrhoids (piles), if there are complication of polydipsia, loss of appetite, pain, excessive

---

प्रभिन्नं प्रस्रुताङ्गञ्च रक्तनेत्रं हतस्वरम् ।
पञ्चकर्म्मगुणातीतं कुष्ठं हन्तीह कुष्ठिनम् ॥७
तृष्णारोचकशूलार्त्तमतिप्रस्रुतशोणितम् ।
शोफातीसारसंयुक्तमर्शोव्याधिर्विनाशयेत् ॥८
वातमूत्रपुरीषाणि क्रिमयः शुक्रमेव च ।
भगन्दरात् प्रस्रवन्ति यस्य तं परिवर्ज्जयेत ॥९
प्रशूननाभिवृषणं रुद्धमूत्रं रुगन्वितम् ।
अश्मरी क्षपयत्याशु सिकताशर्करान्विता ॥१०
गर्भकोषपरासङ्गो मक्कलो योनिसंवृतिः ।
हनुरः स्त्रियं मूढ़गर्भं यथोक्ताश्चाप्युपद्रवाः ॥११
पार्श्वभङ्गान्नविद्वेष-शोफातिसारपीड़ितम् ।
विरिक्तं पूर्य्यमाणञ्च वर्ज्जयेदुदरार्द्दितम् ॥१२
यस्तान्यति विसंज्ञश्च शेते निपतितोऽपि वा ।
शीतार्द्दितोऽन्तरुष्णश्च ज्वरेण म्रियते नरः ॥१२

bleeding, edema and diarrhœa, the patient dies. The anal fistula through which the intestinal gas, urine, feces, microbes and semen are discharged is deadly. In the diseases of hard calculus (*aśmarï*), soft calculus (*śarkarā*) and gravel (*sikatā*-uric acid sands), if there appear edema in umbilical region, testicles, ischuria (retention of urine), and shooting pain, the patient dies quickly. In the transverse presentation, if there is paralysis of the uterus, dull pain (*makkalla*) and spasmic contraction of the vagina, the gravida dies. In abdominal diseases, if there is deplegia, aversion for food, edema, diarrhea and inspite of purgation, the intestine remains inflated, then give up

---

यो हृष्टरोमा रक्ताक्षो हृदि सङ्घातशूलवान् ।
नित्यं वक्त्रेण चोच्छ्वस्यात् तं ज्वरो हन्ति मानवम् ॥१४
हिक्काश्वासपिपासार्त्तं मूढं विभ्रान्तलोचनम् ।
सन्ततोच्छ्वासिनं क्षीणं नरं क्षपयति ज्वरः ॥१५
आविलाक्षं प्रताम्यन्तं निद्रायुक्तमतीव च ।
क्षीणशोणितमांसञ्च नरं क्षपयति ज्वरः ॥१६
श्वासशूलपिपासार्त्तं क्षीणं ज्वरनिपीड़ितम् ।
विशेषेण नरं वृद्धमतीसारो विनाशयेत् ॥१७
शुक्लाक्षमन्नद्वेष्टारमूर्द्ध्वश्वासनिपीड़ितम् ।
कृच्छ्रेण बहु मेहन्तं यक्ष्मा हन्तीह मानवम् ॥१८
श्वासशूलपिपासान्नविद्वेषग्रन्थिमूढ़ताः ।
भवन्ति दुर्बलत्वञ्च गुल्मिनो मृत्युमेष्यतः ॥१९

(treatment). In fevers, if the patient is delirious, unconscious, and is absolutely confined to bed, and while the outside of his body (skin) is cold and inside (in the internal organs) there is hyperaemia, then he dies. In fevers, if there is horripilation, eyes become red, there is an acute shooting pain in the heart, and respiration takes place only through the mouth, the patient is killed by the disease. And in fever, if the patient has hiccup, dyspnea, polydipsia, delirium and wandering eyes, he goes to the abode of death. In fever, if the patient has clouded vision, delirium, paroxysmal somnolence, hydremia (thinness of blood) and emaciation, the fever kills the patient. In diarrhea, if there are the complications of dyspnea, pain, polydipsia, enervation, emaciation and fever, the aged patient never lives, though an infant once in a while might survive. In phthisis, if the patient has glazed eyes, aversion for food, jerky respiration, and hyperalgia in seminal discharge (in prostatic calculus), any of these complications is to be regard-

---

आध्मातं बहुनिष्यन्दं छर्दिहिक्कातृडन्वितम् ।
रुजाश्वाससमाविष्टं विद्रधिर्नाशयेन्नरम् ॥२०

पाण्डुदन्तनखो यस्य पाण्डुनेत्रश्च मानवः ।
पाण्डुसङ्घातदर्शी च पाण्डुरोगी विनश्यति ॥२१

ed critical. In abdominal tumor, if the patient has dyspnea, pain, polydipsia, anorexia, rupture of the tumor and enervation, death takes place. In a deep-seated abscess (*vidradhi*), if there is abdominal tumescence, anuria, vomiting, hiccup, polydipsia, throbbing pain and dyspnea, he does not live. In icterus (jaundice), the patient dies if his teeth, nails and eyes turn yellowish, and he sees everything yellowish. In gastrorrhagia (hemorrhage from the stomach), if the patient repeatedly vomits blood, his eyes become reddish and he sees everything reddish, he perishes." *Suśruta* I. 33. 3-22.

Pains : "*Boring* (*todana* = as caused by the penetration of sewing needle), *terebrant* (*vedana* = to tear out) *lacerating* (*tāḍana* = concussion as a blow from a rod), lancinating (*chhedana* = cutting with a sharp instrument), *dilating* (*āyamana*-radiating), *tensive* (*manthana* = as fire is made by friction of two sticks), *expulsive* (*vikṣepaṇa* = to throw out), *sucking* (*chumuchumāyana* = as a magnet or mustard poultice draws by suction), *burning* (*nirdahana* =

लोहितं छर्द्दयेद् यश्च बहुशो लोहितेक्षणः ।
रक्तानाञ्च दिशां द्रष्टा रक्तपित्तो विनश्यति ॥२२

सुश्रुतसंहिता, सूत्रस्थानम्, ३३, ३—२२ ।

burning), *grinding* (*avabhañjana* = pulverizing), *fulgurant* (*spohtana* = bursting), *shooting* (*vidāraṇa* = penetrating), *evulsive* (*utpāṭana* = to pull up), *throbbing* (*kampana* = tremulous), *dull, sharp, acute, itching, irritant, premonitory* or *after pain* (*vividha-śūla-viśleṣaṇa* = various degrees of pain), *shifting* (*vikiraṇa* = which shifts from place to place as in hysteria), *cramp* or spasmodic (*pūraṇa* = which fills up), *paralyzing* (*stambhana* = which causes insensibility in the adjacent area), *wringing* (*avakuñchana* = to press out), *formication* or itching (*aṅkuśika* = sprouting, a sensation as of ants or similar objects crawling over the body). By the derangement of nerves, these pains manifest in the '*vraṇas*' (abscess, tumor, pustule, boil, carcinoma, eczema, etc.) and if for any reason withot (apparent) cause, different kinds of pain appear, or in certain localities they appear repeatedly, they are to be ascribed to nervous origin.

Unilateral eruption (*oṣa*), cutaneous inflammation (*choṣa*), diffuse eruption (*paridāha*), oppressed feeling (*dhumāyana* = as in smoke suffocation), the sensation as if burning coal were spread over the body with the increase of the subjective sensation of heat, and the similar sensation that is felt if a caustic were applied to a wound,—the pains experienced in these sensations, are of '*pitta*' origin ; pains of the abscesses, originating from the vitiation or poisoning of the blood, are the same.

Pruritus (*kaṇḍū*=itching), heaviness (*gurutva* =heaviness or weight is felt in the chest in hemoptysis, spasmodic asthma, chronic gastritis ; in the head in neurasthenia, hypocondrisis and is occasionally a premonitory symptom of apoplexy ; in the abdomen or pelvis, due to tumors in those regions), somnolence (*suptatva*), tumescence (*upadeha*), numbness (*alpa-vedana*=partial anesthesia), paresis (*stambha*) and chilliness (*śaitya*) are of phlegmatic origin." *Suśruta* I. 22. 9[73].

"The physician should examine first *vitality* (*āyu*=durability of life) of the patient. Even if there is (good) vitality (signs of long life, manifest in the physical organs), *malady*

---

73. तोदनभेदनताडनच्छेदनायमनविक्षेपणचुमुचुमायननिर्दहनावभञ्जनस्फोटनविदारणोत्पाटनकम्पनविविधशूलविश्लेषणविकिरणपूरणस्तम्भनस्वप्नावकुञ्चनाङ्कुशिकाः सम्भवन्ति। अनिमित्तविविधवेदनाप्रादुर्भावो वा मुहुर्मुहुर्यत्रागच्छन्ति वेदनाविशेषास्तं वातिकमिति विद्यात्। ओषचोषपरिदाहधूमायनानि यत्र गात्रमङ्गारावकीर्णमिव पच्यते यत्र चोष्माभिवृद्धिः क्षते क्षारावसिक्तवच्च वेदनाविशेषास्तं पैत्तिकमिति विद्यात्। पित्तवद्रक्तसमुत्थं जानीयात्। कण्डुर्गुरुत्वं सुप्तत्वमुपदेहोऽल्पवेदनत्वं स्तम्भः शैत्यञ्च यत्र तं श्लैष्मिकमिति विद्यात्। सुश्रुतसंहिता, सूत्रस्थानम्, २२, ९।

(etiology and the nature of the pathological manifestation), *season* (of the year in its relation to the disease and its reaction against it), *metabolism* (of the patient ; *agni*=internal combustion, that is oxidation), *age*, *physical strength*, *nervous vitality*, *predispositions*, *characteristics* (of the patient), *remedies* (available and their reaction against the disease) and *the region* (*deśa* : marshy or dry, altitude, low or high land, plain or hilly, salubrity of the climate, prevalence of endemic diseases and of epidemics within the territory).

Signs of longevity : He enjoys long life, who has large hands, feet, sides, back, nipple (papilla mamma), teeth, face, shoulder and forehead ; long phalanx, breath (or respiratory organ), eyes and arms ; wide brows, precordial region (*stanāntara*=the space between the two nipples), and breast ; short crus (*jaṅghā*=the leg, especially the segment between the knee and the ankle), penis and neck ; deep breath (or spiritual force), voice and umbilicus ; the mamma not high but firm ; fleshy, large and hairy ears ; ...... whose joints, veins (vessels) and tendons are hidden, all the bodily parts are healthy and strong, all the senses are steady, and the health has persistently improved, that person will have a long life. He who has never had any sickness from birth and whose body, intelligence and comprehension have progressively been developed, will enjoy a long life. *Suśruta* I. 35. 2-4[74].

"*Life* is (divided) into three periods : infancy, middle-age and senility. Of them, childhood is up to fifteen years (one minus sixteen), divided (further into three sub-divisions) as sustaining on milk (liquid nourishment), milk mixed with other nourishing substances (in liquid or semi-solid form as barley concoction) and (solid) nourishment. A baby up to one year old sustains on milk, up to two years, milk mixed with other substances, and above two years on (solid)

---

74. आतुरमुपक्रममाणेन भिषजायुरादावेव परीक्षितव्यम् । सत्यप्यायुषि व्याध्यृत्वग्निवयोदेहबलसत्त्वसात्म्यप्रकृतिभेषजदेशान् परीक्षेत ॥ २

तत्र महापाणिपादपार्श्व-पृष्ठ-स्तनाग्र-दशन-वदन-स्कन्ध-ललाटं दीर्घाङ्गुलिपर्व्वोच्छ्वासप्रेक्षणबाहुं विस्तीर्णभ्रूस्तनान्तरोरस्कं ह्रस्वजङ्घामेढ्रग्रीवं गम्भीरसत्त्वस्वरनाभिमनुच्चैर्बद्धस्तनमुपचितमहारोमशकर्णं पश्चान्मस्तिष्कं स्नातानुलिप्तं मूर्द्धानुपूर्व्व्या विशुष्यमाणशरीरं पश्चाच्च विशुष्यमाणहृदयं पुरुषं जानीयाद्दीर्घायुः खल्वयमिति ।

गूढ़सन्धिशिरास्नायुः संहताङ्गः स्थिरेन्द्रियः ।
उत्तरोत्तरसुक्षेत्रो यः स दीर्घायुरुच्यते ॥
गर्भात् प्रभृत्यरोगो यः शनैः समुपचीयते ।
शरीरज्ञानविज्ञानैः स दीर्घायुः समासतः ॥४

सुश्रुतसंहिता, सूत्रस्थानम्, ३५, २-३ ।

food. From sixteen up to seventy years of age, is regarded as the middle-age: middle-age is composed of four periods as *pubescence* (*vṛddhi* = growth), *adolescence* (*yauvana* = youth), *adultness* (*sampūrṇatā* = completion of growth), *senescence* (*hāni* = declining period); up to the age of twenty, is the period of growth, up to thirty—youth, up to forty full development or maturity, and from forty to seventy, it slowly and gradually declines. (The skeleton reaches its limit very nearly at the same time as the whole frame reaches its maximum of height, the coalescence of various epiphyses being completed by about the twenty-fifth year. Similarly the mascular system in its increase tallies with the weight of the whole body. The brain, in spite of its increasing complexity of structure and function to which it continues to attain, even in middle life, early reaches its limit of bulk and weight. At about seven years of age it attains what may be considered as its first limit for though it may increase somewhat up to twenty, thirty, or even later years, its progress is more slow after, than before seven. The vascular and the digestive organs as a whole may continue to increase even to a very late period (*Foster's Physiology*, p. 1151). After seventy, elements

(constituent), sense, strength, courage and enthusiasm daily fall off ; at this age, one becomes grey-haired and bald-headed and being subject to dyspnea, bronchitis and other complications, becomes incapacitated for all activities (as before) and becomes like a dilapidated cottage, exposed to the fury of rain, storm and tempests. This is called old age." *Suśruta* I. 35. 26[75].

"Infancy is phlegmatic, youth sanguinary and old-age nervous." *Suśruta* 1. 35. 27[76].

The following diseases may be *congenital* : malformations, syphilis, idiocy, hydrocephalus, hemophilia, infantile hemiplegia, osteomata, nevi, sclerema, pemphigus, dermatitis neonatorum, tetanus neonatorum, ichthyosis, acute fatty

---

75. वयस्तु त्रिविधं, बाल्यं मध्यं वृद्धमिति। तत्रोनषोड़शवर्षीया बालास्तेऽपि त्रिविधाः—क्षीरपाः, क्षीरान्नादाः, अन्नादा इति। तेषु संवत्सरपराः क्षीरपाः, द्विसंवत्सरपराः क्षीरान्नादाः, परतोऽन्नादा इति। षोड़शसप्तत्योरन्तरे मध्यं वयस्तस्य विकल्पो वृद्धिर्यौवनं सम्पूर्णता हानिरिति। तत्राविंशतेर्वृद्धिरात्रिंशतो यौवनमाचत्वारिंशतः सर्व्वधात्विन्द्रियबलवीर्य्यसम्पूर्णता। अत ऊर्द्धमीषत्परिहाणिर्यावत्सप्ततिरिति। सप्ततेरूर्द्धं क्षीयमाणधात्विन्द्रियबलवीर्य्योत्साहमहन्यहनि वलीपलितखालित्यजुष्टं कासश्वासप्रभृतिभिरुपद्रवैरभिभूयमानं सर्व्वक्रियास्वसमर्थं जीर्णागारमिवाभिवृष्टमवसीदन्तं वृद्धमाचक्षते। सुश्रुतसंहिता, सूत्रस्थानम्, ३५, २६।

76. बाले विवर्द्धते श्लेष्मा मध्यमे पित्तमेव तु।
भूयिष्ठं वर्द्धते वायुर्वृद्धे तद्वीक्ष्य योजयेत् ॥२७

सुश्रुतसंहिता, सूत्रस्थानम्, ३५, २७।

degeneration, myotonia congenita, progressive muscular atrophy, icterus neonatorum, atelectasis, hemoglobinuria.

Hereditary diathesis: rheumatism, gout, hepatic disorders, renal disorders, renal calculus, respiratory lesions, diabetes, obesity, adiposis dolorosa, acne, eczema, leprosy, arthritis deformans, hernia, hereditary cerebellar ataxia, hemophilia, alcoholism, pseudo-hypertrophic paralysis, progressive muscular atrophy, cancer.

Diseases peculiar in infancy and childhood: cretinism, infantile paralysis, measles, roseola, scarlatina, cerebro-spinal meningitis, chorea, rachitis, hemophilia, infantile scurvy, hypertrophic cirrhosis of the liver, diarrhœa, adenoids, bronchitis, broncho-pneumonia, spasmodic laryngitis, noma, endocarditis, primary renal sarcoma, eczema, pemphigus, seborrhea, ringworm, diphtheria, hydrocephalus, nodding spasm.

Puberty and adolescence: acne, seborrhea, anemia, chlorosis, chloroma, myxedema, exophthalmic goitre, catalepsy, trance, myoma, myolema, typhoids, meningitis, myocarditis, endocarditis, hysteria, cerebral embolism, epilepsy.

Early adult age: acute tuberculosis, pulmonary phthisis, gastralgia, gastric ulcer, syringomyelia, cerebral abscess, cerebral embolism, myoma, periodic paralysis.

Middle age: exophthalmic goitre, myxedema, diabetes, chronic nephritis, cysts of kidney, myocardial diseases, endocarditis, aneurism, leucemia, pernicious anemia, angina pectoris, ataxic paraplegia, dementia paralytica, paralysis agitans, intraspinal hemorrhage, myelitis, locomotor ataxia, psychosis polyneuritica, carcinoma, gout, cirrhosis of liver, gallstones, mollities ossium.

Old age: pruritus, ecthyma, gout, pephigus, epithelioma, carcinoma, gout, arteriosclerosis, cataract, gangrene, bronchitis, broncho-pneumonia, aneurism, prostatic disease, myocardial disease, angina pectoris, cerebral apoplexy, paralysis agitans, melancholia.

Diseases special or predominant in females: chlorosis, osteomalcia, chorea, floating kidney, lupus erythematosus, gallstones, constipation, chorea, hysteria, neurasthenia, catalepsy, goitre, myxedema, adiposis dolorosa, gastralgia, anemia.

In addition to the above-mentioned constitutional, metabolic or infectious diseases, there are of course countless other infectious diseases which can attack all ages and can bring about by slow or rapid process the cessation of vital activities and their co-ordination of the organism.

But though *death* is inevitable to multicellular life, Sśuruta emphasizes that natural death through degeneration of senescence is a very rare phenomenon: "According to Atharva-veda scholars, deaths are of one hundred and one kinds, of which the natural death (through old age) is one while the rest one hundred are accidental (including infection)." *Suśruta* I. 34. 5[77]. It is an undeniable fact, that protoplasm—the living substance, living a particulate life in unicellular existence and community life in mullicellular existence, under favorable conditions, has not necessarily any limitation of its life, and as every living organism, comes into existence as a protoplasm of a pre-existing living organism protoplasm is potentially immortal. Reproduction among the unicellular creatures is by fission, so in a sense they never die as long as proper conditions are maintained. But life can, also, be preserved under adverse circumstances with arrested vitality as in hibernation of many animals in winter. Even suspended vitality is not incompatible with life as many microb-

---

77. एकोत्तरं मृत्युशतमथर्वाणः प्रचक्षते ।
तत्रैकः कालसंयुक्तः शेषा आगन्तवः स्मृताः ॥५
सुश्रुतसंहिता, सूत्रस्थानम्, ३४, ५ ।

es, or their spores, can be completely desiccated and kept in that state for many years, and after that if they find a favorable medium, they show their full activities again (*anabiosis*). Grains which have been found in ancient Egyptian tombs which have been lying there in a desiccated state for more than one hundred ceturies, have been found to germinate. And many fish can be frozen with water and made an ice block and kept in that condition for any length of time and if it be thawed slowly, the fish can be revivified. Only when protoplasm is coagulated, it loses its vitality. Many trees are known, which according to reliable tradition, have lived more than a thousand years. Death comes to a tree by storm, lightning, fungi and parasitic diseases, improper nutrition from the soil either by the exhaustion or excess of some of the salts or the insoluble combination of others, improper moisture or sunlight ; but these are all accidental and are avoidable. It is asserted that there are authenticated cases of men who have lived more than 152 years. Old age is certainly a disease, brought about by the degenerative changes, caused by microbic infection, absorption of their toxins and unhygienic living. But this will be in future more or less controllable with better knowledge of prophylaxis, dietary, rational living and hygiene. And very few people really die of senile degeneration. What actually happens is this : in the debilitated condition when the resisting power of the organism has been reduced, some infection takes place. Preventive medicine in future will possibly eliminate many of the virulent infections, but it can not impl that death will be preventible. Death is probably nature's economy of life. It eliminates those who are no more capable of reproduction or can not contribute materially to the support and provision of offspring, thus releasing the food-supply to the new-generation for growth, development and progress. Old age (*senility*) is the effect of the cumulative auto-intoxications. Organism in its very functioning—in the metabolic process, produces various toxic products, which, if not thoroughly eliminated, can accumulate in the organism bringing about degenerative changes. According to Metchnikoff toxins are principally absorbed from the putrefactive products of the large intestine and to counteract the activities of the proteolytic bacilli, which can only thrive in alkaline reaction, he proposed the introduction into the large intestine of the most active lactic acid producing bacilli (*bacillus Bulgaricus* or *maya ferment*) in the form of soured and curdled milk,

It is true that the large intestine serves no vital function in the economy of life, and it has been simply developed in animals as an accommodation, so that animals are not compelled to slow the speed and wait for defecation, while running. And animals with comparatively short intestine live relatively longer than the animals with larger intestine. And all the organs of the body do not equally show the signs of senile degeneracy. But the human body is a complex, intricate and delicate machinery. If any of the vital organs is seriously affected, it interferes with the integrity of the organism as all the organs are intimately related and interdependent. A diseased organ like the heart or the kidney can not be replaced like a broken or worn-out part of an auto or aeroplane machinery. They can be only slowly and gradually improved by a regenerating process of relieving them of the burden and tension by proper dietary and rational living. But every disease leaves an indelible mark, every shock an impression and every healed wound a cicatrix. And the effect is cumulative. If all the infections could be controlled, still there would be old age and death brought about by the slow but cumulative effect of the partial retention of the metabolic wastes, defective hereditary inheritance, mental, emotional, and physical shocks and excitements.

Buffon calculated that the duration of life was six to seven times to that of growth, but Flourens estimated it about five times. As the epiphysis closes about twenty five in man, so it can be calculated that the longevity of man should average from 125 years upwards. This is certainly a respectable age compared to the present standard, though some of the animals, lacking intelligence and control over the environment are reputed to live longer as some authenticated records show : salmon one hundred years ; in the case of a carp one hundred and fifty years ; pike two hundred years ; crocodile one hundred years ; tortoise two hundred years ; eagle one hundred years ; parrot eighty years ; swan eighty years; ducks and geese fifty years ; falcons one hundred years. In the records of zoological garden in confinement, the rhinoceros is known to have lived longer than thirty-seven years, and the average duration of the life of horses, asses and zebras from fifteen to thirty years, domestic cattle from twenty-five to thirty years, sheep, goats and antelopes from twelve to fifteen years, llama seventeen years, hippopotamus thirty-seven years, domestic swine twenty years, elephants thirty to forty years, lions, tigers, bears about 25 years, domestic cats from twelve to twenty-three years, dogs from sixteen to eighteen years, hares and rabbits about ten years, mice and rats from five to six years, bats about seventeen years, monkeys eight to thirty years (*Ency. Brit.* Vol XVI. p. 975).

DISEASES AND THEIR CLINICAL STUDIES.

"Ailing (*vyādhi*), disease (*āmaya*), sickness (*gada*), terror (*ātaṅka*), consumption (*yakṣma*) fever (*jvara*), indisposition (*vikāra*), and malady (*roga*) are synonyms. *Etiology* (*nidāna*), *prodrome* (*pūrvarūpa*), *symptoms* (*liṅga*), *remedy* (*upaśaya*) and *sequel* (*samprāpti*) are the *diagnostics* of a disease. That '*etiology*' means the causes of disease, has been previously mentioned. The premonitory symptoms that are observed before the development of a disease, ar termed as '*prodromes*'. The symptom of a developed disease (the disease might stay in a latent state and the incubation of many infections may last for many years in a resisting organism) is called the '*liṅga*'. Characteristic (*ākṛti*), indication (*lakṣmaṇa*), sign (*chihṇa*), lineament (*saṃsthāna*), trait (*vyañjana*), feature (*rūpa*) are synonymous terms with symptom (*liṅga*). Remedy is called that combined action of medicine (*auṣadha*), diet (*āhāra*) and hygienic living (*vihāra*), which cures the disease by counteracting either its causes or symptoms. Sequel (*samprāpti*), outcome (*āgati*) and after-developments (*jāti*) are synonymous." *Charaka* II. 1. 2[78].

"*Fevers* are being mentioned in the beginning of the book of pathology, for fever is the first expression of all physical diseases." *Charaka* II. 1. 6[79].

Fever (pyrexia) in which the normal temperature is markedly exceeded for any length of time above about 37 degree Centigrade or 98. 6 degree Fahrenheiht, is caused by the disturbance of the heat-regulating mechanism. Whatever stimulates the thermogenetic centre or unduly constricts the vaso-dilators so that the excess of heat can not be dissipated, provokes fever. In sun-stroke, the peripheral nervous mechanism is

---

78. तत्र व्याधिरामयो गद आतङ्को यक्ष्मा ज्वरो विकारो रोग इत्यनर्थान्तरम् । तस्योपलब्धिर्निदानपूर्व्वरूपलिङ्गोपशयसम्प्राप्तितश्च । तत्र निदानं कारणमित्युक्तमग्रे । पूर्व्वरूपं प्रागुत्पत्तिलक्षणं व्याधेः। प्रादुर्भूतलक्षणं पुनर्लिङ्गमाकृतिर्लक्षणं चिह्नं संस्थानं व्यञ्जनं रूपमित्यनर्थान्तरमित्यस्मिन्नर्थे । उपशयः पुनर्हेतुव्याधिविपरीतानां विपरीतार्थकारिणाञ्चौषधाहारविहाराणामुपयोगः सुखानुबन्धः। सम्प्राप्तिरागतिर्जातिरित्यनर्थान्तरं व्याधेः।

चरकसंहिता निदानस्थानम्, १ ।

79. इह खलु ज्वर एवादौ विकाराणामुपदिश्यते तत् प्रथमत्वाच्छारीराणाम् ।

चरकसंहिता निदानस्थानम्, १ ।

paralyzed and consequently the body temperature is considerably raised. But when a toxin is introduced into the blood, the auto-defensive mechanism of the body—adrenals and thyroids—are stimulated and their oxidase-secretions are poured into the blood stream, the heat-generating centre is also excited by reflex and sympathetic stimulation, so that by the enhanced metabolism, the toxic products and their agents can be made comparatively harmless to the organism, if not destroyed. Adrenal secretion raises the blood pressure by constricting the vessels so that the toxins and their pathogenic agents are subjected forcibly to the immunizing action of the blood. Thyroid secretion dilates the blood vessels so that the attenuated toxins can be eliminated by sweating to relieve the kidney of its heavy burden, if it has not been equal to the task imposed upon it. Fever is the physiological expression of the severity of the struggle between the invading enemies and the host for self-defence, that is, the reaction that has been set up in the body to make innocuous the toxins and the micro-organisms that produce them. Fever is the index of the resisting power of the organism against the virulence of the infection. It is the nature's healing process, and indicates that the autoprotective mechanism of the body is active. Absence of fever in a toxemia of any kind proves the inability of the body to react, owing to deficient sensitiveness of opsonin of the blood and the immunizing glands, either inherited or acquired, or to the fact that the toxin is itself a very powerful paralyzant or anesthetic of the sensory impressions. Hyperpyrexia (fever above 105° F.) on the other hand indicates the hyper-excitation of auto-defensive mechanism and the consequent over-production of the immunizing principles, and if long continued, might lead to the protoplasmic destruction of the red-corpuscles and the endothelial cells by hemolysis and autolysis. This excessive disintegration of the protoplasm is indicated by the increased excretion of nitrogen, sulphur and phosphorus and in extreme cases, acetone, aceto-acetic and B-oxybutyric acids with the urine. And this is attended with many functional derangements. The activity of the digestive glands is diminished, hence loss of appetite and inanition. On hepatic cells is imposed the heavy task of reducing excessive metabolic wastes, especially the vast number of red-corpuscles, and the consequence of the hepatic hyper-activity is the greatly increased production of the hepatic excretory product—the bile. And if it is continued long, it causes 'bilious remittent fever or malarial hemobloginuric fever' (*paittika jvara*, *Suśruta* VI. 39. 12) in which the urine is brownish yellow in color, containing a good deal of urobilin, less of urea, but more of ammonia, as the excessive quantity of sulphur and phosphorus—the disintegration-productions of abnormal destruction of red corpuscles, become oxidized into sulphuric and phosphoric acids and readily combine with ammonia which otherwise would have been changed into urea. There is of course pronounced jaundice. The liver becomes fatigued and sluggish in its activity. Gradually commences the fatty and granular degeneration of its cells. The kidney also shows its terrible strain by fatty and fibrous infiltration.

I. Fevers.

"Fever is caused by lesions of the body or the mind; for fever otherwise can not be developed in a person without injury." *Charaka* VI. 3. 10[80].

80. तस्य प्रकृतिरुद्दिष्टा दोषाः शारीरमानसाः ।
देहिनं न हि निर्द्दोषं ज्वरः समुपसेवते ॥
चरकसंहिता, चिकित्साथानम्, ३ ।

"Excessive use or abuse of '*snehādi*' [*Sneha* = unguents, *sveda* = sweating through Turkish bath or other sudoriferous means, *vamana* = vomiting, *virechana* = purgation : absorption, retention (of any toxic matter) or exhaustion fever], *traumata* (*abhighāta* = shock or wound fever), *development of disease* (*rogotthāna* = symptomatic fever as a reaction against the pathogenic germs and the toxins elaborated by them), *tumescence* (*prapāka* = coction of tumefaction, that is inflammatory fever), *fatigue* (*śrama* = fatigue fever), *inanition* (*kṣaya* = consumption, that is consumptive or famine fever), *indigestion* (*ajīrṇa* = dyspeptic fever), *toxin* (*viṣa* = toxemia) *mental derangement* (*sātmyarttuparyāya* = hysterical fever), *smell of poisonous flowers* (*oṣadhī-puṣpa-gandha* = coyza or hay fever), *worry* (*śoka* = depression fever), *sudden seasonal changes* (*nakṣatra-prapīḍana* = stellar vexations = spring or autumnal fever), *hypnotism* (*abhichāra* = exorcism : hypnotic fever), *enervation* (*abhiśāpa* = execration : nervous fever), desire or *passion* (*manas or kāma* = unreciprocated and ungratified sensual passion : erotic fever), *hallucination* (*bhūtābhiśaṅkā* = fear of ghosts : hallucinary fever), the unhygienic living of a woman that has miscarried or has given normal birth (*puerperal fever*), the establishment of the secretion of milk following childbirth (*stanyāvataraṇa*= milk fever)—these causing lesion of the nerve etc. produces *fever* in human beings." *Suśruta* VI. 39. 8.[81]

"Excessive consumption of astringent, dry or cold food and drinks , excessive use of vomiting, purgation, sweating and snuffs ; and over-exercise, retention of feces and urine, fasting, traumata, venery, anxiety, sorrow, vigilance—excess of these things irritate the nerves." *Charaka* II. I. 8[32].

"In the erotic fever, there is a good deal of contemplation (of the beloved object) and

---

81. मिथ्यातियुक्तैरपि च स्नेहाद्यैः कर्म्मभिर्नृणाम् ।
विविधादभिघाताच्च रोगोत्थानात् प्रपाकतः ॥
श्रमात् चयादजीर्णाच्च विषात् सात्म्यर्त्तुपर्य्यायात् ।
ओषधीपुष्पगन्धाच्च शोकात् नक्षत्रपीड़नात् ॥
अभिचाराभिशापाभ्यां मनोभूताभिशङ्कया ।
स्त्रीणामपप्रजातानां प्रजातानां तथाहितैः ।
स्तन्यावतरणे चैव ज्वरो दोषैः प्रवर्त्तते ॥८

सुश्रुतसंहिता, उत्तरतन्त्रम्, ३९, ८ ।

82. रूक्षलघुशीतवमनविरेचनास्थापनशिरोविरेचनातियोगव्यायामवेगसन्धारणानशनाभिघातव्यवायोद्वेगशोकशोणितातिषेकजागरणविषमशरीरन्यासेभ्योऽतिसेवितेभ्यो वायुः प्रकोपमापद्यते । चरकसंहिता, निदानस्थानम्, ११ ।

sighing ; in the fever of sorrow, tears ; in the fever of fear, anxiety ; in the fever of anger, excitement ; in the hallucinary fever, delusion ; and in toxemia, unconsciousness, illusion, intoxication and enervation." *Chandika* VI. III. 115.[83]

"In the gastro-intestinal fever, there are anorexia, indigestion, heaviness of the stomach, the irregularity of the heart (beat), semi-consciousness, lassitude, continued fever, unchangeability of the lesion, nausea, salivation, lack of hunger, sliminess of the mouth, fatigue, somnolence and heaviness of the body, polyuria, loose feces and enervation—these are the symptoms in the gastro-intestinal fever." *Charaka* VI. III. 125[84].

---

83. ध्यानं निःश्वासबहुलं लिङ्गं कामज्वरे स्मृतम् ।
शोकजे वाष्पबहुलं त्रासप्रायं भयज्वरे ॥
क्रोधजे बहुसंरम्भं भूतावेशेऽत्वसानुषम् ।
मूर्च्छामोहमदग्लानिभूयिष्ठं विषसम्भवे ॥
चरकसंहिता, चिकित्सास्थानम्, ३ ।

84. अरुचिश्चाविपाकश्च गुरुत्वमुदरस्य च ।
हृदयस्याविशुद्धिश्च तन्द्रा चालस्यमेव च ॥
ज्वरोऽविसर्गी बलवान् दोषाणामप्रवर्त्तनम् ।
लालाप्रसेको हृल्लासः क्षुन्नाशोऽविशदं मुखम् ॥
स्तब्धसुप्तगुरुत्वञ्च गात्राणां बहुमूत्रता ।
न विड्जीर्णा न चाग्लानिर्ज्वरस्यामस्य लक्षणम् ॥
चरकसंहिता, चिकित्सास्थानम्, ३ ।

"Lassitude, watery eyes, yawning, heaviness of the body, fatigue, inclination and disinclination by turn for fire (to sit by the fire side), sun (sun-bath), breeze and water (bath), indigestion, foul taste in the mouth, gradual change of the (physical) strength, complexion and temperament—these are the prodromal symptoms of fever." *Charaka* VI. III. 25[85].

"Excessive internal heat (hyperaemia), thirst, delirium, quick respiration, illusion, pain at the joints, cessation of the perspiration and constipation—these are the symptoms in hyperpyrexia (at the onset of malarial fever the blood is driven from the peripheral to the internal organs, where there is excessive congestion, and while the surface of the body shivers with chills, there is increased high temperature)." *Charaka* VI. III. 35[86].

---

85. आलस्यं नयने सास्रे जृम्भणं गौरवं क्लमः ।
ज्वलनातपवायवम्बुभक्तिद्वेषावनिश्चितौ ॥
अविपाकास्यवैरस्यं हानिश्च बलवर्णयोः ।
शीलवैकृतमल्पञ्च ज्वरलक्षणमग्रजम् ॥
चरकसंहिता, चिकित्सास्थानम्, ३, २५ ।

86. अन्तर्द्दाहोऽधिकस्तृष्णा प्रलापः श्वसनं भ्रमः ।
सन्ध्यस्थिशूलमस्वेदो दोषवर्च्चोविनिग्रहः ॥
अन्तर्व्वेगस्य लिङ्गानि ज्वरस्यैतानि लक्षयेत् ॥
चरकसंहिता, चिकित्सास्थानम्, ३, ३५ !

Though the principle of Hindu medicine is based basically on humoral pathology, it seems, Suśruta formed a vague relationship of malaria with mosquito bites and swampy localities, where mosquitoes are developed. And it was ascribed to a particular kind of mosquito, and not to all classes of them.

"There are five types of *mosquitoes* (*maśaka* belonging to the '*Culicidae*' family, consisting nearly of one hundred genera and eight hundred species), namely '*marine*' (*sāmudra* = coastal mosquitoes), '*globular*' (*parimaṇḍala* = perhaps the mosquitoes belonging to the genus '*migarhininae*' which has strongly curbed proboscis), culex elephanti (*hastimaśaka*), '*dark*' (*kṛṣṇa* = taeniorhynchus) and '*mountainous*' (*pārvvatīya* = anopheles). The biting of the '*mountainous*' mosquito (anopheles) produces an effect like that of deadly insects." *Suśruta* V. 8. 18[87].

"If the part bitten by a spider becomes swollen, white, black, red or bronzed (cyanotic or degenerative changes), and there are symptoms of

87. मशकाः—सामुद्रः परिमण्डलो हस्तिमशकः कृष्णः पार्व्वतीय इति पञ्च। तैर्दष्टस्य तीव्रकण्डूर्दंशशोफश्च। पार्व्वतीयस्तु कीटैः प्राणहरैस्तुल्यलक्षणः। नखावकृष्टेऽत्यर्थं पिड़काः सदाहपाका भवन्ति। जलौकसां दष्टलक्षणमुक्तं चिकित्सितञ्च॥ सुश्रुतसंहिता, कल्पस्थानम्, ८, १८।

fever, burning pain, dyspnea, hiccup and headache, the prognosis is usually bad." *Charaka* VI. 23. 45[88].

"There is a kind of mountainous mosquito whose bite causes symptoms like the bite of deadly spiders (*lūta*—aranea)"[88a].

According to medical experts, tertian(*tṛtīyaka*) and quartan (*chaturthaka*) fevers (of malarial origin) are produced by nervousness ; while the valley or the marsh *aupatyaka*—at the foot-hill of the mountains, that is the swampy Tarai of the Himalayas where anopheles is found in large numbers and malaria is endemic), and drink or intoxication (*madya-samudbhava* = produced by wine) fevers are ascribed to blood-pollution (*pitta-kṛta* = corruption of the bilious principle, which is the blood). Pneumonia (*pralepaka*) and

---

88. शोफाः श्वेताः सिता रक्ताः पीता वा पिड़काज्वरः ॥
प्राणान्तको भवेद्दाहो श्वासहिक्काशिरोग्रहाः ॥
चरकसंहिता, चिकित्सास्थानम्, २३, ४५ ।

88. (a) कण्डूमान् मशकैर्विषच्छोफः स्यान्मन्दवेदनः ।
असाध्यकीटसदृशमसाध्यमशकक्षतम् ॥
चरकसंहिता, चिकित्सास्थानम्, २३, ४५ ।

influenza (*vātavalāsaka*) fevers are said to be of phlegmatic origin. *Suśruta* VI. 39. 25[89].

It has now been definitely proved that the mosquito of the genus of *anopheles* transmits the deadly malaria germ from man to man. It may be possible, however, that there are other carriers of malarial pathogenesis. And anopheles is not the only genus that is guilty. Yellow fever is transmitted by Stegmia calopus, dengue fever by Culex fatigans, filaria bancrofti by Culex fatigans. But all anopheles do not carry malarial protozoa. Anopheles has nearly one hundred species (Culex two hundred), of which only forty species have been proven experimentally to be the hosts in malaria and in India there are only ten of them as follows : Myzomyia culicfactes, Myzomyia listonii, Myzomyia turkhundi, Pyretophorus jeyporensis, Myzorhynchus barbirostris, Myzorhynchus sinensis, Nyssorhynchus theobaldi, Nyssorhynchus stephensii, Nyssorhynchus fuliginosus and Nyssorhynchus maculipalpis. According to Theobald none of the anophelinae species

89. वाताधिकत्वात् प्रवदन्ति तज्ज्ञास्तृतीयकञ्चापि चतुर्थकञ्च ।
औपत्यके मद्यसमुद्भवे च हेतुं ज्वरे पित्तकृतं वदन्ति ।
प्रलेपकं वातबलासकञ्च कफाधिकत्वे न वदन्ति तज्ज्ञाः ।
सुश्रुतसंहिता, उत्तरतन्त्रम्, २, ३४ ।

of Feltinella, Bironella, Aldrichia, Chagasia, Chrystia, Kerteszia, Myzorhynchella and Lephoscelomyia have been found to be the bearers of malarial germs.

But the protozoan parasites of the red blood-corpuscles that cause remittent or intermittent malarial fevers, are not the same, and they appear under four chief forms: tertian is caused by plasmodium vivax, quartan fever by plasmodium malaria, estivo-autumnal fever or subtertian malarial fever by plasmodium falciparum (*lavernia malaria, plasmodium precox*), quotidian fever by plasmodium falciparum quotidianum.

These four kinds of blood-parasites produce different reactions in the organism according to their characteristics. Plasmodium vivax requires forty-eight hours to complete the cycle of schizogony and sporulates principally in the spleen, liberating toxins which are hemolytic, pyrogenous and hemozoanous, and will provoke an attack of fever with single brood in the human host every forty-eight hours, that is on the third day and accordingly it is called '*tertian*' (*tṛtīyaka*), and in the intervening period there is remission of fever. Plasmodium malaria needs seventy-two hours to complete its schizogon, and it principally sporulates in the peripheral blood, and the liberated toxin causes a severe constriction of cutaneous vessels, thus provoking shivering chills on the surface and chattering teeth, though the temperature of the blood is rising rapidly, and driving the blood centripetally, causing congestion of the internal organs; as it takes seventy-two hours for the cycle, that is, the fever appears every fourth day with a single brood of infection, it is called '*quartan*' (*chaturthaka*). Laverania malaria is irregular in its sporulation and needs about from thirty-six to forty-eight hours for schizonomy, and as it sporulates in the red corpuscles of the blood, it causes an immense destruction of them, and as the pathogenic protozoon needs high temperature for its development, the fever takes place in the autumn, and is therefore called '*estivo-autumnal*' (*śāradīya*). This is the most malignant of malarial fevers, for it not only causes a heavy destruction of the red corpuscles of the blood, and it is calculated that there are nearly 25, 000, 000, 000, 000 red corpuscles in an adult human being, and it needs about 3, 000, 000, 000 of them to be affected to cause an acute fever, and if it be below 250, 000, 000, the malarial fever does not manifest and remains in a latent state; but it can also provoke serious lesion in the brain, pancreas, liver, spleen and other internal organs by forming thrombi through blocking the capillary passage by the accumulation of plasmodia, swollen endothelial cells laden with hemozoan and sporules. The bilious remittent fever (bilious hemoglobinuric or *blackwater fever*=*pitta-jvara*) is also caused by it by the excessive destruction of erythrocytes which necessarily imposes a heavy labor on the liver, with the consequent production of excessive quantity of bile, which produces jaundice of the tissues and also appears in the urine with other pigments (*hemozoan*) and the urine looks from brownish yellow to blackish in color. The *quotidian* (*anyedyuṣka*) fever may be produced by plasmodium falsiparum quotidianum which takes twenty-four hours for schizogony, or by three broods of plasmodium malaria, triple quartan fever, the parasites coming to maturity on three successive days), two of plasmodium vivax (*double tertian fever*), or two of laverania malaria (*double estivo-autumnal* or *double subtertian fever*).

At the onset of malarial fever, all these types tend to be irregular, for the simple reason that the pathogenic sporozoa are of different ages and inoculated at different times, and only as the disease proceeds, the fever becomes regular, possibly because the parasites that can not conform to the age period of the majority in their schizogony, when the organism offers least resistance) overwhelmed by the combined attack of the parasites and the toxins liberated by them becomes exterminated by the anti-toxins of the blood) produced as a reaction.

"The fever that lasts for seven, ten or twelve days without interruption, is called *'santata'* (*simple continued fever*, produced by a bacillus, resembling coli communis, or the remittent fever produced by spirocheta carteri, known also as the relapsing fever or typhus recurrens) ; the fever that appears twice in day and night, is called *'satata'* (*doule-quotidian* or *Kala azar*, produced by a protozoan parasite *Leishmania donovani*, and it grows in large numbers by fission, and is principally found in the liver, spleen, bone-marrow, lymphatic glands and to a less extent, in the pancreas, kidneys, suprarenals, lungs and testicles) ; the fever that appears on every third day, is called *'tṛtīyaka'* (*tertian*) ; and which appears on every fourth day, is called the *'chaturthaka'* (*quartan*)." *Suśruta* VI. 39. 31[90].

90. सप्ताहं वा दशाहं वा द्वादशाहमथापि वा ।
सन्तत्यां योऽविसर्गी स्यात् सन्ततः स निगद्यते ।
अहोरात्रे सततको द्वौ कालावनुवर्त्तते ।

"The unhygienic living after the relief from (the primary onset of) the fever, aggravates the lesion, and owing to the low vitality (of the organism) deranges nerves and phlegma, and causes the development of *double-quotidian* (*satata* = kala-azar), quotidian (*anyedyuṣka*), tertian (*tṛtīyakā*), quartan (*chaturthaka*) and pneumonic (*pralepaka*) acute fevers." *Suśruta* VI. 39. 22[91].

"Tremor, irregular onset of fever, congestion of neck, face and lips, insomnia, suppression of sneezing, desiccation of the body, pain especially in the head and the heart, foul taste in the mouth, constipation, flatulence (*ādhmāna* = swelling) and yawning are the symptoms of '*vāta*' (cerebro-spinal estivo-autumnal pernicious) fever.

Onset of fever with rigor, diarrhœa, diminished sleep, vomiting, tumescence of the neck, face, lips and nose, sudoresis, delirium, bitter taste in

---

त्वन्येद्युष्कस्त्वहोरात्रादेककालं प्रवर्त्तते ।
तृतीयकस्तृतीयेऽह्नि चतुर्थेऽह्नि चतुर्थकः ॥३१

सुश्रुतसंहिता, उत्तरतन्त्रम्,, ३९, ३१ ।

91. क्षामाणां ज्वरमुक्तानां मिथ्याहारविहारिणाम् ।
दोषः स्वल्पोऽपि संवृद्धो देहिनामनिलेरितः ॥
सततान्येद्युष्कत्र्याख्य-चातुर्थान् सप्रलेपकान् ।
कफस्थानविभागेन यथासंख्यं करोति हि ॥

सुश्रुतसंहिता, उत्तरतन्त्रम्, ३९, २२ ।

the mouth, semi-consciousness, hyperpyrexia, intoxicated state, polydipsia, the yellowish tinge of the feces, urine and the eyes, and vertigo are the symptoms in '*pitta*' fever (*bilious remittent fever* : known also as malarial hemoglobinuric or blackwater fever).

Heaviness of the body, chills, expectoration, horripilation, excessive sleep, sluggish circulation, mild onset of fever, salivation, sweet taste of the mouth, low fever, vomiting, lassitude of the body, indigestion, acute coryza (*pratiśyāya* = profuse secretion of the watery mucus from the nose), loss of appetite and whiteness of the expectoration and the eyes are the symptoms of '*śleṣma*' (influenza) fever." *Suśruta* VI. 39. 11-13[92].

---

92. वेपथुर्विषमो वेगः कण्ठौष्ठमुखशोषणम् ।
निद्रानाशः क्षवस्तम्भो गात्राणां रौक्ष्यमेव च ॥
शिरोहृद्गात्ररुग्वक्त्र-वैरस्यं बद्धविट्कता ।
जृम्भाध्मानं तथा शूलं भवत्यनिलजे ज्वरे ॥११
वेगस्तीक्ष्णोऽतिसारश्च निद्राल्पत्वं तथा वमिः ।
कण्ठौष्ठमुखनासानां पाकः स्वेदश्च जायते ॥
प्रलापः कटुता वक्त्रे मूर्च्छा दाहो मदस्तृषा ।
पीतविण्मूत्रनेत्रत्वं पैत्तिके भ्रम एव च ॥१२
गौरवं शीतमुत्क्लेशो रोमहर्षोऽतिनिद्रता ।
स्रोतोरोधो रुगल्पत्वं प्रसेको मधुरास्यता ॥
नात्युष्णगात्रता च्छर्दिरङ्गसादोऽविपाकता ।
प्रतिश्यायोऽरुचिः कासः कफजेऽक्ष्णोश्च शुक्लता ॥१३
सुश्रुतसंहिता, उत्तरतन्त्रम्, ३९, १३ ।

Eruptive Fevers : "Feverishness or chilliness by turns ; pains in the bones, joints and the head (headache) ; watery, glazed or reddish, dilated or contracted eyes ; hissing sounds and pain in the ears ; neck as if covered with grains (*śūka*=eruptive typhoid papules) ; somnolence ; illusion ; delirium ; coughing ; dyspnea ; loss of appetite (*anorexia*) ; delusion ; the tongue is rough and has the color of burnt coal (dry, brown, thickly coated, fissured and tremulous) ; inertia of the body ; nasal discharge mixed with blood (nose-bleed) ; bilious sputum (vomiting) ; agitation of the head ; insomnia ; angina pectoris ; scanty perspiration, urination and defecation ; the patient does not look emaciated ; sound in the neck (sonorous or sibilant rales indicating bronchitis) ; appearance of rose-red exanthem (*koṭha*) and rashes (*maṇḍala*) ; aphasia (*mūkatva*) ; lesion in the circulatory system, heaviness of the epigastrium (flatulence) ; and the delay in the coction of the deranged humors (the long duration of the disease and convalescence from it) are the symptoms of the typhoid fever." *Charaka.* VI. 3. 85[93].

---

93. सन्निपातज्वरस्योर्ध्वमतो वक्ष्यामि लक्षणम् ।
क्षणे दाहः क्षणे शीतमस्थिसन्धिशिरोरुजः ।

"Altogether through (varied) lesion, there are thirteen kinds of *typhoid fevers.*" *Charaka* I. 17. 16[94].

It is very probable that all the eruptive fevers have been classified by Charaka, as *typhoid fevers* (*sannipāta jvara*), including in the category typhus, paratyphoid, cerebro-spinal meningitis, measles, mumps, erysipelas, diphtheria, toxemia, septicemia, pneumonia, puerperal fever and small pox. Charaka and Suśruta both mention smallpox as '*masūrikā.*'

"Due to lesion of the phlegma and the biles (circulatory blood), tiny rashes, anorexia, exudative vesicles, called '*romānti*' (varicellaa or chicken

---

साम्रावे कलुषे रक्ते निर्भुग्ने चापि दर्शने ॥
सस्वनौ सरुजौ कर्णौ कण्ठः शूकैरिवावृतः ।
तन्द्रा मोहः प्रलापश्च कासः श्वासोऽरुचिर्भ्रमः ॥
परिदग्धा खरस्पर्शा जिह्वा स्रस्ताङ्गता परम् ।
ष्ठीवनं रक्तपित्तस्य कफेनोन्मिश्रितस्य च ॥
शिरसो लोठनं तृष्णा निद्रानाशो हृदि व्यथा ।
स्वेदमूत्रपुरीषाणां चिराद्दर्शनमल्पशः ॥
कृशत्वं नातिगात्राणां प्रततं कण्ठकूजनम् ।
कोठानां श्यावरक्तानां मण्डलानाञ्च दर्शनम् ॥
मूकत्वं स्रोतसां पाको गुरुत्वमुदरस्य च ।
चिरात् पाकश्च दोषाणां सन्निपातज्वराकृतिः ॥

चरकसंहिता, चिकित्सास्थानम्, ७।

94. सम्मैश्चैको विकारास्ते सन्निपातास्त्रयोदश ॥

चरकसंहिता, सूत्रस्थानम्, १७।

pox) appear with fever, itching and polydipsia. From bile and phlegma (corruption of), the tumescence of the pustules that appear all over the body like lentils (ervum lens : ervum menus), is called the variola or *small pox* (*masūrikā*)." *Charaka* VI. 12. 73[94a].

"The painful, copper-colored, bronzed pustule that appears all over the body and within the mouth with burning fever, is called the *variola* (*masūrikā*)." *Suśruta* II. 13. 30[95].

"The typhoid fevers after passing through a crisis on the seventh, tenth or twelfth day, either become relieved or kill the patient." *Suśruta* VI. 39. 18[96].

As it was believed that disease was due to the derangement or the disharmonious combination of the humors of the body, the cure lay in their

---

94. (a) क्षुद्रप्रमाणा: पिड़का: शरीरे सर्व्वाङ्गगा: सज्वरदाहतृष्णा: ।
कण्डूयुता: सारुचिसप्रसेका रोमान्तिका: पित्तकफात् प्रदिष्टा: ॥
या: सर्व्वगात्रेषु मसूरमात्रा मसूरिका: पित्तकफात् प्रदिष्टा: ।
चरकसंहिता, चिकित्सास्थानम्, १२ ।

95, दाहज्वररुजावन्तस्ताम्रा: स्फोटा: सपीतका: ।
गात्रेषु वदने चान्तर्विज्ञेयास्ता मसूरिका: ॥३०
सुश्रुतसंहिता, निदानस्थानम्, १३ ।

96. सप्तमे दिवसे प्राप्ते दशमे द्वादशेऽपि वा ।
पुनर्घोरतरो भूत्वा प्रशमं याति हन्ति वा ॥१८
सुश्रुतसंहिता, उत्तरतन्त्रम्, ३९, १८

proper combination by coction. The internal heat that was supposed to cause coction of the humors and thus to preserve the balance of the humors, requisite for normal health, was supposed to be dissipated to the peripheral organs by morbid agents and thus to produce fever. Cure from a disease only took place when the internal combustion (metabolism or oxidation) was normalized again. This was brought about by hygienic living and dietary regulation. Medication was but supplementary. It is well known that quinine, the bitter alkaloid of the cinchona bark is a powerful remedy against the malarial plasmodia. Though cinchona is a native of the South American Andes, it belongs to the Rubiaceous family of which there are many members in India. Charaka in the treatment of malarial fever mentions a bitter (*tiktaka*) juice of leaves or bark, or concoction of a dry bark, but it is very hard now to identify what he meant by it :

"In new fever, fasting, sweating, time, barley water and bitter extract (*tiktako rasa*) cause the coction of raw humors (that is, bring about the cure).

"In the cerebro-spinal remittent fever and influenza, when the patient is thirsty, give him hot water to drink. In the bilious remittent fever, cook bitter (bark or root) in water and when it is cooled, give it to drink. Such a concoction is stimulating (*dīpana* = digestive), oxidising (*pāchana* = which causes coction of the humors), (febrifuge (*jvaraghna*), blood-purifying (*srotasāṃ śodhanaṃ* = purifier of the streams, as the blood, lymph, urine), vitalizing (*valya*), appetizing (*ruchi-kara*), sudorific (*gharma-kara*) and is beneficial." *Charaka* VI. 3. 129.[97]

That this treatment was only meant for malarial fevers, is clearly indicated by the following passage: "At the onset of the (malarial) fever fasting is proper. But it should not be followed in consumptive, nervous, phobia, excitement, depression and fatigue fevers. By fasting pathogenic agents (*doṣa*) are destroyed and when metabolism is stimulated, the body

97 लङ्घनं स्वेदनं कालो यवाग्वस्तिक्तको रसः।
पाचनान्यविपक्वानां दोषाणां तरुणे ज्वरे॥
तृष्यते सलिलञ्चोष्णं दद्याद्वातकफज्वरे।
मद्योत्थे पैत्तिके चाथ शीतलं तिक्तकैः श्रृतम्॥
दीपनं पाचनञ्चैव ज्वरघ्नमुभयञ्च तत्।
स्रोतसां शोधनं वल्यं रुचिस्वेदकरं शिवम्॥
चरकसंहिता, चिकित्सास्थानम्, ३।

becomes light and hunger appears. But fasting should not lower vitality (that is fasting for a longer period than is necessary is injurious), for recovery depends on the vitality of the patient, and the object of treatment is recovery." *Charaka* VI. 3. 128[98].

"In all kinds of fever, treat it by counteracting the causative factors. In fatigue, consumption and wound (*abhighāta* = wound or traumatism) fevers, treat the original disease." *Suśruta* VI. 39, 73 [99].

"As long as the fever patient does not regain his strength (i. e. does not completely recover), he should not indulge in shower-bath (*pariṣeka*), plunge-bath (*avagāha*), beverages, vomiting etc. (*saṃśodhana*), inunction, day-sleep, exposure to

---

98. ज्वरे लङ्घनमेवादावुपदिष्टमृते ज्वरात् ।
क्षयानिलभयक्रोधकामशोकश्रमोद्भवात् ॥
लङ्घनेन क्षयं नीते दोषे सन्धुक्षितेऽनले ।
विज्वरत्वं लघुत्वञ्च क्षुच्चैवास्योपजायते ॥
प्राणाविरोधिना चैनं लङ्घनेनोपपादयेत् ।
बलाधिष्ठानमारोग्यं यदर्थोऽयं क्रियाक्रमः ॥
चरकसंहिता, चिकित्सास्थानम्, ३, १२८ ।

99. चिकित्सेच्च ज्वरान् सर्व्वान् निमित्तानां विपर्य्ययैः ।
श्रमक्षयाभिघातोत्थे मूलव्याधिमुपाचरेत् ॥७३
सुश्रुतसंहिता, उत्तरतन्त्रम्, ३९, ७३ ।

cold, exercise and sexual intercourse." *Suśruta* VI. 39. 68 [100].

"If a fever patient suffers from indigestion, old wine and barley broth is beneficial to him. If a fever patient suffers from coryza and anorexia (influenza), let him drink whey mixed with '*trikaṭu*' (a mixture of *śuṇṭhī*—ginger, '*marïcha* black pepper, *pippala*—longpepper; Gr. '*dia trion piperidon*' made of the same ingredients, piperis longum, piperis nigri, and zingiberis). In an exhaustive continuous fever, if the patient is emaciated, on the road to recovery, mentally depressed, in cerebro-spinal or bilious remittent fever, or if the pathogenesis is not well-marked, if the patient is desiccated, has polydipsia and burning sensation, drinking of milk will benefit him. But in new fever, milk should not de drunk, as it might even cause death:" *Suśruta* VI. 39. 63[101].

---

100. परिषेकावगाहांश्च सङ्घान् संशोधनानि च ।
स्नानाभ्यङ्गदिवास्वप्न-शीतव्यायामयोषितः ।
न भजेत ज्वरोत्सृष्टो यावन्नो वलवान् भवेत् ॥
सुश्रुतसंहिता, उत्तरतन्त्रम्, ३९, ६८ ।

101. मद्यं पुराणं मन्दाग्नेर्यवान्नोपहितं हितम् ।
सव्योषं वितरेत् तक्रं कफारोचकपीड़िते ॥
कृशोऽल्पदोषो दीनश्च नरो जीर्णज्वरार्द्दितः ।
विवद्धः सृष्टदोषश्च रूक्षः पित्तानिलज्वरी ॥

*"In a long-standing continuous or remittent fever, if the patient becomes emaciated, he should be treated by light and easily-digestible food for his fever. Broth of a bean (*mudga*= *phaseolus mungo*), red lentil (*masūra* = *ervum hirsutum*), gram pea (*chaṇaka* = *cicer arietinum*), plantain (*musa paradisaica*), and dolichon biflorum. The fever patient that likes meat, can take the partridge (*perdicum cheninensium*), perdicum francolinorum, black antelope (*antioparum nigrarum*), hystricum, small deer, hare (*leporum*), black-tailed deer, golden-colored deer and antiloparum albarum. The crane (*gruidæ*), heron (*ardeidæ*), peacock (*pavo*), chicken (*gallos domesticos*) and heath-cock (*tetraoninnæ*), are hard to digest and very excitant; for this reason they are not prescribed by many physicians. But when the fever patient is nervous, it can be given in a moderate quantity." *Suśruta* VI. 39. 67[102].

पिपासार्त्तः सदाहो वा पयसा स सुखी भवेत् ।
तदेव तु पयः पीतं तरुणे हन्ति मानवम् ।

सुश्रुतसंहिता, उत्तरतन्त्रम्, ३९, ६३

102. सततं विषमं वापि क्षीणस्य सुचिरोत्थितम् ।
ज्वरं संभोजनैः पथ्यैर्लघुभिः समुपाचरेत् ॥
मुद्गान् मसूरांश्चणकान् कुलत्थान् समकुष्टकान् ।
आहारकाले यूषार्थे ज्वरिताय प्रदापयेत् ॥

But Charaka only recommends their broth and not their flesh; however, this meat-broth can be a little acidulated with the admixture of pomegranate (punica granatum) to make it more palatable VI. 3. 165[103].

"Milk boiled together with ginger, raisins and dried dates, and mixed with honey or sugar relieves thirst and fever. Or the milk might be diluted with water four-fold and cooked together; this is beneficial in old fever, and the drinking of hot milk is good in bilious remit-

---

लावान् कपिञ्जलानेणान् पृषतान्शरभाञ्छशान् ।
कालपुच्छान् कुरङ्गांश्च तथैव मृगमातृकान् ॥
मांसार्थे मांससात्म्यानां ज्वरितानां प्रदापयेत् ॥
सारसक्रौञ्चशिखिनः कुक्कुटांस्तित्तिरींस्तथा ।
गुरूष्णत्वान्न शंसन्ति ज्वरे केचिच्चिकित्सकाः ॥
ज्वरितानां प्रकोपन्तु यदा याति समीरणः ।
तदैतेऽपि हि शस्यन्ते मात्राकालोपपादिताः ॥

सुश्रुतसंहिता, उत्तरतन्त्रम्, ३९, ६७ ।

103. लावान् कपिञ्जलानेणांश्चकोरानुपचक्रकान् ।
कुरङ्गान् कालपुच्छांश्च हरिणान् पृषतः शशान् ॥
प्रदद्यान्मांससात्म्याय ज्वरिताय ज्वरापहान् ।
ईषदम्लाननम्लान् वा रसान् काले विचक्षणः ॥
कुक्कुटांश्च मयूरांश्च तित्तिरिक्रौञ्चवर्त्तकान् ।
गुरूष्णत्वान्न शंसन्ति ज्वरे केचिच्चिकित्सकाः ॥

चरकसंहिता, चिकित्सास्थानम्, ३, १६५ ।

tent fever. Milk is restorative in all consumptive fevers; it always produces good result whether drunk hot or cold with whatever medicine prescribed for the particular fever." *Charaka* VI. 3. 196[104].

"The embrace of maidens that are pretty and well-shaped, relieves the chills of (malarial) fevers, by imparting the natural warmth of their body." *Charaka* VI. 3. 208[105].

"In old pneumonic or nervous fever, if the patient suffers from chills, heat should be applied to warm him up, which is very beneficial in such a case ...... (drinking of hot concoction, hot wine, warm bath, hot salve and fomentations are recommended)....The body should be covered with warmed cotton or silken clothes. If the

---

104. सनागरं सम्रद्वीकं सघृतक्षौद्रशर्करम् ।
श्रृतं पयः सखर्ज्जुरं पिपासाज्वरनाशनम् ॥
चतुर्गुणेनाम्भसा वा श्रृतं ज्वरहरं पयः ।
धारोष्णं वा पयः सद्यो वातपित्तज्वरं जयेत् ॥
जीर्णज्वराणां सर्व्वेषां पयः प्रशमनं परम् ।
पेयं तदुष्णं शीतं वा यथास्वैरौषधैः श्रृतम् ॥
चरकसंहिता, चिकित्सास्थानम्, ३, १९० ।

105. चारूपचितगात्राश्च तरुण्यो यौवनोष्मणा ।
आश्लेषाच्छमयन्त्याशु प्रमदाः शिशिरं ज्वरम् ॥
चरकसंहिता, चिकित्सास्थानम, ३, २०८

patient feels fatigued anoint the body with aloes (*aquilaria agallocho*). And well-breasted, pretty and artful maidens in the first inflorescence of their youth, should massage gently his debilitated body. And the maidens with the face like the autumnal moon, eyes like the blue lotus, long-curved tremulous brows, complexion like molten gold, bright-red lips (like the *bimba* fruit = *memordica monadelpha*), narrow abdomen (slender waist) but broad expansive pelvic region, body anointed with delicate fragrance (*croco sativa* and *aquilaria agallocho*), firm, round and elevated breasts, dressed in fine-smelling, washed and white loose dress, as a wild-creeper (entwines round a tree), should embrace him closely. But when the patient seems to be enlivened, then the maidens should be removed. When by the delightful contact of the maidens, the chills have disappeared, the patient should take pleasant and beneficial diet." *Suśruta* VI. 39. 134[106].

106. कफवातोत्थयोश्चापि ज्वरयोः शीतपीड़ितम्।
दिह्यादुष्णेन वर्गेण परश्चोष्णो विधिर्हितः।
सिञ्चेत् कौषेरारनाल-शुक्तगोमूत्रमस्तुभिः।
दिह्यात् पत्राङ्गैरथवा सुरसार्ज्जकशिग्रुजैः॥
क्षारतैलेन चाभ्यङ्गः सशुक्तेन विधीयते।
पानमारग्वधादेश्च क्वथितस्य विशेषतः॥

Prophylaxis in malarial fever can be summed up in these words: (*a*) destruction of mosquitoes; (*b*) the prevention of the entrance of the parasite into the human body; (*c*) increasing resistance of the body against the parasite.

As the mosquitoes require shallow, stagnant water for breeding and development of their larvæ, the first requisite for a determined fight against malaria, is the awakened public sentiment against this pernicious and malignant

---

अवगाहः सुखोष्णश्च वातघ्नक्वाथसंयुतः ।
जित्वा शीतं क्रमैरेभिः सुखोष्णजलसेचितम् ॥
प्रवेश्यौर्णिककार्पास-कौशेयाम्बरसंवृतम् ।
शाययेद् ग्लानदेहञ्च कालागुरुविभूषितम् ॥
स्तनाढ्या रूपसम्पन्नाः कुशला नवयौवनाः ।
भजेयुः प्रमदा गात्रैः शीतदैन्यापहारिभिः ॥
शरच्छशाङ्कवदना नीलोत्पलदलेक्षणाः ।
स्फुरितभ्रूलताभङ्ग-ललाटतटकम्पनाः ॥
प्रलम्बिविलसत्काञ्च्यो विम्बीफलनिभाधराः ।
कृशोदर्य्योऽतिविस्तीर्ण-जघनोरुस्तनालसाः ॥
कुङ्कुमागुरुदिग्धाङ्ग्यो घनतुङ्गपयोधराः ।
सुगन्धिधूपितस्रग्वा-स्त्रस्तांशुकविभूषणाः ॥
गाढमालिङ्गयेयुस्तं नरं वनलता इव ।
प्रह्लादञ्चास्य विज्ञाय ताः स्त्रीरपनयेत् पुनः ॥
तासामङ्गपरिस्पर्श-निवारितहिमज्वरम् ।
भोजयेद्धितमन्नञ्च यथा सुखमवाप्नुयात् ॥१२४

सुश्रुतसंहिता, उत्तरतन्त्रम्, ३९

disease. For without communal co-operation, it can not be accomplished. There should be complete surface and subsoil drainage and the ground should, be so levelled by filling up the ditches and the natural depressions that there can not be any accumulation of water for the breeding of the mosquitoes. All the ponds, lakes, canals and water-ways should be deepened, and the water-plants that usually float on the surface as safe breeding place for mosquitoes, protecting the larvæ from the fish must be regularly and systematically removed. Fish should be cultivated in every pond, lake or canal, especially the '*giradinus poeciloides*' which is a voracious feeder on eggs, larvæ and pupae of mosquitoes. All trees on the bank of the water or near the dwelling house which takes away sunshine or interferes with free current of air, should be felled, for the mosquitoes need a dark place to hide in the day time. Laveran recommends the plantation of castor oil plants (*Prophylaxie du paludism,* p. 134), the odor of which he believes drives away mosquitoes. However the promise held by the Eucalyptus tree has been rather deceptive. Bats appear to be voracious feeders of mosquito larvæ.

The next thing is to protect the inhabitants

against the mosquito bites. Mosquitoes can fly nearly a mile's distance from the breeding place, and many of them go out and bite only in the evening and at night. And it is the females that do the biting. The males live on vegetable and fruit juice. The life of a female mosquito is about a month. It bites any vertebrate it might come across in order to get blood which it needs as nourishment for its eggs. But it is only by biting a malarial patient, it can be infected with the malarial plasmodium, which it transmits to others when biting again. Therefore to prevent the spreading of malaria, it is necessary that the inhabitants be protected from mosquito bites, for in a malarial region, almost every one might harbor malarial germ in the blood, though the disease is in a latent form and there is hardly any apparent symptom, excepting a little malaise and lassitude. The mosquito bite can be easily prevented by using mosquito wire netting in the windows, which does not prevent the circulation of air. Where it can not be done, mosquito-nets must be used in the bed. And if it is necessary to go out at night, one should take care to wrap the body in clothes or smear the body with carbolated vaseline and to use a fine-gauze net round the face and neck.

Quinine is the best prophylactic and curative agent against malaria. In the endemic malarial region, it is a wise policy to take 2 to 4 grains of quinine daily, as a preventive medicine, which seems to be much more effective than larger doses at longer intervals. Chlorhydrate of quinine is preferable in an irritant stomach, or Sulphate of quinine can be given which is much cheaper. During the acute stage of the malarial fever, it is better that quinine be administered in doses not smaller than one gram, nearly four hours before the expectation of the chills, as quinine takes nearly four hours to act, and it should act energetically at the time of the sporulation—when the young broods are liberated and which provokes the chill, and the sporules then should be destroyed, for it is very doubtful how far the old gamets are affected by quinine. Quinine should be given every day, preferably by mouth and in powder form or in solution, and the bitter taste can be covered and neutralised by addition of syrup glycyrrhizae (syrup of licorice) every day when the attack is expected, until the disease is broken, as it may be due to double infection by the tertian, estivo-autumnal and quartan parasites or to the treble infection of the quartan. And with the exception of reinfection, relapses can be usually prevented by giving quinine once a week for four weeks from the occurrence of the last chill.

During the paroxysm, treatment needs simply to be symptomatic: in chills hot drink, warm covers and hot fomentations can be applied to relieve the shivering cold sensation, and during the succeeding hot period cold application on the head to relieve headache and cold drink to relieve thirst. But the sweating period should not be shortened by antipyretics as it might harm the organism by retaining the malarial toxins which perspiration tends to eliminate, and that is why the sweat of a malarial patient has a peculiar odor.

It goes without saying that nourishing food and hygienic living strengthens the resisting power of the organism against any infection.

II.-Diarrhœa.

"Excessive consumption of indigestible (*alimentary diarrhœa* provoked by the irritation of the intestinal mucosa through the indigestible residue), *fatty* (fatty d. or d. adiposa, caused by the splitting of the fat into irritant fatty acids, or as in jaundice with the deficiency of the bile, by the evacuation of the undigested fatty substances), dry (mechanical or *serous d.* caused by an augmentation of pressure within the alimentary canal with exaggerated serous transudation into the intestine), hot (*inflammatory d.*), liquid (*asthenic d.* caused by the fermentation brought by the dilution of the digestive enzymes by an exceedingly large quantity of liquid), coarse (*linteric d.* in which the undigested or half-digested food particles are contained in the dicharges), ice-cold (*congestive d.* is induced by mechanically stimulating the peristalic contractions and possibly glandular secretions by a large quantity of cold water, thereby increasing the amount and fluidity of the intestinal contents, and by diluting the gastro-intestinal secretions which interfering with digestion, provokes fermentation ; the drinking of ice-cold water and beverages cause loose movements for they mechanically bring about contraction of the superficial vessels of the mucosa, followed by reaction and congestion of the membrane, and if long continued to intestinal catarrh), and *improper foods* [diarrhœa is provoked by all kinds of food poisoning, *bromatotoxismus* either putrefactive, fermentative or infective with all toxemic symptoms : meat-poisoning or kreototoxismus arises from decomposed meat (proteus group alone or associated with colon bacilli), meat of diseased animals or infected animals (as tuberculosis); fish-poisoning or ichthyotoxismus arises from eating fish that is venomous, or only at the spawning season or from feeding upon putrefactive substances or from its decomposed ptomaine poisoning as in rotten egg; milk-poisoning or galactotoxismus arises from taking contaminated or spoilt milk: milk may be contaminated from various sources as it is one of the best culture mediums of pathogenic germs, as from tuberculosis from a diseased animal, dust on the animal, filthy hand of the milker, unclean receptacle, or, washed with polluted water, or from exposure when left uncovered for a considerable period, and milk usually contains myriads of bacteria, and in it are frequently observed colon bacilli and bacillus enteritidis, and to a lesser extent bacillus enteritidis sporogenes, staphilococci, paratyphoid and occasionally typhoid germs; grain-poisoning or sitotoxismus arises from using spoilt, contaminated or sprouting grains, as pellagra in the use of diseased maize, or in the spoilt pea, paraplegia or lathyrism (*lupinosis*) in the admixture of the grain with the seeds of the '*lathyrus*'; it is well known that sprouting potatoes contain at the mouth of the sprouts or the greenish surface of the skin exposed to the sun, a glycerid alkaloid-solanine, while many of the mushrooms contain another toxic alkaloid-muscarin], *uncooked food* (uncooked food is not only hard to digest as cooking softens the tissues, but many of the vegetables and fruits might contain fungi, amœba and the eggs of many intestinal worms which are thus introduced into the alimentary canal where they make their habitat, and provoke diarrhœa either by irritating the mucusa, or causing ulceration or impaction), *disharmonious combination of foods* (as milk and acid, or sugar and acid which is apt to cause fermentation in a weak or debilitated stomach), repeated eating before the former meal has been digested (*adhyaśana*=d.ab ingluvie), indigestion (*dyspeptic d.*) excessive use or abuse of purgation, vomiting and sweating (d. cathartica), *poisoning* (in chronic mercurial poisoning perhaps due to the corroding action of its salts, there is an extensive ulceration of the alimentary canal, followed by fetid diarrhœa, anemia, foul breath, falling out of the hair, brittleness of the nails, salivation, stomatitis, buccal ulcers and enteroclitis ; in acute or chronic arsenic poisoning, there is pronounced epigastric and abdominal pain, followed by vomiting and diarrhœa of rice-water and often bloody and offensive stools, suppression of urine or bloody urine, neuralgic pains and paralysis ; in lead poisoning, the gums have a bluish black tinge, progressive anemia, nutritive disturbance, constipation, but often alternating with diarrhœa), anxiety (*emotional d.*) depression (nervous or *neurotic d.*) *polluted water* (water containing dysenteric germs or large amount of earthly alkali as magnesium or sodium, calcium or potassium carbonates, dissolved from the soil) excessive drinking of *spirituous liquor* (in chronic alcoholism diarrhœa results from the thickened, inflamed, congested and often ulcerated intestinal mucosa, imperfect gastro-intestinal indigestion, interference with colonic absorption, disturbance of the biles due to congestion and cirrhosis of the liver, and the effect of alcohol upon the local and cerebro-spinal nerve-centres controlling intestinal nutrition, secretion and motility, thus provoking diarrhœa alternating with constipation), mental derangement (*neurogenic d.*), sudden seasonal changes (thermic or *summer d.* of the hot season : it may be also induced by sun or heat stroke accompanied by enervation, dizziness, cramp, disturbed vision, dry skin, rectal and vesical irritability ; in exposure to cold and dampness, the surface of the body is suddenly chilled with the lowering of the surface temperature, which causes the contraction of the cutaneous blood-vessels, leading to congestion of the internal organs, chiefly the intestine and viscera, and reflexly irritating the motor and secretory nervous mechanism—thus leading to evacuations; in sudden change of climate, diarrhœa may be, also, induced as hill or spruce d..), excessive use of lavage (*mechanical d.*), *obstructive* (due to carcinoma, tumor, calculi, fecal impaction or obstruction of the passage with the tapeworms as tenia solium which is introduced with incompletely cooked pork and might grow from 6 to 12 feet, tenia saginata, from incompletely cooked beef varying in size from 10 to 25 feet, tenia lata from half-cooked fish varying in size from 5 to 25 feet, and tenia nana (dwarf tape) from one-fifth to one and one-fourth inches in length; diarrhœa is provoked by them either because the formed feces can not pass through the obstructed passage and only watery liquid can ooze through, or due to irritation from the mucosa caused by them), and by '*krimis*' [worms uncinariasis or hookworm, ascaris lumbricoides or round worms, oxyuris vermicularis or thread-worm, tricuris trichiura or whipworm, trematodes or flukeworms and strongyloides intestinalis ; microbes : entamebazer rhizapodes in amebic dysentery, flagellates ormastigophores in flagellate dysentery, ciliates (balandium coli, infusoria) in ciliar dysentery, bacillus dysenteriæ in bacillary dysentery, spirillum cholera asiatica in cholera, bacillus typhosus in typhoid fevers, gonococcus among the pedestrians with extensive lesion of the anal mucosa, plasmodium in bilious remittent fever] these causes produce dirrhœa." *Suśruta* VI. 40. 2[107].

"Slow-moving (*ajava* = ascaris). agile (*vijava* = flagellates), creeping (*kipya* = trematodes or flukeworm), stealing (*tripya* = uncinariasis or hookworm), knotted-feet (*gaṇḍū-pada* = tenia), thread-like (*churu* = oxyuris vermicularis or thread-worm)and two mouthed(*dvimukha* = trichuris trichiura or whipworm) are the '*krimi*' (parasites) of the feces ; they are whitish and minute ; they move in the lower intestine and cause (bor-

107. गुर्व्वतिस्निग्धरूक्षोष्ण-द्रवस्थूलातिशीतलैः ।
विरुद्धाध्यशनाजीर्णैर्विषमैश्चापि भोजनैः ॥
स्नेहाद्यैरतियुक्तैश्च मिथ्यायुक्तैर्विषाद् भयात् ।
शोकाद्दुष्टाम्बुमद्यातिपानात् सात्म्यर्त्तुपर्य्ययात् ॥
जलाभिरमणैर्वेग-विघातैः क्रिमिदोषतः ।
नृणां भवत्यतीसारो लक्षणं तस्य वक्ष्यते ॥२

सुश्रुतसंहिता उत्तरतन्त्रम्, ४० ।

ing pain ; and among them there are some that have flagella *puchcua* as in flagellates) and they are broad. These fecal '*krimi*' (worms and other microbic parasites) bring about colics, dyspepsia, jaundice, intestinal obstruction, weakness, overflowing of the watery discharges, heart lesion and non-formation of the feces."

Suśruta VI. 54. 4[108].

"The prodromes of diarrhœa are boring pains in the heart, umbilicus, coccygeal region, abdomen and the groin, lassitude of the body, flatulence, constipation, tympanites and indigestion." *Suśruta* VI. 40. 4[109].

"Abdominal pains, oliguria, sounds in the alimentary canal, prolapsus ani, lassitude of the

---

108. अजवा विजवाः किप्यास्थिप्या गण्डूपदास्तथा ।
चुरवो द्विमुखाश्चैव सप्तैवेते पुरीषजाः ॥
श्वेताः सूक्ष्मास्तुदन्त्येते गुदं प्रति सरन्ति च ।
तेषामेवापरे पुच्छैः पृथवश्च भवन्ति हि ॥
शूलाग्निमान्द्यपाण्डुत्व-विष्टम्भवलसंचयाः ।
प्रसेकारुचिहृद्रोग-विड्भेदास्तु पुरीषजैः ॥४

सुश्रुतसंहिता, उत्तरतन्त्रम्, ४० ।

109 हृन्नाभिपायूदरकुक्षितोद-गात्रावसादानिलसन्निरोधाः ।
विट्सङ्ग आध्मानमथाविपाको भविष्यतस्तस्य पुरःसराणि ॥४

सुश्रुतसंहिता, उत्तरतन्त्रम्, ४० ।

groin, thigh and the knee and the evacuation of mucus-covered (*saphena* = frothy) dark-brownish, hardened scybla in small quantities with gas—these are the symptoms of nervous (dysenteric) diarrhœa.

"Dark-yellowish (in biliary obstruction), greenish (due to the presence of unchanged biliverdin in the discharges as in acute enteritis), or reddish (tarry stools may be due to cancer or ulcer of the intestine or dysentery), unformed, serous (like the juice of pressed meat), foul-smelling and steamy discharges rush forth in bilious diarrhœa (cholera asiatica) ; in this disease the patient becomes exhausted and becomes overpowered by polydipsia, vertigo and hyperemia of the internal organs.

"Whitish (rice-water, or containing undigested fat) and pasty stool appears noiselessly, mixed with mucus in phlegmatic diarrhœa ; in this disease the patient suffers from collapse, somnolence, lassitude and repeated evacuations ; and the patient becomes irritable and there is horripilation (contraction of the peripheral vessels).

"In the typhoid fevers, the above mentioned symptoms appear, but the color of the evacuation is varied and the patient suffers from polydipsia ; it is very hard to cure and the prognosis is especially unfavorable for the infants and for the aged." *Suśruta* VI. 40. 5-8[110]

"If in cholera asiatica (*visūchikā*) and tymphenites (*alasaka*), the teeth (the gum), lips and nails become cyanotic, there is a comatose state, active vomiting, orbits of the eyes are sunk in the sockets, the voice becomes weak and the

---

110. शूलाविष्टः सक्तमूत्रोऽन्त्रकूजी
स्रस्तापानः सन्नकट्यूरुजङ्घः ।
वर्चो मुञ्चत्यल्पमल्पं सफेनं
रूक्षं श्यावं सानिलं मारुतेन ॥५
दुर्गन्ध्युष्णं वेगवन्मांसतोय-
प्रख्यं भिन्नं स्विन्नदेहोऽतिरुग्णः ।
पित्तात् पीतं नीलमालोहितं वा
तृष्णामूर्च्छादाहपाकज्वरार्त्तः ॥६
तन्द्रानिद्रागौरवोत्क्लेशसादी
वेगाशङ्की सृष्टविट्कोऽपि भूयः ।
शुक्लं सान्द्रं श्लेष्मणा श्लेष्मयुक्तं
भक्तद्वेषी निःस्वनं हृष्टरोमा ॥७
तन्द्रायुक्तो मोहमानास्यशोषी
वर्चः कुर्य्यान्नैकवर्णं तृषार्त्तः ।
सर्व्वोद्भूतः सर्व्वलिङ्गोपपत्तिः
कृच्छ्रसाध्यं बालवृद्धेष्वसाध्यः ॥८

सुश्रुतसंहिता, उत्तरतन्त्रम्, ४० ।

joints become relaxed, then the prognosis is very unfavorable." *Suśruta* VI. 56. 8[111] .

"In acute diarrhœa, if the feces is formed or shows symptoms of being formed, and the vitality of the patient is not very low, there has not been much emaciation of flesh nor blood much thinned, appetite and digestion have returned, then the patient can be cured with difficulty. But if the patient has the following symptoms, notwithstanding the above-mentioned presentations, he is to be regarded as incurable. Incurable symptoms are being mentioned : if the stool has the color of concoction (dark-brownish), reddish, like that of the spleen and fat ; or is (in consistency) like water in which meat has been washed, curdled milk (semi-fluid), clarified butter, bone-marrow, oil, butter, milk, condensed milk, or deep bluish (with the development of indican in pronounced putrefaction), reddish, blackish (in bilious remittent or blackwater fever), or transparent like water or the brownish-black color of the banana flowering-stem (clay or chocolate color stool appears in

111. यः श्यावदन्तौष्ठनखोऽल्पसंज्ञश्छर्द्द्यर्द्दितोऽभ्यन्तरयातनेत्रः ।
क्षामस्वरः सर्व्वविमुक्तसन्धिर्य्यायान्नरः सोऽपुनरागमाय ॥८

सुश्रुतसंहिता, उत्तरतन्त्रम्, ५६ ।

absence in *urobilin,* that is in the deficiency of the biliary secretion in the intestine), very fatty, pale-greenish or dark-greenish (due to unchanged biliverdin), or multi-colored ; or is turbid, lubricous or mixed with thread-like substance (*oxyuris vermicularis* or thread-worms), mucus or like the ocellate spots on the tail-feather of a peacock (flakes) ; the odor is like that of a decomposed corpse (cadaverous), putrid, pyogenous or like raw fish (fishy) ; if the feces attracts quickly the flies, or various viscid substances are observed in it (the stool may contain undigested food, blood, mucus, pus, membranes, fat ; calculi from the gall-bladder, intestines, stomach, salivary glánds ; intestinal parasites, exfoliated polypi and nerotic sloughs), or the discharge contains very little feces (a normal stool should have hard but flexible consistency, golden-brownish in color, cylindrical in form, nearly an inch in diameter, three to four inches in length ; but if it is of small calibre, it is indicative of prolapsus ani or an annular stricture of the rectum ; ribbon-shaped or flattened stool of stricture or cancer of the rectum ; roundish masses of hardened feces (*scybala*) may shoot out in dysentery or is indicative of the gastric ulcer, gastric dilatation, cancer of the rectum or chronic constipation) or is free from it (*serous*) and the patient suffers from polydipsia, hyperemia of the internal colics or its insensibility to pain ; if there is anal fistula or ulceration, or hemorrhage of the pile or the pile does not go back to its own place, stricture of the anus, emaciation of the body, thinning of the blood (anemia due to the reduction of the red corpuscles), pain in the lumbar region, anorexia, morbid delirium and coma, or the diarrhœa suddenly ceases, that patient is to be regarded as incurable." *Charaka* VI. 19. 11[112]

"In the first stage sf diarrhœa, fasting is beneficial. After fasting, for relief from diarrhœa barley water should be given with (astringent) concoction (*pāchana*). If patient still suffers

---

112. महद् ग्रथितमामं शकृदपि वा पक्वमनतिक्षीणमांसशोणितबलो मन्दाग्निविहतमुखरसश्च तादृशमातुरं कृच्छ्रसाध्यं विद्यात्। एभिर्वर्णैरतिसार्यमाणं सोपद्रवमातुरमसाध्योऽयमिति प्रत्याचक्षीत। तद्यथा—पक्वशोणिताभं यकृत्पिण्डोपमं मेदोमांसोदकसदृशं दधिघृतमज्जतैलवसाक्षीर-वेशवाराभमतिनील-मतिरक्तमतिकृष्णमुदकमिवाच्छं पुनर्मेचकाभमतिस्निग्धं हरिताभं नीलकषायवर्णं कर्बुरवर्णमाविलं पिच्छिलं तन्तुमदामं चन्द्रकोपगतमतिकुणपपूतिपूयगन्ध्याममत्स्यगन्धि मक्षिकाक्रान्तं क्वथितबहुधातुस्रावमल्पपुरीषमपुरीषं वातिसार्यमाणं तृष्णादाहज्वरभ्रमतमोहिक्काश्वासानुबन्धमतिवेदनमवेदनं वा स्रस्तपक्वगुदं पतितगुदवलिं मुक्तनालमतिक्षीणबलमांसशोणितं सर्वपर्वास्थिशूलिनमरोचकारतिप्रलापसंमोहपरीतं सहसोपशान्तविकारमतिसारिणमचिकित्स्यं विद्यादिति सन्निपातातिसारः।

चरकसंहिता, चिकित्सास्थानम्, १९।

from colics and flatulence, give him an emetic with piper longum (which is carminative) and rock salt, dissolved in water. After vomiting light food can be given, barley water and piper longum. But if this does not relieve diarrhœa then every morning a concoction of turmerics (*curcuma longum*) or *sweet flag* (*acorum calamum*) should be given to drink." *Suśruta* VI. 40.16[113].

"In morbid diarrhœa (dysentery) and strangury, a (rectal) enema (*vasti*=clyster) of concoction of liquorice root (*glycyrrhiza glabra*) and blue lotus (*nyphaca cacrulea*) mixed with milk, clarified butter and honey (for irrigation) should be given ; hemorrhagia proctica, aesus and fever are also relieved by this enema. If there is bloody stool an oily enema of soothing and honeyed herbs should be given daily either

---

113. तत्र लङ्घनमेवादौ पूर्व्वरूपेषु देहिनाम् ।
तत: पाचनसंयुक्तो यवागूदिक्रमो हित: ॥
अथवा वामयित्वा तु शूलाध्माननिपीड़ितम् ।
पिप्पलीसैन्धवाम्भोभिर्लङ्घनाद्यैरुपाचरेत् ॥
कार्य्यञ्च वमनस्यान्ते प्रायशो लघुभोजनम् ।
खड़यूषयवागूषु पिप्पल्याद्येव योजयेत् ॥
अनेन विधिना चामं यस्य वै नोपशाम्यति ।
हरिद्रादिं वचादिं वा पिवेत् प्रात: स मानव: ॥१६

सुश्रुतसंहिता, उत्तरतन्त्रम्, ४०, १६ ।

at day or at night. An oily enema relieves the nervous irritation where it is administered; and if the nerves are subdued, the dysentery is also cured." *Suśruta* VI. 40. 90[114].

Rectal irrigation with soothing oil or sterilizing medical solution or their combined emulsion is certainly one of the best means known to combat pernicious, ulcerated and resistant diarrhœa and is very effectively utilized in advanced modern treatment Enemata serve to dislodge or to prevent fecal impaction where ulcers have healed and a stenosis has formed in the lower bowel, and for evacuating gas, putrefying matter, toxic discharges and other irritants within the rectum. An enema is generally given in constipation. And in an enema the fluid administered has to be limited to two to three quarts or it might cause distension, pain, ptosis

---

114. महारुजे मूत्रकृच्छ्रे भिषग्वस्तिं प्रदापयेत् ।
पयोमधुघृतोन्मिश्रं मधुकोत्पलसाधितम् ॥
स वस्तिः शमयेत् तस्य रक्तं दाहमथो ज्वरम् ।
मधुरौषधसिद्धश्च हितं तस्यानुवासनम् ।
रात्रावहनि वा नित्यं रुजार्तो यो भवेन्नरः ॥ ९०
यथा यथा सतैलः स्यादातशान्ति तथा तथा ।
प्रशान्ते मारुते वापि शान्तिं याति प्रवाहिका ॥
सुश्रुतसंहिता, उत्तरतन्त्रम्, ४० ॥

or paresis of the intestine and in severe cases even the rupture of its membrane. While in irrigation, there is no limit to the quantity of fluid, for the solution is allowed to flow into and out of the gut through a double or return-flow tube (*irrigator*) or by making the fluid flow into the bowel by way of an artificial opening (*appendiceal or cecal*) and making it flow out at the anus through a proctoscope or a pipe introduced for the purpose, thus escaping as fast as the solution enters into the bowel. Therefore irrigation serves by the soothing and antiseptic properties of its content to heal the local ulcerated lesions, prevent the formation of impacted fecal masses, to wash out the sores and to neutralize the toxins, to remove toxins, irritating pus, blood, mucus, tissue debris and feces, to dislodge and wash away parasites, and to relieve enterospasm, colics and tenesmus. By *vasti* is meant to include the functions of an enema and irrigator according to the needs.

Improvement invariably follows *daily irrigation* of the intestine. But it is not so much due to the medicaments as to the dissolvent and cleansing quality of water and washing away the toxins, so that the organism does not suffer so much from their absorption. Undoubtedly antiseptic, deodorant, soothing and stimulating medicaments exert beneficial influence, especially in inflammatory, ulcerative and obstructive lesions of the intestine, but they are only of secondary value. The only thing that is important is to irrigate the intestine as often as possible with body temperature of the solution. Positive good result is obtained by daily irrigation with warm saline solution, camomile, flax-seed, oak-bark tea, pinas canadensis (1 p. c.), borolyptol, potassium permanganate, glyco-thymolin or listerin (3 p. c.), salicylic acid, alum, zinc sulphate or silver nitrate (1 p. c.), boric acid or Carlsbad salt (2 p. c.) or thymol (1 : 2000). In advanced cases of deep-seated ulceration and erosions, it is better to use the above solutions a little stronger or ichthyol or balsam of Peru (2 to 5 p. c.), salicylate of soda (3 to 5 p. c.) and bisulphate of quinine (1 :1000) especially in entamebic and bacillary dysentery. Oils named according to the degree of their proven usefulness, olive, sesame, sweet almond, cotton seed, liquid vaselin and neutralol, either alone or in emulsion with the above-mentioned medicaments, can be used with marked result.

Propyhlaxis : As water seems to be the principal source of infection of cholera asiatica, typhoids and dysentery, and in water spirillum cholera asiatica, bacillus typhosus and pathogenic agents of dysentery (*entameba dysenteria, bacillus dysenteria, bälantidium coli*) can all live and thrive for a long time, it is essential that all drinking water must be thoroughly boiled and filtered. Milk also must be boiled before it is drunk, as it is often contaminated by water from suspicious sources. All dejecta from the victim of any of these diseases must be dis-infected with a five per cent solution of carbolic acid, one per cent of chloride of lime or one-fortieth per cent of corrosive sublimate, so that all the pathogenic microbes be destroyed and they can not enter into the soil, especially if it be saturated with moisture where they can multiply, and retain their vitality and virulence for years. This also applies to urine and sputum. Nor should any vegetable or fruit be eaten raw or not thoroughly cooked which might have grown on the soil or fallen upon it, where there is the least possibility that the soil has been fertilized by human feces. And all coarse vegetables and unripe fruits which might leave a good deal of irritant residue, should be avoided. It is true that these germs have been found living in harmless, inert vegetative state without provoking any lesion in the gastro-intestinal tract where they have been harboured, and the predisposing cause of their development is the malnutrition, fatigue, over-work and exhaustion of the organism. Yet it must be admitted that it is very dangerous to sustain such potential enemies.

In the treatment of *typhoid and choleraic diarrhœa*, there are two fundamentally opposed theories. One is the destruction and removal of the vibrios and to neutralize the toxins by a powerful antiseptic purgative like calomel (3 to 5 grains with 6 to 12 grains of sodium bicarbonate) and after this initial dose to administer small doses (one-tenth to one-twentieth grain), every half or quarter hour until the symptoms improve or the patient passes into algide stage. Some strongly recommend the administration of castor oil (half an ounce emulsified with chloroform) before giving calomel. And to inject saline solution (1. 25 per cent solution of salt, prepared by dissolving 2 drachms of salt in one pint of water) at blood temperature, ten to fifteen ounces every half an hour to counteract the circulatory disturbance through the evacuations.

The other theory is to spare the vitality of

the patient which is seriously dissipated by repeated evacuations, and for this purpose a strong astringent like tannic acid (*kino, catechu, rhatania* are to be preferred to pure tannic acid) should be introduced into the rectum one to two litters daily in one per cent solution at a little above the body temperature. This seems to have shown good result. And if there are evidences of toxic accumulation and fecal retention, calomel is to be given every two hours in doses of 0.03 to 0.05 gram. The patient must be confined to bed. The body should be kept warm by fomentation. To quench thirst, sterilized water should be given, preferably acidulated with the juice of pomegranate, but any other fruit juice or milk under no circumstances. During convalescence pigeon, dove or chicken broth with rice, with aromatic but non-irritant spices is to be preferred, but all coarse and irritant food should be avoided.

In *puerperal diarrhœa* (*sutikā*) which is usually caused by the invasion of the blood by the streptococci, staphilococci, united with gonococci, coli bacilli and other micro-organisms through a wound of the uterus at child-birth or in miscarriage by careless, septic handling and spreading of the germs, treatment should be more or less confined to increase the resisting power, bacteriolytic and agglutinative functions of the blood by dietary and hygienic regulations. The . symptom-complex of septicemia (*sutikā*) commences usually within a week after infection. At the onset there is chilliness with low and moderate fever, but which rises and tends to become of continued type with decided daily remission. If however pyogenic germs have also got admission into the blood, the fever sets in with rigor, there is high temperature with steep curve and daily remission with sweating like malarial remittent fever. However, the fever runs an irregular course. But it may be complicated by previous or post malarial infection. As compared with septicemia, pyemia exhibits recurring chills, deeply remitting fever and sweats, rapid wasting and moderate icterus ; while in septicemia the chilliness is only felt at the onset of the fever which runs a mild continuous type with no sweats and jaundice is much lighter. Headache, marked anorexia, nausea and diarrhœa are the usual symptoms of septicemia (*sutikā*). The pulse is rapid, small and compressible. The spleen may be palpably swollen ; petechial spots are not uncommon ; rashes or herps might also appear. Slight toxemic jaundice is also usually seen. The urine usually contains albumin, leucocytes, red-cells and tube casts. The leucocytes are increased and there is an immense destruction of the red-corpuscles of the blood, leading often to hemoglobinemia and hemoglobinuria. Loss of appetite is very pronounced and there is no desire to partake of any kind of food and there is a special disgust to meat. The stool is emptied with severe tenesmus and consists of mucus mixed with blood. Often the joints become painful and swollen, and the skin of those parts reddish. Respiration is rapid but there is no dyspnea. But there may be complications of bronchitis or pneumonia.

Prognosis is not very favorable except in cases where within 6 to 8 weeks the temperature, respiration and pulse slowly tend to be normal. The treatment should chiefly consist ef hygiene and dietary. The patient must be confined to bed. All movements should be restricted as much as possible, as movement tends to spread the infection. Even after convalescence has set in, the patient shall remain in bed, at least for four weeks and all physical motion and mental excitement should be forbidden. However it is very desirable that the room is airy, bright and cheerful, so that there is no oppressive dullness and monotony. Food should be varied, easily digestible, appetizing and nutritious. However, all irritating spices must be avoided though aromatic and sweet-smelling substances can be added with advantage, with only exception to old wine which is very well tolerated in '*sutikā*'. Meat broth of pigeon, dove, chicken, tender goat or lamb (from lamb, fat should be taken out) is very useful in fighting this tragic malady which pitilessly transforms the long-dreamt happy motherhood into painful suffering and sad struggle for life. Lean, light fish can be given in any appetizing way, but fatty and heavy fish should be avoided.

Antistreptococcic serum which is calculated to destroy the bacteria either by producing agglutins or phagocytosis can be injected three times daily with promising result unless there is pyomia, in which case it is apt to do positive harm according to Menzer whose serum has good reputation for its efficacy. The inunction of unguentum is claimed by Crede to be beneficial. But none of these preparations have given completely satisfactory results. They are more or less empirical. The antipyretics are recommended by some.

But as fever is the expression of the bodily

reaction against the toxic products of the invading micro-organisms, suppression of fever is apt to do rather more harm than good unless absolutely necessary to reduce the temperature and relieve certain nervous symptoms. Moreover all the antipyretics—antipyrin, phenacetin, acetanilid, malakin, kryofene, lactophenin and others are all coal-tar products. And the use of these drugs is followed by depression and sometimes serious collapse. Therefore its repeated use in continued and prolonged fever might endanger the life of the patient by heart failure which is seriously damaged by this disease, though the temperature of fever is thereby reduced. Quinine of course in non-malarial septicemia, is hardly of any value. Only it is very useful when *'sutikā'* is complicated by malarial infection.

Prophylaxis in *'sutikā'* is the absolute aseptic handling at every child-birth, for otherwise with least wound or abrasion of the female genital organs which is inevitable, circulatory system may be invaded by pathogenic micro-organisms through lymph channel or veins. All the instruments must be thoroughly sterilized, and sterilized glove should be used. Genital organ also should be carefully examined before delivery for any infectious disease, especially gonorrhea. In case of gonorrhea all precautions must be taken and the baby's eyes should be washed with one to two per cent silver-nitrate solution, or better still—Argyrol in 1-50 to 1-20 solution to prevent the affection of the eyes with its virus (*ophthalmia neonatorum*).

III-Diabetes.

"The causes, lesions and the organs that are affected which provoke temporary (alimentary) diabetes are as follows : too often an excessive consumption of various kinds of new cereals, bean-broths (of new *pisum sativum* and *phaseolus roxburghi*) seasoned with clarified butter, meat of animals and amphibious creatures, vegetable-leaves, sesame-seeds, rice or wheat cakes, rice-pudding, rice and lentil curry, puff-corn, sugar-cane-juice, milk, fermenting milk, fluid-food, sweet-meats and the intemperate eating of other products which are phlegmatic (reduces metabolism), fattening and diuretic—they are etiologic factors of diabetes (that is, the excessive consumption of carbohydrates in various forms above the assimilative power of the organism). Excessive liquid phlegma is the pathological production and abnormal accumulation of fat, flesh, perspiration, (production of) semen, blood, marrow, lymph, chyle and lecithin (*oja*) are the predisposing causes (become affected)" *Charaka II. 4.* 3[115].

There are *various kinds of diabetes*: "The urine is whitish, painless (micturition) and aquatic in '*udaka-meha*' [*diabetes insipidus*, in which the quantity of urine is enormously increased (10 to 30 pints), it is light-pale in color and the specific gravity is low (1.002 to 1.007); the total urea output is slightly increased, but it does not contain albumin, sugar or casts; only inosite (muscle-sugar) is met with on rare occasions. Except excessive thirst and loss of fluid, the patient otherwise might be in apparent good health. This disease is supposed to be of nervous origin]; the urine is (sweetish) like the

---

115. तत्रेमे त्रयो निदानादिविशेषाः श्लेष्मनिमित्तानां प्रमेहाणामाश्वभिनिर्वृत्तिकरा भवन्ति, तद् यथा हायनकयवकचीनकोद्दालकनैषधेत्कटमुकुन्दक-महाव्रीहि-प्रमोदकसुगन्धकानां नवान्नानामतिवेलमतिप्रमाणेन चोपयोगः, तथा सर्पिष्मतां नवहरेणु-माषसूप्यानां ग्राम्यानूपौदकानाञ्च मांसानां शाकतिलपललपिष्टान्नपायसकृशरविलेपीक्षु-विकाराणां क्षीरमन्दकदधिद्रवमधुरतरुणप्रायाणामुपप्रयोगः, मृजाव्यायामवर्ज्जनं, स्वप्न-शयनासनप्रसङ्गो यः कश्चिद्विधिरन्योऽपि श्लेष्ममेदोमूत्रजननः स सर्वो निदानविशेषः। बहुद्रवः श्लेष्मा दोषविशेषो, बहुबद्धं मेदो मांसं शरीरजक्लेदः शुक्रम् शोणितं वसा मज्जा लसीका रसश्चौज इति संख्याता दूष्यविशेषाः।

चरकसंहिता, निदानस्थानम, ४

sugar-cane juice in '*ikṣu-meha*' (*diabetes mellitus* or glycosuria in which the urine contains one to ten per cent of glycose, is pale, acid and has a sweetish odor ; the quantity of urine is greatly increased (5 to 20 pints) and is usually of high specific gravity (1.030 to 1.045) ; urea is increased and in advanced stage of the disease acetone, diacetic and B-oxybutyric acid may be present. This disease is due to the lesion of the pancreas which seems to control the carbohybrate metabolism) ; the urine is like spirituous liquor in '*surā-meha*' [*acetonuria* in which a large amount of acetone is excreted with the urine, indicating incomplete oxidation of albumines and fats, especially in absence of carbohydrate which is needed for their complete combustion. Acetonuria is met with in inanition, typhoid fever, pneumonia, acute miliary tuberculosis, acute rheumatic fever, cancerous cachexia, intestinal auto-intoxication, septicemia and in diabetes, especially when sugar is completely withdrawn from diet for some time or sugar metabolism is disturbed. Acetone is a colorless mobile liquid of pleasant odor, produced commercially by the destructive distillation of acetates (whence the name '*pyroacetic spirit*'), and of sugar, cellulose and various organic compounds.

Acetone is the simplest representative of the aliphatic ketones and is known as '*demethyl-ketone*'. It has some anesthetic quality and smells as ether. Pure alcohol when ingested in excess or under certain pathological condition of the alimentary canal passes with the urine (A. Ronchese : *L'analyse des urins*, p. 306) ; urination is painful and the urine contains sand-like minute but hard and angular crystals (uric acid sands) in '*sikatā-meha*' (*gravel*—very small concretions, usually of uric acid, calcium oxalate or phosphates, are formed in the kidney and pass through ureter with the urine) ; repeated micturition of phlegmatic (colorless, jellylike) and viscous substance in *śanairmeha*' [*fibrinuria* in which a colorless sticky sediment (*coagulum*), or if much febrin is present, the conversion of the urine into a jellylike mass upon standing takes place. It is due to the presence of fibrinogen and a ferment capable of forming fibrin. It occurs in cases where the plasma of the blood enters some portion of the urinary tract, as in chyluria, croupous inflammation of the tract, villous growths in the bladder] ; the urine is clear and saline in '*lavaṇameha*' (*chlorides* are normally present in the urine and are daily excreted from 8 to 10 grams ; but a persistent increase of 15 to 30 grams occurs in the prodromal stage of general paresis and diabetes insipidus, during convalescence from lobar pneumonia and post convulsive stage of epilepsy) ; there is horripilation (peripheral contraction) and the urine is whitish like thick rice-paste water (*albuminuria* occurs in acute nephritis, chronic parenchymatous nephritis and urethritis) ; the discharge is turbid and thick in '*sāndra-meha*' (*gleet* in chronic urethritis causes a thin whitish discharge, but becomes, also, thick and yellowish under various causes. The origin of the discharge is the numerous mucous follicles, lining that portion of the urethra corresponding to the site of the chronic inflammation. When congested, granular or abraded patches exist, there is a constant hyper-secretion of mucus or muco-pus with exfoliation of the epithelium upon the surface of the lesion. In this condition the current of urine, as it passes over the diseased portion of the canal, rolls up into strings or threads the desquamated epithelium and muco-purulent deposit upon the surface and this appears in the urine as the delicate thready filament which is a familiar occurrence in chronic gonorrhea) ; the discharge is like the semen in '*śukra-meha*' (*spermatorrhea* is indicative of self-abuse, excessive coitus, sexual neurasthenia as cause or consequence, and prodrome of locomotor ataxia. Sedentary habits, an habitually loaded rectum, ascarides, and the too free use of condiments and liquors may be responsible for the slighter degree of the symptom. In a continent individual involuntary emissions during sleep, if occurring at intervals of 2 to 6 weeks, are quite normal. But if it be much more frequent and if the emissions occur without erection, unconsciously to the patient, in the day time or while straining at stool, their pathological character is marked. Spermatozoa are found in the first urine passed after emission in men. They occur also in some cases of injury or disease of the spinal cord. Occasionally a small amount of semen is expressed from the vesiculae seminales by the pressure of hard fecal masses, during severe expulsive efforts accompanying obstinate constipation. The persistent presence of spermatozoa in the urine is symptomatic of spermatorrhea) ; scanty foamy urine in '*phenameha*' (in renal congestion, the urine is scanty, acid, of high specific gravity and usually cloudy with urates).

The urine is frothy, transparent and bluish (*indicanuria* in which indican is found in large quantity. When albuminous substances undergo bacterial putrefaction in the intestine, or are rapidly decomposing in any part of the body, as in the putrid pus of septic peritonitis, or in empyema, indol is formed. When the indol is absorbed, it is oxidized, forming indoxyl, and the latter combines with the preformed potassium sulphate to become the conjugate potassium indoxyl-sulphate, or as it is more commonly termed '*indican*'. If indican which is itself colorless comes in contact with acids or oxidizing agents, it is decomposed with the formation of indigo blue. An excessive formation of indican is indicative of abnormal intestinal putrefaction. As a rule, it is usually associated with hypochloro-hydria, as hydrochloric acid exerts restraining influence on proteolytic bacteria. An excess of indican is found in gastric cancer and peritonitis) ; the micturition is painful and the urine has the color of turmeric (curcuma has yellowish-brown color) in '*haridrā-meha*' (*choluria* in which the urine is yellowish-brown or greenish-yellow due to the presence of bilirubin in the urine. It occurs in many diseases in which an excessive quantity of bile is excreted as bilious remittent fever and part of it appears unchanged in the urine); sour odor and sourish taste in '*amla-*

meha' (*oxaluria* in which there is a persistent excretion of oxalates. Normally oxalic acid is excreted daily from 0. 010 to 0. 020 gram (one-sixth to one-third grain), but exists in combination as calcium oxalate, and is held in solution by the acid sodium phosphate of the urine, and when the latter is deficient, the oxalates are precipitated. Oxalic acid is increased by certain foods, as cabbage, rhubarb, tomato, and to a lesser extent by asparagus, spinach, carrots, string beans and celery. Oxalic acid may also result from oxidation of uric acid or an incomplete oxidation of carbohydrates, in which case the intermediate product is oxaluric acid. A persistent increase in the excretion of oxalates is usually associated with the disorders of the gastro-intestinal tract or neurasthenia); the urine is like pressed alkaline water from (laundry) cloth, in smell, color, taste and touch in '*kṣāra-meha*' (*phosphaturia* in which a considerable amount of earthy phosphates mixed with fixed alkali is excreted with the urine. It is found in dyspepsia and neurasthenia. Occasionally the fixed alkali and the earthly phosphates deposit their sediments in the bladder, and the few whitish drops passed at the end of urination like semen, may be their symptomic expression. The urine is decidedly alkaline. Normally phosphoric acid is daily excreted from 2 to 3 grams (30 to 45 grains) in combination as alkaline and earthly phosphates, the alkaline salts predominating. It is derived from the food and partly from the decomposition of lecithin and nuclein. The excretion is greatly increased in leucemia, pernicious anemia, nervous dyspepsia and considerably diminished in intermittent malaria, pulmonary tuberculosis with high temperature, typhoid, nephritis, chronic rheumatism and yellow atrophy of the liver) ; the urine is like the water of Indian madder (*mañjiṣṭhā =rubia munjista*, which has bright red color in '*mañjiṣṭhā-meha*' (*hemoglobinuria* in which the urine contains the blood-coloring matter '*hemoglobin*' and its oxidation product '*methemoglobin*'. Hemoglobinuria occurs in cases where there is such an extensive destruction of the erythrocytes that it exceeds the power of the hepatic activity to transform the whole of the liberated hemoglobin into bilirubin, and the excess escapes by way of the kidney with the urine. It is found in pernicious bilious remittent malarial fever, especially after excessive doses of quinine, syphilis, yellow fever and severe form of jaundice) ; and the urine is like the blood in '*sonita-meha*' (*hematuria* in which the red-corpuscles of the blood appear in the urine. It occurs in cases where there is an acute congestion of the kidney and the number of erythrocytes indicates the severity of the lesion. Bloody urine may be voided in leucemia, hemophilia, purpura, and in renal cancer, tuberculosis, abscess and lithiasis).

The discharge is like clarified butter in '*sarpi-meha*' (*pyuria* in which the pus appears in the urine. It may be due to different causes, but often it is associated with the gonorrheal urethritis. The urine containing the pus from any renal lesion is usually acid and from the bladder alkaline); the urine is fatty in '*vasā-meha*' (*lipuria* in which the fat is present in the urine in such quantities as to enable its identification by the unaided eye. The fat may appear in the urine due to the ingestion of excessive amounts of fat (fat meat, or in cases of fracture involving the bone marrow and causing fat embolism, in long-continued suppurative processes, in the lipemia of diabetes mellitus, from the fatty degeneratiou of the renal epithelium in chronic nephritis, of pus cells, in pyonephrosis or neoplasm along the urinary tract, or in the fatty degeneration in phosphorus poisoning. If the urine is so crowded with minute fat globules as to present a milky appearance to the naked eye, it is called '*chyluria*' or '*galacturia*'. Chyluria is usually due to parasitic origin, especially due to the presence of 'filaria, sanguinis hominis'); the urine is in taste and color like honey-sugar (*kṣaudra* = fruit-sugar, that is levulose) in *kśaudra-meha*' (*levulosuria* in which levulose appears in the urine. It seems that the pancreas does not regulate the metabolism of levulose, for when there is intolerance for dextrose as in glycosuria, a good deal of fruit sugar can be assimilated. Probably the liver synthetizes the fruit sugar and in the severe hepatic lesion or in the presence of toxins in the blood which causes irritation to the muscles, which possess a considerable power to utilize sugars, levulose is abnormally excreted with the urine, though its permeability through the kidney is nearly four times less than that of maltose); the urine flows like that of a mad elephant in '*hasti meha*' (*polyuria* or the diabetes insipidus in which 10 to 20 quarts of pale urine is discharged daily). *Suśruta* II. 6. 10[116].

---

116. तत्र श्वेतमवेदनमुदकसदृशमुदकमेही मेहति ; इक्षुरसतुल्यमिक्षुमेही, सुरामेही सुरातुल्यं, सरुजं सिकतानुविद्धं सिकतामेही, शनैः सकफं सतन्तुं शनैर्मेही, विशदं लवणतुल्यं लवणमेही, हृष्टरोमा पिष्टरसतुल्यं पिष्टमेही, आविलं सान्द्रं सान्द्रमेही, शुक्रतुल्यं शुक्रमेही, स्तोकं स्तोकं सफेनं फेनमेही मेहति ॥१०

"Any one who repeatedly urinates ink-colored (blackish) warm urine, suffers from '*kāla-meha*' (*alkaptonuria* in which the urine darkens on standing, due to the presence of alkapton (glycosuric acid) or related oxyacids, or melanin from melanotic cancer; or in hemoglobinuria as in pernicious remittent bilious fever, due to the destruction of large amounts of erythrocytes, the blood-pigment may undergo change and appear in the urine as brownish-black or blackish, and for this reason the fever is called '*black-water-fever*')." Charaka II. 4. 17.[117].

Prognosis: "If one has acquired diabetes mellitus (*madhu-meha*) by hereditary transmission, he is incurable. It is not only hereditary glycosuria that is incurable, but all hereditary

---

अत ऊर्द्ध' पित्तनिमित्तान् वक्ष्यामः। सफेनमच्छं नील' नीलमेही मेहति ; सदाहं हरिद्राभं हरिद्रामेही, अम्लरसगन्धमम्लमेही, स्तुतक्षारप्रतिम' क्षारमेही, मञ्जिष्ठोदकप्रकाशं मञ्जिष्ठामेही, शोणितप्रकाशं शोणितमेही मेहति ॥११

अत ऊर्द्ध' वातनिमित्तान् वक्ष्यामः। सर्पिःप्रकाशं सर्पिर्म्मेही मेहति ; वसाप्रकाशं वसामेही, क्षौद्ररसवर्ण क्षौद्रमेही, मत्तमातङ्गवदनुप्रबद्ध' हस्तिमेही मेहति ॥१२

सुश्रुतसंहिता, निदानस्थानम्, ६।

117. मसीवर्णमजस्रं यो मूत्रमुष्णं प्रमेहति।
पित्तस्य परिकोपेण तं विद्यात् कालमेहिनम्॥

चरकसंहिता, निदानस्थान, ४।

predispositions are hard to remedy." *Charaka* VI. 6. 41[118].

"As birds easily take shelter in low trees, so glycosuria rapidly attacks those who are addicted to gluttony, but averse to bathing and walking (physical exercise and exertion). Glycosuria proves fatal for one who lacks energy, is very fleshy, fat and extremely corpulent. He who eats only to cover his metabolic needs, recovers his health." *Charaka* II. 4. 32. [119].

"If the diabetes lasts for a long time, then there are complications of polydipsia, fever, diarrhœa, hyperaemia, weakness, anorexia, indigestion and putrefying boils, abscesses and gangrenes." *Charaka* II. 4. 30[120].

---

118. जातप्रमेही मधुमेहिनो वा
न साध्य उक्तः स हि बीजदोषात्।
ये चापि केचित् कुलजा विकारा
भवन्ति तांश्च प्रवदन्त्यसाध्यान् ॥ चरकसंहिता, चिकित्सास्थानम्, ६, ४१।

119. गृध्नमभ्यवहार्येषु स्नाने चंक्रमणद्विषम्।
प्रमेहः क्षिप्रमभ्येति नीडद्रुममिवाण्डजः ॥
मन्दोत्साहमतिस्थूलमतिस्निग्धं महाशनम।
मृत्युः प्रमेहरूपेण क्षिप्रमादाय गच्छति ॥
यस्त्वाहारं शरीरस्य धातुसाम्यकरं नरः।
सेवते विविधाश्चान्याश्चेष्टाः स सुखमश्नुते ॥
चरकसंहिता, निदानस्थानम्, ४।

120. उपद्रवास्तु खलु प्रमेहिनां तृष्णाज्वरातिसारदाहदौर्बल्यारोचकाविपाकाः, पूतिमांसपिड़कालजीविद्रध्यादयश्च तत्प्रसङ्गाद् भवन्ति।
चरकसंहिता, निदानस्थानम्, ४।

"If a diabetic has boils then an expert surgeon shall treat him by cleaning and restoring (*cicatrizing*) them by his instruments. *Charaka* VI. 6. 42[121].

Prophylaxis: In diabetes mellitus, it is necessary to know whether the disease is acquired or inherited. In lesions affecting the pons medulla, cerebellum, liver, thyroid and especially the pancreas, diabetes may be provoked. But in other diseases which do not seriously damage the pancreas, as in syphilis, acute infection, traumatic and surgical neurasthenia, physical and mental excesses, there usually exists a predisposing cause. The predisposing cause consists of metabolic deficiency of assimilating carbohydrates. It might lie in some inherent weakness of the hepatic and principally the pancreatic cells or that of the organism to burn the carbohydrates or that of the nervous mechanism controlling the process. Susruta did not fail to distinguish them. He says :

121. प्रमेहिणां याः पिडका मयोक्ताः
रोगाधिकारे पृथगेव सप्त।
ताः शल्यविद्भिः कुशलैश्चिकित्स्याः
शस्त्रेण संशोधनरोपणैश्च॥

चरकसंहिता, चिकित्सास्थानम्, ६, ४२।

"Diabetes is either inherited or acquired (alimentary). Inherited diabetes is due to improper dietary. The hereditary diabetic is very lean, dry (skin), has weak appetite (*anorexia*), polydipsia and is very nervous ; the alimentary diabetic is fleshy, has voracious appetite (*bulimia*), adiposis and is addicted to sedentary habits (fond of bed, seat and sleep. The lean diabetic should be treated by dietetic regulation, and the fat diabetic by '*apa tarpaṇa*' (exercise and fasting). *Suśruta* IV. 11. 2[122].

Prophylaxis should begin with children, especially when children of hereditarily predisposed parents are found with tendencies to neurosis, gout or obesity, and they should not intermarry with families of the same diathesis, nor over-indulge in sugars or excess of carbohydrates. Adults with hereditary tendencies should avoid taking sugar and should not exceed in the carbohydrate diet beyond the physiologic

---

122. द्वौ प्रमेहौ सहजोऽपथ्यनिमित्तश्च भवतः। तत्र सहजो मातृपितृबीजदोषकृतः। अहिताहारजोऽपथ्यनिमित्तः। तयोः पूर्व्वेणोपद्रुतः कृशो रूक्षोऽल्पाशी पिपासुर्भृशं परिसरणशीलश्च भवति। उत्तरेण स्थूलो बह्वाशी स्निग्धः शय्यासनस्वप्नशीलः प्रायेणेति। तत्र कृशमन्नपानप्रतिसंस्कृताभिः क्रियाभिश्चिकित्सेत्, स्थूलमपतर्पणयुक्ताभिः ॥२

सुश्रुतसंहिता चिकित्सितस्थानम्, ११।

and metabolic needs. Rather it would be wise to partly replace the carbohydrates with fat and protein. Tendency to obesity should be combatted by regular exercise and frugal diet. When obesity has developed, it should be reduced by a slow process of moderate daily outdoor exercise and a slight undernutrition, especially in carbohydrates and fat.

Treatment : Glycosuria can be successfully fought only by rational dietary. It is a safe policy in the beginning of the treatment to eliminate all carbohydrates from the diet. It may be said against this, that the excretion of sugar in the urine is but a symptom of the lesion, and the elimination of the sugar can not remedy the cause of the lesion, and moreover even in a sugar-free diet, sugar is synthetically prepared and excreted out of the protein and fat molecules. This may be all true, but the clinical experience shows that in a sugar-free diet, the patient soon develops carbohydrate tolerance. And the presence of an excessive quantity of sugar in the circulation and tissues which can not be metabolized, causes various pathological changes and manifestations. Von Noorden finds the use of oatmeal gruel once a week proves very beneficial. But on the oatmeal day he forbids the use of any protein, even not egg or milk. Only a little butter is permitted. And the day before the oatmeal diet, he gives only vegetables and fat. Levine finds that potato is just as efficacious as the oatmeal. Fruits containing minimum of glucose like the lemon and orange can be given, as there is certain tolerance for levulose. The alternating constipation and diarrhœa which is symptomatic of diabetes due to gastro-intestinal disorders, should be remedied by laxative and constipative food according to the needs. Strong purgatives should be avoided. If this is not sufficient, in constipation Carlsbad or Epsom salts can be given and in diarrhœa irrigation should be applied. Special attention should be given to the cleanliness of the skin as many skin lesions are apt to take place in glycosuria. Mild antiseptic neutral soaps, containing tar, boric acid or eucalyptus have proved beneficial. When an infective process has already begun, great care should be taken that the surrounding tissues or other parts do not become infected and for local use, iodoform, iodol or aristol can be used with advantage.

Diabetes insipidus : The pathology of this disease is not yet well understood. It occurs in cases where there is lesion in the pons, medulla or the cerebellum. It may be caused by many diseases, but syphilis is the principal cause. And in that case its principal remedy is antisyphilic treatment.

IV.—Diseases of the Bladder.

"There are twelve kinds of lesions of the bladder as follows:—annular swelling (*vāta-kuṇḍalikā=pericystis*), hard globular tumor (*mūtrasṭhīlā=myoma*), swelling of the mouth of the bladder (*vātavasti=prostatic hypertrophy*), difficult and scanty repeated urination (*mūtrātīta =vesical tenesmus*), abdominal bladder (*mūtra-jaṭhara*=over-distension and *hypertrophy of the bladder* with contraction and obstruction of the cavity), obstruction to the passage of urine (*mūtrotsaṅga=urethritis*), *uremia* (*mūtra-kṣaya*), *fibroma* (*mūtra-granthi*), *spermatorrhea* (*mūtra-śukra*), *cystitis* (*uṣṇa-vāta*) and gangrenous or suppurative *cystitis* (*mūtraukasāda*).

"If the urine is concentrated and is not evacuated (in time), the humor '*vāyu*' becomes vitiated and it circulates at the mouth in circular form (that is causes annular inflammation). This causes much pain and there is repeated painful scanty micturition. This difficult disease is known as '*vāta-kuṇḍalikā* (*pericystitis*, which implies inflammation of the tunica advenitia of the bladder. Inflammation of the bladder (*cystitis*) may be provoked by various causes as follows: (*a*) Cystitis may occur during the course of many acute infectious diseases as acute articular rheumatism, typhoid fever, small-pox, measles, influenza, cholera, diphtheria. This complication may set in during the height of the disease, or may appear during convalescence. Toward its cause, a number of factors probably contribute. The chemical constituents of the urine are often profoundly altered: the urine is concentrated; it contains abnormal substances of disturbed metabolism which are more or less irritant and moreover may contain the pathogenic germs of specific infections. The tissues of the bladder are deprived of proper nutrition and lack their full power of resistance. (b) In constitutional diseases as gout and diabetes in which the urine is irritant. (c) In general septicemia as pyemia or internal suppuration of any organ in which the suppuration foci may be brought to the bladder. (d) From irritating food and drink as excessive consumption of strong and irritant pepper and alcoholic drinks. (e) Infections from the adjacent organs as the kidney and the urethra. The bladder may be affected by the kidney either directly by the urine, or by the lymph channel or by contiguity of the tissues. Urethritis is a common cause of which gonorrhea is an important factor. In acute gonorrhea the passage of gonococci is favored through spincter vesicae in its ascent during vesical congestion under sexual excitement or under the stimulation of alcohol or irritating spicy food. Chronic prostatic hypertrophy is also often a causative factor of the congestion of the base of the bladder. The cystites are of two kinds—simple aseptic and septic. The simple aseptic inflammation may be provoked by the irritating substances in the urine, metabolic or ingested, by the disturbances in the function of micturition or by the disturbances in the circulation incident to vascular or nervous conditions. It is well known that ammonia, oxalates, urates and sugar, if they are concentrated in the urine are active irritants of the bladder. And the primary role of the irritants can be ascribed to the uric acid sands and calculi. They by their mechanical irritation cause congestion and inflammation and if the pathogenic germs are present, ulcerous gangrenes. Disturbances in the functions of the urine cause more or less hyperemia and inflammation. Over-distension of the bladder either voluntary or pathological, the too frequent and too forceful contractions in the act of urination bring about this condition. When the causes of the over-distension, retention and obstruction are organic, septic infection takes place. Various micro-organisms have been found to be related with the suppurative process as the staphylococcus pyogenes aureus, albus and citreus which can decompose urea, streptococcus pyogenes, bacterium coli, proteus vulgaris (which possesses the power of decomposing urea with the production of ammoniacal reaction), gonococcus and tubercle bacillus.

"Unusual frequency of micturition is present in all cases, except in the beginning and in mild cases when the urine remains acid. The causes of frequency are threefold, The reflex influences of an inflammation of the vesical mucous membrane are alone able to provoke frequent urination. In an analogous manner, the irritation of ammoniacal urine and of precipitated salts effects contraction of the organ. In cases of obstruction, the partial retention of the irritant urine powerfully excites the detrusors. Thus the condition of the frequent micturition is usually worse in the contracted bladder of prostatic obstruction. In calculous cystitis, violent movement usually aggravates the condition. Tenesmus is frequently present. In some cases it becomes so exaggerated and remains almost constant, that the patient in order to get relief from the exasperating pain, constantly attempts to urinate, to force a few drops, though the bladder may be almost empty).

"'*Vāyu*' causes in the intermediate region of the lower intestine and the bladder, a hard, immovable and tough tumor. This causes the obstruction of the passage of the feces, urine and intestinal gas. This provokes tympanitis and pain. This (disease) is known as '*vātāṣṭhīlā*' (*myoma* is usually a hard interstitial tumor, producing a globular induration of the bladder wall. It is generally located at the orifice of the bladder, and it has been noted from the size of a cherry up to such dimension as fill half of the cavity. The tumor is divided into lobules by connective tissue ; its main bulk is composed of unstriped muscle-cells, in some places arranged in fasciculi, in others irregularly grouped).

"In any one who retains urine, the '*vāyu*' of the bladder becomes vitiated and closes the mouth of the bladder, and consequently the urine is obstructed. And this vitiated *'vāyu'* remains in the bladder and the prostrate (*kukṣi* = groin) as an oppressor (in intumescence). This disease is very hard to cure and it is called *'vāta-vasti'* (*obstructive hypertrophy of the prostate* which may range in size from an orange to that of a cocoanut. The hypertrophy may be general, affecting the whole organ symmetrically or the enlargement is confined within the capsule of the gland and may extend a considerable distance, pushing the capsule and remain only connected with the prostate by a glandular and fibrous tissue. As the internal spincter may be considered as an integral part of the prostate, hence any alteration of the structure of the latter would be followed by the interference of the function of the former. In addition, as the prostate is limited in front and below by dense fascia, it tends to grow upward and backward as it hypertrophies, elongating and narrowing or deflecting the urethra, according to whether the enlargement is symmetrical or irregular, but always raising the vesical outlet to a higher level than normal. The urine therefore left after each micturition (residual urine) settles at the bottom, causing the formation of calculi by precipitation and sedimentation of the mineral constituents. And an early effect of the prostatic hypertrophy is congestion and later inflammation of that portion of the mucous membrane of the bladder in contact with the tumor. The inflammation spreads in time, aggravated by the sluggish venous return. And as the passage of the urine is reduced, the bladder can only be incompletely evacuated and a small quantity at a time by slow dribbling from the distended bladder. And in this condition, the mucous membrane offers but slight resistance to microbic invasion).

"If for a long time the urine is retained, then when an attempt is made for its evacuation, there is no micturition, or it appears but slightly. If strained, the urine appears with slight pain and in small quantities. This disease is caused by the suppression of the urine, and is called '*mūtrā-tīta*' (*vesical tenesmus*).

"If the urine is suppressed, it causes distension; distension vitiates '*vāyu*' and provokes painful tympanites. This is called '*mūtra-jaṭhara*' and this disease contracts the downward channel (*hypertrophy of the bladder* with contraction of the cavity and obstruction of the passage).

"In the disease in which the flow of the urine is interfered with either at the neck of the urethra or near the glans penis, or under tenesmus bloody urine appears with pain, or without pain it dribbles little by little, this is known as '*mūtrot-saṅga*' (*urethritis*). This disease is caused by a qualified (special) '*vāyu*'.

"In an emaciated and tired body, '*pitta*' and '*vāyu*' absorb the urine. It causes hyperemia and pain. This disease is called '*mūtrakṣaya*' (*uremia*) This is very troublesome. (Uremia occurs in the course of acute or chronic nephritis, puerperal eclampsia, some cases of obstructed renal calculus, and occasionally in patients with pronounced vascular changes. The symptoms are general malaise, nausea, vomiting, insomnia, amaurosis, mania, delirium. dyspnea, increased arterial tension. In complete uremia, the patient lives about 10 to 12 days).

"The tiny, globular and firm tumor that is formed at the interior part of the neck of the bladder, is called '*mūtra--granthi* (*fibroma* generally occurs in the adult and is usually located single upon the base and trigonum. The size is like that of a nut. It may be sessile or prediculated, hard or soft. The surface is lobulated and covered with normal or inflamed mucous membrane, which may or not be firmly attached to the growth. On section the tumor is white and glistening, and there may be patches of myxomatous or areas of calcification). This tumor is painful, nonulcerative and narrows the mouth of the bladder. It resembles pain like that of calculus.

"If any one indulges in sexual intercourse with full bladder, then the semen is displaced and becomes mixed with urine, and pale watery semen appears just before urination or after it. It is called '*mūtra-śukra*' (*prostatorrhea*).

"'*Pitta*' becomes vitiated in heavy exercise, long journey or exposure to the sun, and mixed with the '*vāyu*' brings about the inflammation of the bladder, urethra and the pelivic region (sympathetic) and causes discharge. In this yellowish, slightly reddish (pinkish) or pure reddish urine is excreted with tenesmus. This disease is called by the specialists as '*uṣṇa-vāta*' (in non-suppurative *cystitis*, the urine is pale yellow, or according to the extent of bleeding, the color will vary from the faintest pink to a deep dark-red).

"The disease in which the urine is excreted with burning sensation, is turbid, dark-brownish and concentrated, and if dried (by the sun or evaporated), leaves a residue like powdered granite, is called the bilious '*mūtraukasāda*'.

(*suppurative cystitis*, in which the urine is turbid, containing tenacious flocculi of altered pus and there is a large amount of precipitated salts and detritus. On standing, a heavy sediment forms, but the supernatant urine does not become clear. The crystalline sediment consists of a moderate amount of amorphous phosphates, amorphous ammonium urates and large quantities of triple phosphates. The crystals of ammoniun urate are dark balls which may be spiculated ; the triple phosphate commonly appears in the form of slab-shaped crystals ; there may however, be needles, squares and many forms of irregular crystallization). The disease in which the urine is whitish, concentrated and appears with tenesmus, and when dried, it is pale-colored like the conch-shell powder and is slimy, is to be known as phlegmatic *'mūtraukasāda'* (*cystitis* and tumor of the bladder in which the urine is pale-whitish, opalescent, with a heavy deposit of pus, phosphates and detritus. It is alkaline in reaction. The benign tumors are in themselves quite compatible with long life: in several carefully observed subjects, they existed, ten, twenty or more years. The course of papilloma is largely determined by the hemorrhage and the complications. The malignant tumors are usually fatal within one or two years, particularly of the base or the neck. The fatality of the disease of course depends upon the site affected, the variety of growth present, the clinical course, and complications of cystitis and nephritis. The causes of death are indirect. Rarely profuse hemorrhrge has been the direct cause. In the cachectic debility which follows prolonged hemorrhage, the system becomes vulnerble, and any intercurrent disease may prove fatal). "*Charaka* VI. 58, 2-13[123].

---

123. वातकुण्डलिकाष्ठीला वातवस्तिस्तथैव च ।
मूत्रातीतः सजठरो मूत्रोत्सङ्गः क्षयस्तथा ॥
मूत्रौकसादौ द्वौ चापि रोगा द्वादश कीर्तिताः ॥ ४
रौक्ष्याद्वेगविघाताद्वा वायुर्बस्तौ सवेदनम् ।
मूत्रं संगृह्य चरति विगुणः कुण्डलीकृतः ॥
सृजेदल्पाल्पमथवा सरुजस्कं शनैः शनैः ।
वातकुण्डलिकां तान्तु व्याधिं विद्यात् सुदारुणम् ॥ ३
शकृन्मार्गस्य वस्तेश्च वायुरन्तरमाश्रितः ।
अष्ठीलावद्घनं ग्रन्थिं करोत्यचलमुन्नमम् ॥
विण्मूत्रानिलसङ्गश्च तत्राध्मानश्च जायते ।
वेदना जायते वस्तौ वाताष्ठीलेति तां विदुः ॥ ४
वेगं विधारयेद्यस्तु मूत्रस्याकुशलो नरः ।
निरुणद्धि मुखं तस्य वस्तेर्वस्तिगतोऽनिलः ।
मूत्रसङ्गो भवेत् तेन वस्तिकुक्षिनिपीड़ितः ।
वातवस्तिः स विज्ञेयो व्याधिः कृच्छ्रप्रसादनः ॥ ५

"In these thirteen kinds of urinary troubles use remedial medicines which will relieve strangury. In all these lesions bougie and irrigations are applicable.

The cylinder of the bougie is to be made of

वेगं सन्धार्य्य मूत्रस्य यो भूयः स्रष्टुमिच्छति ।
तस्य नाभ्येति यदि वा कथञ्चित् संप्रवर्त्तते ॥
प्रवाहतो मन्दरुजमल्पमल्पं पुनः पुनः ।
मूत्रातीतन्तु तं विद्यान्मूत्रवेगविघातजम् ॥ ६
मूत्रस्य विहते वेगे तदुदावर्त्तहेतुना ।
अपानः कुपितो वायुरुदरं पूरयेद्भृशम् ।
नाभेरधस्तादाध्मानं जनयेत् तीव्रवेदनम् ।
तं मूत्रजठरं विद्यादधःस्रोतोनिरोधकम् ॥ ७
वस्तौ वाप्यथवा नाले मणौ वा यस्य देहिनः ।
मूत्रं प्रवृत्तं सज्जेत सरक्तं वा प्रवाहतः ।
स्रवेच्छनैरल्पमल्पं सरुजं वाथ नीरुजम् ।
विगुणानिलजो व्याधिर्मूत्रोत्सङ्गः स संज्ञितः ॥ ८
रूक्षस्य क्लान्तदेहस्य वस्तिस्थौ पित्तमारुतौ ।
सदाहवेदनं कृच्छ्रं कुर्य्यातां मूत्रसंक्षयम् ॥ ९
अभ्यन्तरे वस्तिमुखे वृत्तोऽल्पः स्थिर एव च ।
वेदनावाननिष्यन्दी मूत्रमार्गनिरोधनः ।
जायते सहसा यस्य ग्रन्थिरश्मरिलक्षणः
स मूत्रग्रन्थिरित्येवमुच्यते वेदनादिभिः ॥ १०
प्रत्युपस्थितमूत्रस्तु मैथुनं योऽभिनन्दति ।
तस्य मूत्रयुतं रेतः सहसा संप्रवर्त्तते ॥

gold or silver. The aperture of the cylinder made of gold should be like that of the jasmine flower stem, and that of the silver like a mustard seed. It should have the shape like a cow's tail (slightly curved and graduated in dimension), with two rings (so that it can not be pushed farther than is necessary, or it might wound the bladder) and twelve digits long." *Charaka* VIII. 9. 28-29[124].

पुरस्ताद्वापि मूत्रस्य पश्चाद्वापि कदाचन ।
भस्मोदकप्रतीकाशं मूत्रशुक्रं तदुच्यते ॥ ११
व्यायामाध्वातपैः पित्तं वस्तिं प्राप्यानिलावृतम् ।
वस्तिमेढ्रगुदञ्चैव प्रदहन् स्रावयेदधः ॥
मूत्रं हारिद्रमथवा सरक्तं रक्तमेव वा ।
कृच्छ्रात् प्रवर्त्तते जन्तोरुष्णवातं वदन्ति तम् ॥ १२
विशदं पीतकं मूत्रं सदाहं वहलं तथा ।
शुष्कं भवति यच्चापि रोचनाचूर्णसन्निभम् ।
मूत्रौकसादं तं विद्याद्रोगं पित्तकृतं बुधः ॥
शुष्कं भवति यच्चापि शंखचूर्णप्रपाण्डुरम् ।
पिच्छिलं संहतं श्वेतं तथा कृच्छ्रं प्रवर्त्तते ।
मूत्रौकसादं तं विद्यादामयञ्चापरं कफात् ॥ १३

सुश्रुतसंहिता, उत्तरतन्त्रम्, ५८ ।

124. दोषाधिक्यमवेक्ष्यैतान् मूत्रकृच्छ्रहरैर्जयेत् ।
वस्तिमुत्तरवस्तिञ्च सर्व्वेषामेव योजयेत् ॥
पुष्पनेत्रन्तु हैमं स्यात् सूक्ष्ममौत्तरवस्तिकम् ।
जातीपुष्पस्य वृन्तेन समं गोपुच्छसंस्थितम् ॥
रौप्यं वा सर्षपच्छिद्रं द्विकर्णं द्वादशाङ्गुलम् ॥

चरकसंहिता, सिद्धिस्थानम्, ९ ।

The underlying principles in the treatment of acute or chronic cystitis are (a) to render the urine bland and slightly antiseptic ; (b) to put the bladder at rest and to relieve pain ; (c) to lessen pelvic congestion. With healthy kidney and in non-suppurating cystitis of the bladder, the urine may be made bland by drinking a good deal of whey or butter-milk or plenty of pure water. Hot baths, particularly hot sitz-baths are revulsive and counter-irritant. They relieve pain and congestion. To relieve congestion leeches may also be applied to the peritoneum and above the pubis. To make the urine slightly antiseptic, salol can be administered three times a day, in small doses of five grains.

But in chronic cystitis, irrigation is the best curative means known. Irrigation removes mechanically decomposing discharges, diminishes the quantity of pus and mucus, renders the urine bland and unirritating, lessens the severity of the inflammation, lessens further fermentation and decomposition, and exerts a stimulating and healing influence upon the diseased membrane. The main symptoms of cystitis, frequency, urgency, tenesmus and strangury are chiefly dependent upon inflammation located about the vesical neck. Though irrigation can not disinfect the entire diseased and suppurating tissues, this part can be easily reached, and the healing influence of a disinfectant and soothing lotion can be easily exerted on it. This can be accomplished by irrigations, instillations or drainage, or all these combined. For irrigation, a weak, non-irritating, antiseptic solution is preferable as silver nitrate 1: 5000 to 500, potassium permanganate 1 ; 5000 to 2000, carbolic acid 1 : 500, boric acid 1 : 50, normal saline solution 0. 7 per cent. Irrigation is only recommended when the patient urinates easily and empties his bladder completely. But bladder should not be distended to the point of causing pain and spasm. Usually one daily irrigation is sufficient, but in severe cases, it can be repeated. When urination is extremely painful, irrigation can be done by a soft catheter. The catheter is attached to a fountain syringe. The lotion is allowed to flow through, and while it is flowing, the catheter is slowly passed into the bladder. Three to five ounces are injected and the tube leading to the fountain syringe is discontinued, and the injection is allowed to flow out.

Instillations are applied by means of an

instillator, which is a silver or hard rubber cylindrical catheter about 18 Fr. caliber, provided with a fine canal. To the end of the shaft of the catheter is fitted a hypodermic syringe with a capacity for forty minims and is filled with a choice lotion, silver nitrate 1 to 5 per cent in gonorrheal cystitis, iodoform emulsion in tubercular cases with ten per eent glycerine. The catheter is lubricated with glycerin or boroglyceride, and is introduced into the urethra until its tip is within the grasp of the compressor urethrae muscle. The piston of the syringe is then driven down, causing the injection to flow along the membraneous and prostatic urethra into the bladder.

The simplest and the safest form of drainage is that by continuous catheterization. A soft catheter of medium caliber should be selected. Important points to observe are that the eye of the catheter lies just within the bladder and that the instrument thoroughly and continually drains this viscus. To determine the eye of the catheter in relation to the neck of the bladder, the instrument is introduced and the bladder is emptied. Four to six ounces of boric acid solution are then injected, and the catheter is withdrawn until the fluid ceases to flow. It is then passed in until the fluid begins to flow, and is held in this position until the bladder is empty. This continuous catheterization may be kept up from one to three weeks. It usually causes a mild traumatic urethritis. This is treated by withdrawing the catheter slightly at each irrigation until its end lies without the compressor urathræ muscle. By forcing an antiseptic solution into the catheter, it will then flash out the entire anterior urethra. In case of intense pain, suprapubic drainage can be also performed with advantage.

The method adopted by the Charaka School is as follows :—

"The patient after his bath, shall take meat broth or milk. And he shall be seated on a soft, easy and comfortable cushion, after he has evacuated his bladder when there is natural call. Then his penis should be massaged with ointment. After that a sound (*śalākā*) should be introduced for the urethral exploration. If the sound passes without any obstruction, then it should be withdrawn, and the eye of the bougie introduced. All the regulations recommended for anal irrigation (*enema*) are to be observed. If the lotion is allowed to flow at great speed, it causes inflammation of the base, and if it be not sufficient, it does not spread all over the surface, so with a steady hand (not trembling), the bougie is to be introduced and withdrawn." *Charaka* VII. 9.3[125].

Prodrome of lithiasis : "Bladder-irritability, anorexia, strangury, lacerating pain at the neck of the bladder, scrotum and the urethra, fever, lassitude, and the goat-smell of the urine are the prodromes of lithiasis. Moreover, before the calculus formation, the color of the urine becomes unnatural and micturition is painful. The urine is concentrated and cloudy (with urates). The urine becomes corrupt with *'vāyu'* (ammoniacal decomposition).

Symptoms :—With the calculi formation, there are pains in the umbiculus, bladder, scrotum,

---

125. स्नातस्य भुक्तभक्तस्य रसेन पयसापि वा।
सृष्टविण्मूत्रवेगस्य पीठे जानुसमे मृदौ॥
ऋजोः सुखोपविष्टस्य हृष्टे मेढ्रे घृतान्विते।
शलाकयान्विष्य गतिं यद्यप्रतिहता व्रजेत्॥
ततः शेफःप्रमाणेन पुष्पनेत्रं प्रवेशयेत्।
गुदवन्मूत्रमार्गेण प्रणयेदनु सेवनीम्॥
हिंस्याद्व्यतिगतं बस्तिमूने स्नेहो न गच्छति।
सुखं प्रपीड्य निष्कम्पं निष्कर्षेन्नेत्रमेव च॥

चरकसंहिता, सिद्धिस्थानम् ९।

urethra and their adjacent regions at the time of micturition, sudden interference with the flow of the urinal stream (by the spasmodic closing of the voluntary muscles when a small stone is forced into the vesical orifice), bloody urine (the blood is invariably present in the vesical calculus, though the hemorrhage from the bladder is never profuse; the quantity of blood and the degree of pain depends on the nature of ulcerated surface and the contour of the stone), splashing urine, the color of the urine like that of a gem (reddish), clear urine containing sand (uric acid crystals) and pain is much increased by running, jumping, riding and long journeys (violent movements are apt to cause friction of the stone with the vesical surface)." *Suśruta* II. 3. 4-6[126]

---

126. तासां पूर्व्वरूपाणि वस्तिपीड़ारोचकौ मूत्रकृच्छ्रं वस्तिशिरोमुष्कशेफसां वेदना कृच्छ्रा ज्वरावसादौ वस्तगन्धित्वं मूत्रस्येति ॥ ४

यथास्वं वेदनावर्णं दुष्टं सान्द्रमथाविलम्।
पुर्व्वरूपेऽश्मनः कृच्छ्रान्मूत्रं सृजति मानवः ॥ ५

अथ जातासु नाभिवस्तिसेवनीमेहनेष्वन्यतमस्मिन् मेहतो वेदना मूत्रधारासङ्गः सरुधिरमूत्रता मूत्रविकिरणञ्च गोमेदकप्रकाशमनाविलं ससिकतं विसृजति धावनलङ्घनप्लवनपृष्ठयानाध्वगमनैश्चास्य वेदना भवति ॥ ६

सुश्रुतसंहिता, निदानस्थानम्, ३।

"As gallstone is formed in a cow by desiccation of the bile, so calculus is formed. *Calculi* are formed in various shapes like that of the flower of '*nuclea cadamba*' (the oxalate-of-lime calculus is the hardest, often orange-dark in color, more or less spherical in form and studded with nodules, whence it derives its name as mulberry calculus); like stone (finely laminated stones are often found among the vesical calculi, with alternate layers of distinctly crystalline oxalates and urates ; the urates are yellow-reddish in color) ; smooth (pure uric-acid stones are the softest, are yellow, red or brown in color and generally present a smooth surface); like pea (*custin*) or soft (amorphous phosphates). If the calculus is pushed against the vesical orifice, then the passage of urine is obstructed, and it provokes great pain (the stone is grasped and forced against the sensitive neck either by the flow of urine or in violent motion as jolting over a rough road or riding). This exasperates the patient and he makes repeated attempts to urination. There is defecation with tremor. There is lancinating pain in the scrotum, urethra and the bladder, and if the urethra is wounded, the urine comes mixed with blood. But when the calculus is dislodged from the vesical neck, the urine again flows with ease. If the calculus is split into fragments, it passes through the urethra and is called *'śarkarā'* (gravel)." *Charaka* VI. 26. 21[127].

"*Gravel* (*śarkarā*), *sand* (*sikatā*—uric acid brick dust, a fine yellow reddish sediment) and *amorphous phosphates* (*bhasmākhya-meha*) are varieties of lithiasis. The symptoms and pain of gravel resemble that of calculus. If the calculi (concretions) are tiny, they are excreted with the urine, with favorable *'vāyu'*. If the calculus is split up into minute fragments by *'vāyu'*, it is called the gravel. The gravel causes heartache, fatigue of the thighs, pain in the perineum, tremor, polydipsia, nausea, cyanosis, anemia, weakness, anorexia and indigestion, if the gravel be obstructed in the passage through the urethra.

---

127. यदा तदाश्मर्य्युपजायते तु क्रमेन पित्तेष्विव रोचना गोः ॥
कदम्बपुष्पाकृतिरश्मतुल्या श्लक्ष्णा त्रिपुट्यप्यथवापि मृद्वी ।
मूत्रस्य चेन्मार्गमुपैति रुद्ध्वा मूत्रं रुजां तस्य करोति वस्तौ ॥
मृद्नाति मेढ्रं स तु वेदनार्त्तो मुहुः शकृन्मुञ्चति वेपते च ।
ससीवनीमेहनवस्तिशूलं विशीर्णधारञ्च करोति मूत्रम् ॥
क्षोभात् क्षते मूत्रयतीह सास्रं तस्याः सुखं मूत्रयति व्यपायात् ।
एषाश्मरी मारुतभिन्नमूर्त्तिः स्याच्छर्करा मूत्रपथात् क्षरन्ती ॥
चरकसंहिता, चिकित्सास्थानम् २६ ।

"*The bladder* is situated in the midst of umbilicus, back-bone, pubic bones, scrotum, rectum, groin and the urethra. The bladder has only one orifice or outlet (urethra) and its base is downward, its skin (muscular coating) is thin. The bladder is like bottle-gourd (*alābu-lagenaria vulgaris ser*) in shape and is covered with nerves, arteries and veins. The bladder is situated in the pelvis, between the pubic bones in front and the rectum (in woman, the uterus) behind. During the fetal and infantile life, it is usually situated above the pubes. It is a flattened, more or less horizontal body, when empty, but when distended, it becomes an oval bag and rises so as to occupy more or less the hypogastrium. It is attached below, but free to expand above. It is essentially a muscular organ, lined with mucous membrane and covered except in its lower portion with a loosely attached peritoneal coat. Into its lower and posterior portion, the ureters empty, and from its neck the urethra arises. When not over-distended, it holds about a pint of urine—somewhat more in woman than in man. It is a hollow organ, serving as a receptacle for the urine and has a strong muscular investment of unstriped muscles in several layers, which are innervated by branches from the sacral nerves).

The bladder, the bladder-neck, (perhaps including the prostates) urethra, testicles and rectum are all united in one system (genito-urinary) and is situated within the pelvis. The other name of the bladder is the *'receptacle for the excretory product'* (*malādhāra*), and it is a vital organ. As rivers discharge their waters into the ocean, so the tubules in the digestive canal (*the kidneys* are bean-shaped organs, about 4½ inches in length and 2 inches in width and 1½ inches in thickness, lying on either side of the spinal column, behind the peritoneum, about opposite the twelfth thoracic and first three lumbar vertebrae. At the inner edge of each kidney is a concave depression, the *'hylus'*, where the vessels and the nerves enter and leave the organs and where the ureter emerges. The kidney is enclosed in a fibrous envelope, the *'capsule'*, which dips into the sinus at the hylus. The substance of the organ is divided into cortex and medulla. The former is darker colored and more granular in appearance than the latter; it contains the Malphigian corpuscles and most of the convoluted tubules. The medulla is lighter in color and striated and contains the majority of the straight tubules; it is formed of the pyramids whose bases rest in the cortex and whose aspices are the renal papillæ at which point the central collecting tubule opens into a calyx, this in turn emptying into the pelvis of the kidney from which the water with the waste products of metabolism dissolved into it passes into the ureter and thence into the urinary bladder, discharges the urine into the bladder. These tubules are thousands in number and because of their minuteness, they are invisible. Awake or asleep they trickle down by osmosis (*niṣyanda*) and fill up the bladder, as a new earthen pot (porous) is filled up by the surrounding water, if pressed down into it up to its neck." *Suśruta* II. 3. 13-14[128].

"Calculus is hard to cure and is dangerous.

---

128. शर्करा सिकता मेहो भस्माख्योऽश्मरिवैकृतम्।
अश्मर्याः शर्करा ज्ञेया तुल्यव्यञ्जनवेदना॥
पवनेऽनुगुणे सा तु निरेत्यल्पा विशेषतः।
सा भिन्नमूर्त्ति र्वातेन शर्करेत्यभिधीयते॥
हृत्पीड़ा सक्थिसदनं कुक्षिशूलं सवेपथु।
तृष्णोर्द्ध्वगोऽनिलः कार्श्यं दौर्व्वल्यं पाण्डुगात्रता॥
अरोचकाविपाकौ तु शर्करार्त्ते भवन्ति च।
मूत्रमार्गप्रवृत्ता सा सक्ता कुर्य्यादुपद्रवान्॥
दौर्व्वल्यं सदनं कार्श्यं कुक्षिशूलमरोचकम्।
पाण्डुत्वमुष्णवातञ्च तृष्णां हृत्पीड़नं वमिम्॥ १२

When it is young (tender), it may be controllable by medicines, but when it is mature (hard), it has to be extracted by operation.

"In the preliminary stage of lithiasis oleaginous potions are beneficial and remove the cause of its formation. A decoction of Plectranthus scutellaroides, Aeschynomene grandiflora, Pothus officinalis, Oxalis, Asparagus racemosus, Flacourtia cataphracta, Solanum jacquini, Flacourtia sapida, Columba domestica, Solanum melongena, Barleria caerulia, Pentaptera arjuna,

---

नाभिपृष्ठकटीमुष्क-गुदवङ्क्षणशेफसाम् ।
एकद्वारस्तनुत्वक्को मध्ये वस्तिरधोमुखः ॥
अलाव्वा इव रूपेण शिरास्नायुपरिग्रहः ।
वस्तिर्वस्तिशिरश्चैव पौरुषं वृषणौ गुदम् ॥
एकसम्बन्धिनो ह्येते गुदास्थिविवरस्थिताः ।
मूत्राशयो मलाधारः प्राणायतनमुत्तमम् ॥
पक्वाशयगतास्तत्र नाड्यो मूत्रवहास्तु याः ।
तर्पयन्ति सदा मूत्रं सरितः सागरं यथा ॥
सूक्ष्मत्वान्नोपलभ्यन्ते मुखान्यासां सहस्रशः ।
नाड़ीभिरुपनीतस्य मूत्रस्यामाशयान्तरात् ।
जाग्रतः स्वपतश्चैव स निष्यन्देन पूर्य्यते ॥
आ मुखात् सलिले न्यस्तः पार्श्वेभ्यः पूर्य्यते नवः ।
घटो यथा तथा विद्धि वस्तिर्मूत्रेण पूर्य्यते ॥ १४

सुश्रुतसंहिता, निदानस्थानम्, ३ ।

Andropon muricatus, Trapa bisponosa, Hedysarum gangeticum, Bballuca, Capparis trifoliata, Tectonae grandis fructus, Hordeum hexastichon, Dolichos biflorus, Zizyphus jujuba and Strychni potatorum fructus,seasoned with clarified butter, and sprinkled with alkaline earth, if drunk in proper doses, causes fracture of the calculi. And in addition, in this treatment alkalies, barley-water, soup, astringents and milk should be drunk for the amelioration of *'vāta'*. *Suśruta* IV. 7. 3[129].

---

129. अश्मरी दारुणो व्याधिरन्तकप्रतिमो मतः ।
औषधैस्तरुणः साध्यः प्रवृद्धश्छेदमर्हति ॥ २
तस्य पूर्व्वेषु रूपेषु स्नेहादिक्रम इष्यते ॥
तेनास्यापचयं यान्ति व्याधेर्मूलान्यशेषतः ॥
पाषाणभेदो वसुको वशिराश्मन्तकौ तथा ।
शतावरी श्वदंष्ट्रा च वृहती कण्टकारिका ॥
कपोतवङ्काऽऽर्त्तगलः ककुभोशीरकुब्जकः ।
वृक्षादनी भल्लुकश्च वरुणः शाकजं फलम् ॥
यवाः कुलत्थाः कोलानि कतकस्य फलानि च ।
ऊषकादिप्रतीवापमेषां क्वाथैर्घृतं कृतम् ॥
भिनत्ति वातसम्भूतामश्मरीं क्षिप्रमेव तु ।
क्षारान् यवागूर्यूषांश्च कषायाणि पयांसि च ।
भोजनानि च कुर्व्वीत वर्गेऽस्मिन् वातनाशने ॥ ३

सुश्रुतसंहिता, चिकित्सितस्थानम्, ७ ।

Spontaneous fracture of stone has been observed by many in the bladder (*Ord, Debout d' Estrees, Fenwick, Martin,* etc),either by radical cleavage from the centre to the periphery or by splitting in concentric laminae. It has been demonstrated that spheres of carbonate of lime, which had formed in solutions of gum, split radially and disintegrate, if placed in a solution of different specific gravity. It is possible that in a similar way, the urinary calculi split and disintegrate under the influence of varying specific gravities and reactions of the urine, which causes molecular tension and cleavage, and consequently spontaneous cure takes place at some famous springs (as Carlsbad or Contrexeville) which enjoy special reputation for this curative property. Uric acid or oxalate of lime calculi can be formed only in strongly acid urine while in the alkaline urine phosphates of ammonia and magnesia are precipitated. Therefore if in the uric acid or oxalate of lime calculus, the urine can be made and kept alkaline for some time, it is likely to create molecular instability of the calculi and split them into fragments, gravel or brick dust. And vice versa in phoshate calculi, Carbonate of potash, acetate of potash, piperine, common and lithia salts are also reputed to exercise a solvent action upon uric acid crystals in the urine.

"If emulsion, alkalies (carbonate of potash), astringent infusion, milk and bougie do not relieve the calculi, then operation is the only remedy. *Suśruta* IV. 7. 11[130].

"Place the patient upon the lap af a strong man (to hold in position) seated on a knee-high table. The patient with courage and determination stretches his upper part on his back and his pelvis raised by a cushion underneath it ; the legs are to be flexed (to about a right angle with the table) and supported by a man (on each side), or held in position by a cloth crutch. Then the umbilical region should be massaged and pressed with unguents by hands as long as the calculus does not come below the umbilicus. Next after manicuring and lubricating the fingers with oil, the fore and the middle-fingers of the left hand should be introduced in the rectum towards the raphe scroti. When the calculus has been found, it should be carefully forced down between the

130. घृतैः क्षारैः कषायैश्च क्षीरैः सोत्तरबस्तिभिः ।
यदि नोपशमं गच्छेच्छेदस्तत्रोत्तरो विधिः ॥
सुश्रुतसंहिता, चिकित्सितस्थानम्, ७ ।

middle of pubis and the urethra, and placed in an even, medium-sized and polished staff, and pressed so hard that the calculus appears like a tumor.···Incision should be made about third of an inch to the left of the raphe scroti (and an inch and half from the anus) of the size of the calculus. According to some (authorities), if it facilitates the operation, incision can also be made at the right side. But care should be taken that the calculus be not broken (into fragments) by the instruments or pulverized, for if even a minute fragment remains (in the bladder), the calculus grows (round it as nucleus). Therefore for extracting calculi, use forceps with curved blades (serrated and concave in the inner side).

"In woman, the uterus is situated by the bladder, therefore do not make long incision, nor deep incision, as it might wound the sphincters (*mūtra-srāvï*). If the incision is made at the proper place (by distending the bladder upward and forcing the calculus downward), it might also result in the incontinence of urine in man by severing the sphincters (by the lateral perineal incision). Without lithotomy, there cannot be any break in the bladder, but if it does (in rupture by over-distension), the patient dies. If however in the extraction of the calculus, the bladder is penetrated, the patient might survive, for the medicines that are used for the healing of the incision wound, can be also applied for the cicatrization of the other wound. And the penetration of the bladder (sphincters ?) is not in violation of the (medical) code. Moreover, the urine causes the formation of the calculus, and the little incontinence of the urine can not do much harm, and though the barley-water is diuretic, it is found beneficial (in lithiasis). After the extraction of the calculus, the patient should be given hot sitz bath (hip bath), for in hot water, the bladder can not be filled with blood. But if it takes place, the bladder shall be irrigated with astringent effusion of Ficus glomaratæ." *Suśruta* IV. 7. 13-15[131].

"Prostatolith or phosphatic crystals (prosta-

---

131. ततो वलवन्तमविक्लवमाजानुसमे फलके प्रागुपवेश्य पुरुषञ्च तस्योत्सङ्गे निषण्णपूर्व्वकायमुत्तानमुन्नतकटीकं वस्त्रधारकोपविष्टं सङ्कुचितजानुकूर्परमितरेण सहावबद्धं सूत्रेण शाटकैर्वा ततः स्वभ्यक्तनाभिप्रदेशस्य वामपार्श्वं विमृद्य मुष्टिनावपीड़येदधोनाभेर्यावदश्मर्य्यधः प्रपन्नेति। ततः स्नेहाभ्यक्ते कृत्तनखे वामहस्तप्रदेशिनीमध्यमे पायौ प्रणिधायानुसेवनीमासाद्य प्रयत्नबलाभ्यां पायुमेढ्रान्तरमानीय निर्व्यलीकमनायतमविषमञ्च वस्तिं सन्निवेश्य भृशमुत्पीड़येदङ्गुलिभ्यां यथा ग्रन्थिरिवोन्नतं शल्यं भवति।

tic calculi are of two kinds—those formed in the kidney or bladder and lodging in the prostatic sinus, and those which originate in the gland itself), if they are dislodged from their own cavities and are locked up in the passage through the urethra, they should be extracted (by forceps) through the urethral passage. If it can not be done then an incision should be made in the urethra (*median perineal urethrotomy*) and the calculus extracted by hook-forcep. And though the wound is cicatrized for a year, sexual intercourse, riding horses and elephants, tree-

---

स चेद् गृहीतशल्यं तु विवृताक्षो विचेतनः।
हतवक्षश्शीर्षश्च निर्विकारो मृतोपमः॥
न तस्य निर्हरेच्छल्यं निर्हरेत् तु म्रियेत सः।
विना त्वेतेषु रूपेषु निर्हर्त्तुं समुपाचरेत्।

सव्ये पार्श्वे सेवनीं यवमात्रेण मुक्त्वावचारयेत् शस्त्रमश्मरीप्रमाणं ; दक्षिणतो वा क्रियासौकर्य्यहेतोरित्येके। यथा च न भिद्यते चूर्ण्यते वा तथा प्रयतेत, चूर्णमल्पमप्यवस्थितं हि पुनः परिवृद्धिमेति, तस्मात् समस्तामग्रवक्रेणाददीत॥ १३

स्त्रीणान्तु वस्तिपार्श्वगतो गर्भाशयः सन्निकृष्टः, तस्मात्तासामुत्सङ्गवच्छस्त्रं पातयेत अतोऽन्यथा खल्वासां मूत्रस्रावी व्रणो भवेत्। पुरुषस्य वा मूत्रप्रसेकक्षणनान्मूत्रक्षरणम्। अश्मरीव्रणादृते भिन्नो बस्तिरेकधा न भवति, द्विधाभिन्नवस्तिराश्मरिको न सिध्यति॥

अश्मरीव्रणनिमित्तमेकधाभिन्नवस्तिर्जीवति क्रियाभ्यासात् शास्त्रविहितच्छेदान्निःस्यन्दपरिवृद्धत्वाच्च शल्यस्येति। उद्धृतशल्यन्तु क्षीरोदकद्रोण्यामवतार्य्य स्वेदयेत्, तथा हि वस्तिरसृजा न पूर्य्यते। पूर्णे वा क्षीरवृक्षकषायं पुष्पनेत्रेण विदध्यात्॥

सुश्रुतसंहिता, चिकित्सितस्थानम्, ७।

climbing, mountaineering, charioteering and swimming should not be indulged in; heavy indigestible food should also be avoided.

Make incision so that the prostate, vesicula seminalis, vas deferens, ureter, raphe scroti, vagina, rectum or the bladder are not hurt. If the prostates are severed, death takes place by the accumulation of urine in the bladder (the passage for the discharge of the urine into the urethra being blocked by the tumorous or hypertrophic growth of the prostate); by the severance of the vesicula seminalis, death or eunuchism takes place; by the severance of vas deferens, impotence; by the severance of the ureter, dispersion of the urine (to the contiguous tissues by percolation); wound in the raphe scroti causes intense pain; and if the bladder and the rectum are wounded, all the symptoms due to their penetration, mentioned before, appear. *Suśruta* IV. 7. 19-20[132].

Modern lithotomi hardly differs much from that of the Suśruta school, especially when lateral

132. मूत्रवहशुक्रवहमुष्कस्रोतोमूत्रप्रसेकसेवनीयोनिगुदवस्तीन् परिहरेत्। तत्र मूत्रवहच्छेदान्मरणं मूत्रपूर्णवस्तेः शुक्रवहच्छेदान्मरणं क्लैब्यं वा। मुष्कस्रोतउपघाताद्ध्वजभङ्गः। मूत्रप्रसेकक्षणनान्मूत्रप्रक्षरणम्। सेवनीयोनिच्छेदाद्रुजः प्रादुर्भावः। वस्तिगुदविद्धलक्षणं प्रागुक्तमिति॥

incision is made, except that before operation, the bladder is drained off and distended by hot boracic lotion, and kept in that condition during operation by plugging the spigot of the silver catheter by which the injection has been introduced. But generally now-a-days supra-pubic operation is preferred, but below the peritoneum, as higher up serous membrane is met. After the bleeding has stopped, the wound is closed by sutures.

However, litholapaxy seems to be the favorite means adopted for the removal of vesical calculus. And when the urethra is not roomy enough to admit an instrument of adequate calibre, or the stone is very large or hard (oxalate of lime calculus), and if under these circumstances, litholapaxy can not be practised, lithotomy is adopted for the removal of the stone. Lithotrity consists of crushing the stone within the notched and fenestrated inside surface of very hard steel

---

भवतश्चात्र

मर्म्माण्यष्टावसम्बुध्य स्रोतोजानि शरीरिणाम्।
व्यापादयेद्वहून् मर्त्त्यान् शस्त्रकर्म्मा पटुर्भिषक्॥
सेवनी शुक्रहरणी स्रोतसी फलयोर्गुदम्।
मूत्रसेकं मूत्रवहं मूत्रवस्तिस्तथाष्टमः॥

सुश्रुतसंहिता, चिकित्सितस्थानम्, ८।

blades under a severe and continuous pressure into a very fine powder, and the removal of the detritus by flushing out through a full-sized hollow metal catheter and an India-rubber wash bottle.

V Diseases of the mouth.

"There are sixty-five diseases of the mouth. The centers of their origin are seven, namely, lips, gum, tooth, tongue, palate, throat and the buccal cavity. Of these the lips have eight kinds of diseases, gum fifteen, teeth eight, tongue five, palate nine, throat seventeen, and the buccal cavity three". *Suśruta* II. 16. 2-3[133].

"In the '*vāta*' affections, the lips are asperous (herpes upon the lips are common in malaria, fevers, pneumonia, acute coryza as well as other febrile diseases ; cracks or fissures —*rhagades*—or the scars resulting from them, if occurring in infants or children, are indicative

133. मुखरोगाः पञ्चषष्टिः सप्तस्वायतनेषु। तत्रायतनान्योष्ठौ दन्तमूलानि दन्ता जिह्वा तालु कण्ठः सर्व्वाणि चेति॥

तत्राष्टावोष्ठयोः पञ्चदश दन्तमूलेषु। अष्टौ दन्तेषु। पञ्च जिह्वायाम्। नव तालुनि। सप्तदश कण्ठे। त्रयः सर्व्वेष्वायतनेषु॥

सुश्रुतसंहिता, निदानस्थानम्, १६।

of congenital syphilis ; the vertical crack in the middle of the lower lip, as occasionally seen, may be due to defective nutrition or may be associated with stomatitis), dry (associated with herpes or gastro-intestinal disorders, numb (labial paralysis or bulbar palsy), blackish (cyanosis associated with open and dry lips is indicative of dyspnea, due to disease of the heart or lungs, especially the chronic forms as emphysema or failing compensation in valvular lesions ; otherwise it may be associated with the associated local diseases of the mouth as stomatitis, glossitis, cacrum oris, phlegmonous tonsilitis, or some form of nasal stenosis), pressed and beated (loose and pendulous lips are suggestive of diphtheritic paralysis, chronic bulbar palsy ; and associated with open lips it is observed in various conditions of prostration, in idiocy and in cases of insanity).

"In the *'pitta'* affections of the lips, the lips are bluish (*cyanosed*), bronzed (in Addison's disease), and are covered with many vesicles like mustard seeds which give burning sensation, rupture and exudate (in aphthous or follicular stomatitis, small vesicles appear on the inner surface of the lips, or cheeks or edges of the tongue and soon rupture, leaving small and very sensitive superficial grayish ulcers with red areolae).

"In the '*kapha*' affections of the lips, the lips are covered with mucous patches like the color of the skin, and they are painless, pruritic, edematous, slippery, tepid and heavy (flattened, warty outgrowths, strictly delimited, coated with a gray matter, and found at the angles of the mouth, are the mucous patches of the secondary stage of syphilis ; congenital hypertrophy —*macrocheilia*—is caused by distension of the lymphatic space).

"In the vitiation of the three humors, the lips are sometimes blackish (cyanosed), sometimes bronzed (in Addison's disease), or pallid (in anemia), and are covered with various kinds of eczemas.

"In the labial diseases, originating from the derangement of the blood (vessels), the lips are covered with tumors which have color like dates (reddish brown), and they contain blood and bleeding takes place from them (*angioma*).

"In the labial diseases, from the corruption of flesh, the lips become heavy and swollen, and the tumors appear like meat balls and germs from the edges enlarge the ulceration (a somewhat irregular ulcer, usually upon the lower lip, gradually enlarging, recurrently scabbing over and becoming denuded, is probably an epithelioma).

"In the adipose labial affection, the lips are pruritic, numb, soft and heavy, and they are bright like the outer layer of clarified butter; and from them there is a clear exudation like clear crystal (congenital hypertrophy, *macrocheilia*, is caused by distension and dilatation of the lymphatic spaces, the lower lip being frequently affected).

"In the traumatic lesions of the lips, there is a terebrant pain, or like that of a wound from an axe, and it becomes like the color of blood (inflamed), tumorous (inflammatory swelling) and pruritic." *Suśruta* II. 16. 5-12[134].

---

134. कर्कशौ परुषौ स्तब्धौ कृष्णौ तीव्ररुगन्वितौ ।
दाल्येते परिपाट्येते ओष्ठौ मारुतकोपतः ॥ ५
आचितौ पिडकाभिस्तु सर्षपाकृतिभिर्भृशम् ।
सदाहपाकसंस्रावौ नीलौ पीतौ च पित्ततः ॥ ६
सवर्णाभिस्तु चीयेते पिडकाभिरवेदनौ ।
कण्डूमन्तौ कफाच्छूनौ पिच्छिलौ शीतलौ गुरू ॥ ७
सकृत्कृष्णौ सकृत्पीतौ सकृच्छ्वेतौ तथैव च ।
सन्निपातेन विज्ञेयावनेकपिडकाचितौ ॥ ८
खर्जूरफलवर्णाभिः पिडकाभिः समाचितौ ।
रक्तोपसृष्टौ रुधिरं स्रवतः शोणितप्रभौ ॥ ९

Diseases of the Gum.

In *'śitāda'* the gums are bleeding, ulcerative with foul-smelling exudation, and soft (spongy) ; this disease is due to the vitiation of the blood and the *'kapha'* (*gangrenous stomatitis*).

In *'danta-pupputaka'* there is an intense pain and swelling at the root of one or two teeth for a time ; this is due to the vitiation of the *'kapha'* and the blood. (*Gum boils* are usually formed round a foreign particle, especially with the tartar deposit encrusted with the pyogenic bacteria, but their outlet of discharge being closed).

The disease in which the teeth become loose, and from the tooth-sockets blood and pus come out, is called *'danta-veṣṭaka'* (in *pyorrhea alveolaris,* the teeth become loosened as the gum

---

मांसदुष्टौ गुरू स्थूलौ मांसपिण्डवदुद्गतौ ।
अन्तवश्राव मूर्च्छन्ति सृक्कस्योभयतो मुखात् ॥ १०
मेदसा घृतमण्डाभौ कण्डूमन्तौ स्थिरौ मृदू ।
अच्छस्फटिकसंकाशमास्रावं स्रवतो गुरू ॥ ११
क्षतजाभौ विदीर्येते पार्श्वे ते चाभिघाततः ।
ग्रथितौ च समाख्यातावोष्ठौ कण्डूसमन्वितौ ॥ १२

चरकसंहिता, निदानस्थानम् १६ ।

recedes or the pus socket causes necrosis of the tissues at the root. The affection is probably due to streptococcal infection of the periosteum of the alveoli. Usually it is associated with an excess of tartar deposit or the carious condition of the teeth).

The disease in which the gum has a pruritic and painful inflammation, and salivation, is called the *'śauṣira'* (*gingivitis*).

The disease in which the teeth are loose in their sockets, the palate is falling (*uvula descendens*) and ulceration in the gum and pain in the buccal cavity, is called the *'mahā-śauṣira* (*gangrenous gingivitis*).

The disease in which there is ulceration and bleeding of the gum, is called the *'paridara'* (*phlegmonous gingivitis*).

The disease in which there is necrosis of the tissues in the sockets, and for this reason the teeth become loose, there is bleeding at the slight pressure of the teeth, but slight pain, and with the bleeding the mouth becomes foul-smelling, is called the *'upakuśa'* (*chronic hypertrophic gingivitis*).

If strong inflammation follows the traumatism of the gum, and the teeth become loose, it is called *'vaidarbha'* traumatic interstitial *ulitis*).

If an extra tooth appears due to the influence of '*vāyu*' with intense pain, it is called the '*varddhana*' (*wisdom tooth* or dens serotinus, the most posterior of the molar teeth appear about the eighteenth year). The pain ceases after the tooth comes out.

"The disease in which in the gum of the lower posterior tooth, there is a large neoplasm with intense pain and salivation, is called the '*adhimāṃsa*' (epithelioma or *epulis*. Epulis is a fibrous growth and develops in the peridontal membrane ; it is often found near a decayed tooth, grows slowly and forms a more or less pedinculated tumor of the same color as the gum).

The tumors of the gum are of five kinds with symptoms similar to those that have been described of the tubular vessels, by the corruption of '*vāyu, pitta, kapha*, their morbid combination or infection' and they are known as '*pañcha-nāḍī*' (*alveolar abscesses* are nearly always due to sepsis originating in a decayed tooth. (1) The pus may be limited to the margin of the gum, forming a tumor. (2) The pus may be slow in forming and there may be a great inflammatory infiltration of the cheek with the edema of the face and spasm of the masseter and pterygoid muscles. (3) The pus may extend widely beneath the periostenum and cause necrosis of the jaw. (4) A persistent sinus or sinuses may be present if the abscess has burst spontaneously or has been opened externally; there is either a dead tooth, a portion of a fang or a piece of necrosed bone which keeps open the sinus. (5) The pus may burst into the antrum of the upper jaw or extend deeply and widely in the neck)". *Susruta* II. 16. 14-24[135].

---

135. शोणितं दन्तवेष्टेभ्यो यस्याकस्मात् प्रवर्त्तते ।
दुर्गन्धीनि सकृष्णानि प्रक्लेदीनि मृदूनि च ॥
दन्तमांसानि शीर्य्यन्ते पचन्ति च परस्परम् ।
शीतादो नाम स व्याधिः कफशोणितसम्भवः ॥ १४
दन्तयोस्त्रिषु वा यस्य श्वयथुः सरुजो महान् ।
दन्तपुप्पुटको ज्ञेयः कफरक्तनिमित्तजः ॥ १५
स्रवन्ति पूयरुधिरं चला दन्ता भवन्ति च ।
दन्तवेष्टः स विज्ञेयो दुष्टशोणितसम्भवः ॥ १६
श्वयथुर्दन्तमूलेषु रुजावान् कफरक्तजः ।
लालास्रावी स विज्ञेयः कण्डूमान् शौषिरो गदः ॥ १७
दन्ताश्चलन्ति वेष्टेभ्यस्तालु चाप्यवदीर्य्यते
दन्तमांसानि पच्यन्ते मुखञ्च परिपीड्यते ।
यस्मिन् स सर्व्वजो व्याधिर्महाशौषिरसंज्ञकः ॥ १८

Diseases of the Teeth.

"The disease in which the tooth becomes blackened and perforated by microbes, due to the vitiation of the blood, and the tooth becomes loose accompanied by inflammation of the gum, pain and salivation; is called the '*krimi-dantaka*' *dental caries* : it is a fact of common observation that caries begin only at spots protected from friction or left uncleansed as (a) pits, grooves and fissures in the enamel ; (b) proximal surfaces just above the contact points ; (c) surfaces which for any cause are habitually

---

दन्तमांसानि शीर्यन्ते यस्मिन् ष्ठीवति चाप्यसृक् ।
पित्तासृक्कफजो व्याधिर्ज्ञेयः परिदरो हि सः ॥ १९
वेष्टेषु दाहः पाकश्च तेभ्यो दन्ताश्चलन्ति च ।
आघट्टिताः प्रस्रवन्ति शोणितं मन्दवेदनाः ॥
आध्मायन्ते स्रुते रक्ते मुखं पूति च जायते ।
यस्मिन्नुपकुशः स स्यात् पित्तरक्तकृतो गदः ॥ २०
घृष्टेषु दन्तमूलेषु संरम्भो जायते महान् ।
भवन्ति च चला दन्ताः स वैदर्भोऽभिघातजः ॥ २१
मारुतेनाधिको दन्तो जायते तीव्रवेदनः ।
वर्धनः स मतो व्याधिर्जाते रुक् च प्रशाम्यति ॥ २२
हानव्ये पश्चिमे दन्ते महाञ्छोथो महारुजः ।
लालास्रावी कफकृतो विज्ञेयः सोऽधिमांसकः ॥ २३
दन्तमूलगता नाड्यः पञ्च ज्ञेया यथेरिताः ॥ २४

सुश्रुतसंहिता, निदानस्थानम्, १६ ।

unclean; (d) necks of the teeth at or near the junction of the cementum and the enamel. In these localities, the oral bacteria, protected from friction, attach themselves to the enamel, forming microbic plaques which are sufficiently adherent to attach themselves, obtaining their food supply from the carbohydrate and the albuminous particles that adhere to those spots and are not thoroughly cleansed. From carbohydrate fermentation, lactic acid is produced and this is prevented from being diluted and washed away; the slightly alkaline salivary secretion by the bacterial plaques and added to it, the enzymes secreted by the bacteria, attack the inorganic matter of the enamel following first the interprismatic cement substance between the prisms, later dissolving the transverse cement substance of the globules. The effect is to 'produce an irregular and roughened surface, and in the process of enamel dissolution and decalcification, the bacteria enter into the crevices and gradually gain access to the dentine. The leptothrix buccalis maxima is invariably associated with more or less streptococci and bacillus buccalis maximus in rapid dental caries).

The disease in which the teeth are very

sensitive to cold or heat (paroxysms of pain induced by thermal stimuli), is called the '*danta-harṣa*' (*hyperemia of the dental pulp* : the most common cause of active hyperemia of the pulp is a lessening of the non-conducting covering of the organ—enamel and dentine, through abrasion, erosion, fracture or caries, leading to an increased response and continued irritation of the pulp through the thermal stimuli).

The disease in which the face becomes misshaped (either by caving in through necrosis of the jaw-bone or with odontomes which are neoplasms composed of dental tissues in varying proportions and different stages of development), the teeth become eroded and painfnl, is called the *bhañjanaka* (*necrosis of the jaw* with odontones and erosion of the teeth).

If the solids (*mala*=the mineral constituents and the mucus of the saliva) are dried up and become sugar-like hard on the teeth, by '*vāyu* and *pitta*' it is called the '*śarkarā*' (*salivary calculus* or *tartar* : the deposition of the tartar is perhaps activated by the bacterial fermentation, causing the precipitation of the mineral salts, chiefly calcium phosphate enclosing with them the epithelium and the bacteria, especially the leptothrix forms).

If this tartar scales out with the dentine, it is called the *kapālikā* (large tartar formations); it is very destructive to teeth.

If by the vitiated blood and the '*pitta*', the enamel of the teeth become burnt (stained) dark-brownish or greenish, it is called the '*śyāva-dantaka*' (*the green stain of the enamel*: these most common green deposits upon enamel occur upon both the temporary and the permanent teeth, particularly of young persons; the deposits usually have a concentric form and are mainly upon the labial faces of the anterior teeth. The green stain is usually preceded by a lack of oral hygiene and superficial decalcification of the enamel, as it is found slightly roughened, indicating the action of the acids upon it by fermenting food particles sticking to it. The green stain is the more advanced stage of the dark-brownish coloring).

If the jaw is fractured by the source of '*vāyu*' through loud talking, chewing of hard substances or yawning, it is called '*hanu-mokṣa*' (fracture of the jaw); it gives all the symptoms of tetanus (the fracture of a healthy jaw is only possible through traumatism. But if it is eaten up by necrotic process as in the tertiary stage of syphilis, tubercular caries, phosphorus poisoning or local sepsis, and made very brittle, it may be easily fractured by any slight sudden tension as chewing any hard substance or movement). *Suśruta* II. 16. 27-33[136].

Treatment: "Without injuring the gum, all the tartar deposits have to be carefully scaled out (by scalers) ; then those parts of the teeth are to be polished with the powder of Butea frondosa (*lākṣā*) mixed with honey. (The modern treatment for the tartar is just the same, except that to secure the smoothness of the

---

136. कृष्णश्छिद्री चलः स्रावी संरम्भी महारुजः ।
अनिमित्तरुजो वाताद्विज्ञेयः क्रिमिदन्तकः ॥ २७
दशनाः शीतमुष्णं च सहन्ते स्पर्शनं न च ।
यस्य तं दन्तहर्षं तु व्याधिं विद्यात् समीरणात् ॥ २८
वक्त्रं वक्रं भवेद्यस्मिन् दन्तभङ्गश्च तीव्ररुक् ।
कफवातकृतो व्याधिः स भञ्जनकसंज्ञितः ॥ २९
शर्करेव स्थिरीभूतो मलो दन्तेषु यस्य वै ।
सा दन्तानां गुणघ्नी तु विज्ञेया दन्तशर्करा ॥ ३०
दलन्ति दन्तवल्कानि यदा शर्करया सह ।
ज्ञेया कपालिका सैव दशनानां विनाशिनी ॥ ३१
योऽसृङ्मिश्रेण पित्तेन दग्धो दन्तस्त्वशेषतः ।
श्यावतां नीलतां वापि गतः स श्यावदन्तकः ॥ ३२
वातेन तैस्तैर्भावैस्तु हनुसन्धिर्विसंहतः ।
हनुमोक्ष इति ज्ञेयो व्याधिरर्दितलक्षणः ॥ ३३

सुश्रुतसंहिता, निदानस्थानम्, १६ ।

scaled surface, so that no nucleus is left for the new tartar deposit, pumice-powder on a piece of wood is used, instead of the powder of Butea frondosa with honey)." *Suśruta* IV. 22-23[137].

"The alveolar abscesses should be treated in the same way, as an ordinary abscess, with this difference, that the tooth with the sepsis of which the abscess has been formed, must be extracted. If it can not be done, then after cleansing (an incision is made, large enough to open the abscess cavity fully, inside the mouth, all the pus is thoroughly drained off, and the abscess cavity is repeatedly washed with antiseptic and astringment infusion or decoction), the abscess cavity should be cauterized either by caustic or cautery. If the alveolar abscess is neglected, it is sure to cause necrosis of the jaw. Therefore the tooth should be uprooted (thus cure may be effected in light cases, by causing the abscess drainage through the tooth socket). If the bone has

137. अस्मिन् दन्तमूलानि शर्करामुद्धरेद्भिषक् ।
लाक्षाचूर्णैर्मधुयुतैस्ततस्ताः प्रतिसारयेत् ।

सुश्रुतसंहिता, चिकित्सितस्थानम्, २२ ।

been affected (necrosized), it should be also scraped off." *Suśruta* IV. 22. 18[138].

"The disease in which the teeth seem to be rent asunder with pain, is called '*dālana*' (odontalgia of neuralgic character or due to caries or periodonitis)." *Suśruta* II. 16. 26[139].

The Diseases of the Tongue.

"The disease in which the tougue becomes inflamed, due to the derangement of '*vāyu*', loses its sensibility to taste, and becomes fissured like that of the leaves of '*tectona*', is the '*vāta*' disease of the tongue (glossitis desiccans or chronic superficial glossitis may be induced by

---

138. सामान्यं कर्म्म नाड़ीनां विशेषश्चात्र मे शृणु ।
यं दन्तमभि जायेत नाड़ी तं दन्तमुद्धरेत् ॥
छित्त्वा मांसानि शस्त्रेण यदि नोपरिजो भवेत् ।
शोधयित्वा दहेद्वापि क्षारेण ज्वलनेन वा ॥
भिन्नत्वापेचिते दन्ते हनुकास्थिगतिध्रुवम् ।
समूलं दशनं तस्मादुद्धरेद्भग्नमस्थि च ॥ १८

सुश्रुतसंहिता, चिकित्सितस्थानम, २२ ।

139. दाल्यन्ते बहुधा दन्ता यस्मिंस्तीव्ररुगन्विता: ।
दालन: स इति ज्ञेय: सदागतिनिमित्तज: ॥ २६

सुश्रुतसंहिता, निदानस्थानम्, १६ ।

persistent and excessive use of tobacco, spirits and highly spiced foods; it is characterized by the slow formation of a number of deep fissures and indentations, in the depth of which there are ulcers and excoriations).

"The tongue is dark-yellowish, congested and is convered with blood-red fissures in the *'pitta'* disease of the tongue (the raspberry tongue has a pale-red surface, from which project greatly swollen and bright-red fungiform papillæ, as it appears in the first stage of the scarlet fever or in other acute specific infections).

"The tongue is swollen, heavy and is covered with a fur, resembling the thorns of *'Bombacis heptaphylli'* in the *'kapha'* derangement of the tongue (the tongue is flabby, swollen, indented and covered with a uniform, yellow pasty fur in catarrhal gastritis or gastro-duodenitis).

"The severe inflammation that is caused in the tongue by the corrupt *'kapha'* and the blood, is called the *'alāsa'* (glossitis); in severe cases paralysis of the tongue and ulceration at its root, (*cellulitis* or parenchymatous inflammation of the tongue is due to the infection of streptococcus; while acute glossitis may be the result of a burn or wasp-sting).

The disease in which the tongue is inflamed and on the tip of the tongue, there is a salivating, pruritic and painfully congestive tumor, is called '*upajihvikā*' (secondary syphilitic sore, usually as condylomata, accompanied by subacute glossitis, arising from the primary hard or tender ulcerating nodule that is seen on the tip of the tongue in a syphilitic lesion ; or it may be carcinoma of the tongue.)" ***Suśruta*** **II. 16. 37**[140].

The Diseases of the Palate.

"The elongated tumor that develops and spreads from the bottom of the palate like a leathern bag filled with air, is called *galaśuṇḍikā*' (angioma of the palate) ; it causes polydipsia, bronchitis and dyspnea (in uvulutis).

"The tumor that develops at the bottom of

140. जिह्वानिलेन स्फुटिता प्रसुप्ता भवेच्च शाकच्छदनप्रकाशा ।
पित्तेन पीता परिदह्यते च चिता सरक्तैरपि कण्टकैश्च ।
कफेन गुर्वी बहुला चिता च मांसोद्गमैः शाल्मलिकण्टकाभैः ॥ ३५
जिह्वातले यः श्वयथुः प्रगाढः सोऽलाससंज्ञः कफरक्तमूर्त्तिः ।
जिह्वां स तु स्तम्भयति प्रवृद्धो मूले तु जिह्वा भृशमेति पाकम् ॥ ३६
जिह्वाग्ररूपः श्वयथुर्हि जिह्वामुन्नम्य जातः कफरक्तयोनिः ।
प्रसेककण्डूपरिदाहयुक्ता प्रकथ्यतेऽसावुपजिह्विकेति ॥ ३७
सुश्रुतसंहिता, निदानस्थानम्, १६ ।

the palate (an acute abscess from a carious tooth in the upper jaw may spread inwards and raise the muco-peristeum of the hard palate) like the (fruit of) '*Memordica monadelpha*'; it causes pricking pain and *hyperæmia* and it suppurates (*septic tumor of the palate*).

"The reddish and the benumbing tumor that develops in the palate, is called the '*adhruṣa*' (the *peritonsilar abscess* is liable to burrow in the soft palate) ; it causes high fever and intense pain.

"The slightly painful and pale tumor that develops slowly for a long time like the tortoise shell, due to the corruption of '*phlegma*' is called the '*māṃsa-kachchhapa* (*endotheliomal tumor of the palate*).

"The tumor that appears in the palate like the lotus bud, is called the '*arvvuda*' (*angioma*) ; it has all the characteristics of the angioma as mentioned before.

"At the base of the uvula, the malignant and painless carcinoma that grows, is called the '*māṃsa-sanghāta*' (*papilloma of the uvula*).

"The painless and the chronic tumor that grows in the palate like a plum, due to the corruption of the '*phlegma and fat*', is called the '*tālu pupputa*' (*cyst* or *gumma ofthe palate*).

There is much edema and lacerating pain in the palate, and dyspnea, due to the derangement of *pitta associated with vāyu* which causes *tālu-śoṣa*' when the syphilitic gummata break, septic infection follows, and thus there is usually much edema of the surrounding tissues.

There is malignant ulceration of the palate due to the derangement of '*pitta*', which causes '*tālu-pāka*' (*syphilitic ulceration* of the palate which may lead to its perforation, usually circular or oval in shape, and finally to its necrosis and destruction of its major part)". *Suśruta* II. 16. 39-47[141].

---

141. श्लेष्मासृग्भ्यां तालुमूलात् प्रवृद्धो
दीर्घः शोफो ध्मातवस्तिप्रकाशः ।
तृष्णाकासश्वासकृत् संप्रदिष्टो
व्याधिर्वैद्यैः कण्ठशुण्डीति नाम्ना ॥ ३९
शोफः स्थूलस्तोददाहप्रपाकी
प्रागुक्ताभ्यां तुण्डिकेरी मता तु ॥ ४०
शोफः स्तब्धो लोहितस्तालुदेशे
रक्ताज्ज्ञेयः सोऽध्रुषो रुग्ज्वराढ्यः ॥ ४१
कूर्म्मोत्सन्नोऽवेदनोऽशीघ्रजन्मा-
ऽरक्तो ज्ञेयः कच्छपः श्लेष्मणा स्यात् ॥ ४२
पद्माकारं तालुमध्ये तु शोफं
विद्याद्रक्तादर्व्वुदं प्रोक्तलिङ्गम् ॥ ४३

The Diseases of the Throat.

'The gummata that are produced in the pharynx, causing its stricture, due to the vitiated action, either individual or collective, of '*vāyu, pitta, kapha and the blood,*' are called the '*rohiṇī*' (*syphilitic gummata*); due to the pharyngeal stenosis, life is lost (unless it is treated by the regular passage of bougies for the rest of the patient's life, and in some intractable cases gastrostomy may be necessary).

The painful gummata, causing stricture of the pharynx, also appear at the dorsum of the tongue in the '*vāta*' gummatous affection of the pharynx; and it has all the complications of the '*vāta*'.

The *gummata* appear and ulcerate rapidly

दुष्टं मांसं श्लेष्मणा नीरुजञ्च
ताल्वन्तःस्थं मांससङ्घातमाहुः ॥ ४४
नीरुक्स्थायी कोलमात्रः कफात् स्या-
न्मेदोयुक्तात् पुप्पुटस्तालुदेशे ॥ ४५
शोषोऽत्यर्थं दीर्य्यते चापि तालु
श्वासो वातात् तालुशोषः स पित्तात् ॥
पित्तं कुर्य्यात् पाकमत्यर्थघोरं
तालन्येनं तालुपाकं वदन्ति ॥ ४७
सुश्रुतसंहिता, निदानस्थान,म् ११

with high fever in the *'pitta'* affection of the disease.

The gummata (or syphilitic nodes) are hard and ulcerate freely in the *'kapha'* affection of the disease, and they cause stricture of the pharynx.

The gummata ulcerate deeply and are very intractable and have all the triple complication in the *'sānnipāta'* (acute) affection of the disease.

The gummata have all the symptoms of the *'pitta'* affection of the disease, and are covered with the abscesses in the blood lesion of the *'rohiṇī'* ; it is incurable.

A plum-stone like (zizyphus jujubæ), rough and hard tumor that develops and causes terebrant pain, is called *'kaṇṭha-śālūka'* (*carcinoma of the pharynx*) ; it is curable by operation. *Suśruta* II. 16. 49-55[142].

142. गलेऽनिलः पित्तकफौ च मूर्च्छितौ
पृथक् समस्ताश्च तथैव शोणितम् ।
प्रदूष्य मांसं गलरोधिनोऽङ्कुरान्
सृजन्ति यान् सासुहरा तु रोहिणी ॥ ४९
जिह्वां समन्ताद्भृशवेदना ये
मांसाङ्कुराः कण्ठनिरोधिनः स्युः ।
तां रोहिणीं वातकृतां वदन्ति
वातात्मकोपद्रवगाढयुक्ताम् ॥ ५०

If a tumor (syphilitic or tuberculous cancer) appears at the root of the tongue due to the vitiation of the *'kapha and the blood'* as it appears on its tip, it is called *'adhi-jihvā'* (*cancer of the tongue*) ; and if it suppurates, it is incurable.

The tumescence that develops like a bracelet and causes the stricture of the esophagus, is called the *'valaya'* (*hypertrophic* thickening in the phreno-cardiac portion of the *gullet*) ; it is intractable and incurable.

The inflammation that causes dyspnea, pain and devitalising, due to the derangement of *'kapha and vāyu'* is the *'valāsa'* (*stenosis of the trachea*, caused by acute edematous inflammation from diphtheria and specific fevers, sometimes leading to perichondritis and erysipe-

---

क्षिप्रोद्गमा क्षिप्रविदाहपाका
तीव्रज्वरा पित्तनिमित्ततः स्यात् ॥ ५१
स्रोतो निरोधिन्यपि मन्दपाका
गुर्वी स्थिरा सा कफसम्भवा वै ॥ ५२
गम्भीरपाकाप्रतिवारवीर्य्या त्रिदोषलिङ्गा त्रयसम्भवा स्यात ॥ ५३
स्फोटाचिता पित्तसमानलिङ्गाऽसाध्या प्रदिष्टा रुधिरात्मिकेयम् ॥ ५५
कोलास्थिमात्रः कफसम्भवो यो ग्रन्थिर्गले कण्टकशूकभूतः ।
खरः स्थिरः शस्त्रनिपातसाध्यस्तं कण्ठशालूकमिति ब्रुवन्ति ॥ ५५
सुश्रुतसंहिता, निदानस्थानम्, १६ ।

las spreading down the throat or spreading to the mucosa through a tracheal wound); this is hard to cure.

The globular, elevated, congestive, pruritic, slightly suppurative, sweetish and heavy inflammation that is developed in the tonsils, due to the vitiation of '*kapha and the blood*', is called the '*eka-vṛnda*' (phlegmonous or suppurative tonsilitis).

The elevated and the globular inflammation that develops with high fever and 'hyperæmia'; is called the '*vṛnda*' (follicular or *lacunar tonsilitis*); if it be of '*vāta*' origin, it causes pricking pain.

The hard tumor that develops causing stricture of the esophagus, due to the corruption of the humors, resembling '*Śataghnī*' which is a stone covered with iron pikes, and likewise the tumor that is covered with papillæ, is called the '*śataghnī*' (*papilloma*); it is an incurable disease, and it has all the complications of the three corrupt humors (malignant papilloma of the esophagus).

The hard and slightly painful tumor that develops in the esophagus, causing dysphagia, and resembles in appearance and shape the stone of '*Emblic myrobalan*', is called the '*gilāyu*'(benign fibroma of the esophagus). It is curable by operation.

The tumescence that develops throughout the throat, due to the corruption of the three humors, is called the '*gala-vidradhi*' (*parenchymatous goitre* in which there is a general and uniform enlargement of the thyroids and the vesicles are over-distended with colloid secretion, which however does not escape freely into the lymphatics) ; it causes all kinds of pain of the corrupt humors, as pricking pain, hyperæmia and pruritis, and has all the complications of an acute abscess (parenchymatous goitre may be provoked by septic absorption from a local septic lesion as carious tooth, an ulcer, suppurative tumor or drinking water from a contaminated source).

If such a large tumor develops in the esophagus, due to the corruption of the '*kapha and the blood*,' as to cause aphagia, dyspnea and high fever, it is called the '*galaugha*' (a large *epithelioma* that causes the stricture of the esophagus and the trachea).

The disease in which, due to the stenosis of the trachea, the patient suffers from dyspnea and falls into a swoon, the voice is broken, the throat becomes dry and the patient collapses, is called the *'svaraghna'* (*stenosis of the trachea* may be caused by many diseases as : (1) enlargement or neoplasm of the thyroids ; (2) enlargement and the tumor of the thymus ; (3) mediastinal tumors or abscesses ; (4) pressure stenosis by aneurism ; (5) tertiary syphilitic lesions).

The disease in which there is an extensive, very painful and continuous inflammation which gradually causes stenosis of the throat, is called *'māṃsa-tāna'* (*syphilitic ulceration of the throat*); it is deadly and arises from the corruption of the three humors.

The disease in which there is a bleeding inflammation with pricking pain and hyperæmia and which ulcerates with cadaverous odor, especially on the side the patient sleeps, is called the *'vidārī'* (syphilitic *gangrenous ulceration of the throat*). *Suśruta* II. 16. 56-67[143].

---

143. जिह्वाग्ररूपः श्वयथः कफात् तु जिह्वाप्रबन्धोपरि रक्तमिश्रः ।
ज्ञेयोऽधिजिह्वः खलु रोग एष विवर्ज्जयेदागतपाकमेनम् ॥ ५६
बलास एवायतमुन्नतञ्च शोफं करोत्यन्नगतिं निवार्य्य ।
तं सर्व्वथैवाप्रतिवारवीर्य्यं विवर्ज्जनीयं वलयं वदन्ति ॥ ५७
गले च शोफं कुरुतः प्रवृद्धौ श्लेष्मानिलौ श्वासरुजोपपन्नम् ।
मर्म्मच्छिदं दुस्तरमेतदाहुर्बलाससंज्ञं निपुणा विकारम् ॥ ५८
वृत्तोन्नतो यः श्वयथुः सदाहः कण्ड्वन्वितोऽपाक्यमृदुर्गुरुश्च ।
नाम्नैकवृन्दः परिकल्पितोऽसौ व्याधिर्बलासक्षतजप्रसूतः ॥ ५९

Diseases of the Buccal Cavity.

The buccal cavity is covered with ulcers with pricking pain in the *'vāta sarvva-sara'* (*ulcerative stomatitis* or putrid sore of the mouth occurs in oral sepsis, especially associated with carious tooth or pyorrhea).

The buccal cavity is covered with small reddish or dark-yellowish vesicles (small, slightly raised whitish plaques starting as vesicles, surrounded by a red areola) in *'pitta sarvva-sara'* (*aphthous* or *follicular stomatitis*, which is very

---

समुन्नतं वृत्तममन्ददाहं
तीव्रज्वरं वृन्दमुदाहरन्ति।
तञ्चापि पित्तक्षतजप्रकोपाद्
विद्यात् सतोदं पवनात्मजं तम्॥ ६०
वर्त्तिर्घना कण्ठनिरोधिनी या
चितातिमात्रं पिशितप्ररोहैः।
नानारुजोच्छ्रायकरी त्रिदोषाज्
ज्ञेया शतघ्नीव शतघ्न्यसाध्या॥ ६१
ग्रन्थिर्गले त्वामलकास्थिमात्रः
स्थिरोऽल्परुक् स्यात् कफरक्तमूर्त्तिः।
संलक्ष्यते सक्तमिवाशनञ्च
स शस्त्रसाध्यस्तु गिलायुसंज्ञः॥ ६२
सर्व्वं गलं व्याप्य समुत्थितो यः
शोफो रुजो यत्र वसन्ति सर्व्वाः।

common in infants and young children associated chiefly with indigestion, but also prevails in adults when the general health is impaired).

The buccal cavity (especially on the tongue and the inner margins of the lips) is covered with pruritic, slightly painful and skin-colored

---

स सर्व्वदोषो गलविद्रधिस्तु
तस्यैव तुल्यः खलु सर्व्वजस्य ॥ ६३
शोफो महानन्नजलावरोधी
तीव्रज्वरो वातगतेर्निहन्ता ।
कफेन जातो रुधिरान्वितेन
गले गलौघः परिकीर्त्यतेऽसौ ॥ ४
योऽतिप्रताम्यन् श्वसिति प्रसक्तं
भिन्नस्वरः शुष्कविमुक्तकण्ठः ।
कफोपदिग्धेष्वनिलायनेषु
ज्ञेयः स रोगः श्वसनात् स्वरघ्नः ॥ ६५
प्रतानवान् यः श्वयथुः सुकष्टो
गलोपरोधं कुरुते क्रमेण ।
स मांसतानः कथितोऽवलम्वी
प्राणप्रणात् सर्व्वकृतो विकारः ॥ ६६
सदाहतोदं श्वयथुं सरक्त-
मन्तर्गले पूतिविशीर्णमांसम् ।
पित्तेन विद्याद्वदने विदारीं
पार्श्वे विशेषात् स तु येन शेते ॥ ६७

सुश्रुतसंहिता, निदानस्थानम्, १६ ।

patches in '*kapha sarvva-sara*' (*mycotic or parasitic stomatitis* in which small, sl elevated, pearly white spots are devel through '*saccharomyces* (*oïdium*) *albicans*' in debilitated children and old people).

All the symptoms of aphthous stomatitis appears in stomatitis from blood vitiation, and by many authorities, it is called the '*mukha-pāka*' (*acute or catarrhal stomatitis* in which the mucosa membrane of the mouth is more or less extensively reddened, dry and hot, with associated salivation and swelling of the tongue, due to gastro-intestinal disturbances or due to irritants as alcohol or tobacco)" *Suśruta* II. 16. 69-72[144].

144. स्फोटैः सतोदैर्वदनं समन्ताद्
यस्याचितं सर्व्वसरः स वातात् ॥ ६९
रक्तैः सदाहैस्तनुभिः सपीतै-
र्यस्याचितं वापि स पित्तकोपात् ॥ ७०
कण्डूयुतैरल्परुजैः सवर्णै-
र्यस्याचितञ्चापि स वै कफेन ॥ ७१
रक्तेन पित्तोदित एक एव
कैश्चित् प्रदिष्टो मुखपाकसंज्ञः ॥ ७२
सुश्रुतसंहिता निदानस्थानम्, १६ ।

VI. Tumors.

"*Tumor* (*granthi*), *abscess* (*vidradhi*), *neoplasm* (*alaji* perhaps means edema, as *arvvuda* has been definitely defined as neoplasm), all develop from *inflammation* (*Śotha*). They have all their own individual charateristics, and tumors are of various kinds. The swelling that is extensive, slightly elevated, of even or uneven surface, in the skin (including mucous membrane) and the tissues, confined to a part of the body due to a lesion, is called the '*śotha*' (inflammation)." *Suśruta* I. 17. 2[145].

"'*Śotha*' is of three varieties, '*vāyu*, *pitta and kapha*'. Either they originate from internal causes (in the process of eliminating toxins produced as a metabolic reaction, or, introduced into the economy) or external lesions (as traumatism, microbic invasion or local irritants). Cutting, penetrating, crushing, lacerating, pressing, beating, binding and all kinds of wound and oppression of the tissue cause inflammation ; as well as the contact of the (toxic or irritant sub-

---

145. शोफसमुत्थाना ग्रन्थिविद्रध्यलजीप्रभृतयः प्रायेण व्याधयोऽभिधास्यन्ते अनेकाकृतयः, तैर्विलक्षणः पृथुर्ग्रथितः समो विषमो वा त्वङ्मांसस्थायी दोषसङ्घातः शरीरैकदेशोत्थितः शोफ इत्युच्यते ।

सुश्रुतसंहिता, सत्रस्थानम्, १७ ।

stances) flower, fruit or juice of '*Semecarpus anacardium*', sting of insects (mucuna pruritus) and (penetration) of microbes (*krimi*), at the contact of injurious leaves, vines and bulb (as that of the poison ivy, *Rhus radicans*), the perspiration, or excreta of a poisonous creature, a wound of a poisonous or non-poisonous creature by tooth, horn or nail, poisonous gas (*viṣa vāta*) and fire—all these cause inflammation." *Charaka* I. 18. 1[146].

"Vomiting, tympanites, cholera, dyspnea, asthma, diarrhœa, tuberculosis, anemia, gastro-intestinal troubles, menorrhagia, fistula-in-ano, and piles by osmosis (*ati-karṣaṇa*=excessive pressure) cause (edematous) inflammation." *Charaka* I. 18. 4[147].

When the tissues are injured by mechanical

---

146. त्रयः शोथा भवन्ति वातपित्तकफनिमित्ताः। ते पुनर्द्विविधाः निजागन्तुभेदेन। तत्र आगन्तवश्छेदनभेदनक्षणनभञ्जनपिच्छनोत्पेषणवेष्टन प्रहारवधबन्धनव्यधनपीड़नादिभिर्वा। भल्लातकपुष्पफलरसात्मगुप्ताशूकक्रिमिशूकाहितपत्रलतागुल्मसंस्पर्शनैर्वा स्वेदपरिसर्पणावमूत्रणैर्वा विषिणां। सविषाविषप्राणिदन्तविषाणनखनिपातैर्वा सागरविषवातहिमदहनसंस्पर्शनैर्वा शोथाः समुपजायन्ते॥ चरकसंहिता, सूत्रस्थानम्, १८।

147. छर्द्यलसकविसूचिकाश्वासकासातीसारशोषपाण्डुरोगोदरप्रदरभगन्दरार्शोविकारातिकर्षणैर्वा। चरकसंहिता, सूत्रस्थानम्, १८।

agents, or, by cnemical, thermic or bacterial irritants or their toxins, inflammation sets in as a restorative process of the tissue repair.

When a mechanical agent has produced a cut, the edges of the wound are slightly separated, and the open vessels are bleeding. The first reactions will arrest the hemorrhage. On the one hand, the calibre of the vessels will contract in consequence of the direct excitation of the nonstriated muscular fibers entering into the structures of their walls, and on the other hand as the result of reflex constriction. The blood flowing with less force, will coagulate ; fibrine will be formed, and its effect will be to occlude the vessel, to assure hemostasis and to unite the edges of the wound, and then serve as a nutrition and as a guide to cells which will insure reparation. This commences when the cellular elements lining the wound begin to proliferate and form a cicatrix. To facilitate the work, the leucocytes rush in, some to take part in the formation of the tissues and others to carry away the dead cells. This causes *inflammation.*

The same phenomenon occurs, with a chemical irritant or toxin ; if it be weak and diluted, it might be absorbed and neutralized without any perceptible local reaction. But if it is strong enough to destroy a few cells, then there is a vaso-dilatation, a serous exudation (*edema*) to dilute the toxin and to prevent its absorption.

But if these wounds are not kept in aseptic condition, the ubiquitous pus coccus (*staphylococcus* or *streptococcus*), finding favourable medium, starts a colony. It not only multiplies rapidly, but also engenders toxins which cause death of the cells of the region, thus creating a necro-biotic area, surrounded by a proliferative zone of the healthy tissues. Struggle now begins between the invading hosts and the healthy tissues. If the victory is quick with the latter, then the inflammation gradually subsides. But if the tissues lack the resisting power and the bodily defensive mechanism is not powerful or prompt in its response, then leucocytes circumscribe the infection, round the dead cells, so that the general economy can not be affected, and they can fight more conveniently against the microbes and replace the fallen defenders. Coincidently the nervous terminations are aroused by the microbic toxins and their excitation gives rise to a series of reflex acts which ending in the active dilatation of the vessels of the invaded area, are followed by migrations of the leucocytes and the formation of the serous exudate. If the pus cocci gain the upper hand, the cells that are killed undergo liquefaction and are converted into the *pus*, so that an *abscess* results. This soon coagulates and a creamy substance is formed which softens towards the centre. And if it be not now evacuated, the softened area increases in size, the skin over it is thinned and mortified, and a small slough is formed, through which the pus escapes and the tension is relieved. If the pus cavity contains a ropy fibrile core, as in a boil or carbuncle, it indicates that the cells have been destroyed in mass by a virulent agent, and of the dead cells, the core is composed. After the escape of the pus, a space—the abscess cavity, is left, the walls of which are lined with vascular or granulation tissues, which escaped destruction, and which slowly fill the contracting cavity and obliterate it by forming interstitial *scar-tissues*. But if the abscess be deeply situated and be not able to open on to a free surface, thus allowing the pus to be drained off, the phagocytes mobilize all their forces, surround the necrotic area and make an advance from all sides. The vanguard of the advancing army is composed of a more or less compact layer of the mono-nuclear phagocytes (*polyblasts*) accompanied by numerous new vessels which bring the food-supply for the phagocytic scavengers who voraciously ingest all the enemy microbes as well as the injured and dead cells, and carry out their removal from the fighting zone. They also drain off the toxic fluid of the disintegrating cells. Behind the polyblasts, are seen in mighty battle array, the fibroblasts or connecting tissue cells in active proliferation, and with their fibrous laminæ shut off the abscess from the healthy tissues, and with the absorption of the pus, encroach on the pus area. With the absorption of the pus, the abscess cavity is replaced by the fibrous tissue, forming the cicatrical scar. But in case the phagocytes lack the necessary vitality for the operation, the abscess burrows through and forms a dangerous fistula (*visarpa nāḍī*).

Tumors are developed in these eight places : skin (pustular inflammations : acne, ecthymoses, variola ; subcutaneous inflammation : erysipelas, eczema; vesicular lesions (herpes) or bullæ varicella, pempigus), flesh (*myxoma* = tumor of mucous tissue ; *fibroma* = tumor of fibrous tissue; *lipoma* = tumor of adipose tissue ; *myoma* = tumor of muscular tissue), vessels (*angioma*—tumor composed of blood vessels ; *endothelioma*—tumor originating from the endothelium or lining cells of the vascular tissue ; *hemangioendothelioma* = tumor of endothelium of the blood-vessel ; *lymphangioendothelioma* = tumor of the endothelium of the lymphatic vessel ; *endothelioma* = tumor composed of both endothelial and muscular elements ; *lymphangioma* = tumor of the lymphatic vessels ; *aneurism* = a blood-containing tumor connecting directly with the lumen of the artery or formed by circumscribed enlargement either axial or lateral, of an artery) ligament (*snāyu* perhaps included soft cartilage: *chondroma* = cartilaginous tumor), bone (*osteoma* = bony tumor ; odontoma = tumor of dental structure), joints (*arthromeningitis* = inflammation of the joints ; synovitis = inflammation of the synovial membrane, especially that of a joint), nerve (*snāyu* : *neuroma* = tumor in connection with nerves ; glioma = neuroglial tumor), viscera (*papilloma*, *adenoma* = epithelial tumors ; carcinoma is maligant) and in vital organs." *Suśruta* I. 22. 2[148] .

---

148. त्वङ्मांसशिरास्नाय्वस्थिसन्धिकोष्ठमर्म्माणीत्यष्टौ व्रणवस्तूनि, अत्र सर्व्वव्रणसन्निवेशः ॥ २ सुश्रुतसंहिता, सूत्रस्थानम्, २२ ।

"Now we shall describe the exudation of tumors. If the skin is bruised or lacerated, or in skin-tumors (varicella, acne, eczema etc.), whether spontaneously or when lanced, an aquatic, slightly acid-smelling and light-yellowish exudation (serous fluid mixed with sebaceous secretion) comes out. The evacuation of an abscess in the flesh, is like clarified butter, thick, whitish and slimy (*caseous or cheesy pus*—a very thick, almost solid pus resulting from the absorption of the liquor puris). In a recent incision of a blood vessel there is an excessive bleeding from the vascular swelling ; if it suppurates, the pus flows from it as from a water-pipe (*toya-nāḍi*), thin, unmixed, viscous, flaky (caseous flakes consisting of necrosed or sphacelated cells and fatty acids, floating upon the serous fluid) and has a pale brownish color (*serous or curdy pus*). The exudation from a '*snāyu*' (nerve or ligament tumor) is creamy, thick, mixed with blood and is like the mucous from the nose (*phlegmonous* or *laudable pus* which is a yellowish-white, creamy, thick and odorless liquid). If a bone is wounded or fractured, a kind of pearly white exudation comes out ; but that of an osseous tumor is mixed with bone-marrow, blood and fat (the pus of osseous origin contains fat and often small splinters of bone). If an inflammatory joint (tumous joint) is pressed, no exudation comes out ; but on contraction, extension, standing on the toes, sitting low, pressure sitting, spasmic tension brings out an exudation which is viscous, flaky, foamy and is mixed with blood and pus (suppurated synovia). From the visceral tumors, are evacuated blood, urine, fecal matters, pus and serous fluid (there may be found in pus foreign bodies, tissue fragments, elastic fibers, animal or vegetable parasites, hydatids, actinomycets, organic liquids, bile, milk, urine, fecal matters and alimentary fragments. Their finding is of great importance from a semiological standpoint, indicating as to the origin of pus and as to the possibility of organic fistula). As to the exudations of the tumors of the vital organs, nothing is mentioned, for they belong to the same category of tumors of the skin and flesh (mucous membrane and the muscular and adipose tissues). *Suśruta* I. 22. 6[149].

---

149. अत ऊर्द्ध्वं सर्व्वस्रावान् वक्ष्यामः। तत्र घृष्टासु छिन्नासु वा त्वक्षु स्फोटेषु भिन्नेषु बिदारितेषु वा सलिलप्रकाशो भवत्यास्रावः किञ्चिद्विस्रः पीतावभासश्च। मांसगतः सर्पिःप्रकाशः सान्द्रः श्वेतः पिच्छिलश्च। शिरागतः सद्यश्छिन्नासु शिरासु रक्तातिप्रवृत्तिः पक्कासु च तोयनाड़ीभिरिव तोयागमनं, पूयस्यास्रावश्चात्र तनुर्विच्छिन्नः पिच्छिलोऽवलम्बी श्यावोऽवश्याय-

The color of the pus is no less variable (*Suśruta* IV. 1. 8-17). Usually yellowish, it may be of orange, brownish red or greenish color. There is no suppuration presenting blue color, but it is occasionally seen due to the pigment produced by bacillus pyocyaneus which is not pyogenic by itself. However, there is no relation between the color of the pus and the cause which develops it, but on the locality where it is formed and imbibe the coloring matter, with the only exception of the suppuration of the pneumococcic origin, which is thick, greenish and rich in fibrine, often having the aspect of the false membrane. In subcutaneous or pleural collections the pus is phlegmonous, thick ; in meningeal membranes of the brain, it is greenish ; in the liver, of the chocolate color ; and reddish in the

---

प्रतिमश्च । स्नायुगतः स्निग्धो घनः सिंहाणकप्रतिमः सरक्तश्च । अस्थि-
गतोऽस्थन्यभिहते स्फुटिते भिन्ने दोषावदारिते वा दोषभक्षितत्वादस्थि
निःसारं शुक्तिधौतमिवाभाति । आस्रावश्चात्र मज्जमिश्रः सरुधिरः स्निग्धश्च
सन्धिगतः पीड्यमानो न प्रवर्त्तते, आकुञ्चनप्रसारणोन्नमनविनमनप्रधावनोत्-
कटासनप्रवाहणैश्च स्रवति । आस्रावश्चात्र पिच्छिलोऽवलम्बी सफेनपूय-
रुधिरोन्मथितश्च । कोष्ठगतोऽसृङ्मूत्रपुरीषपूयोदकानि स्रवति । मर्म्मगता-
स्त्वगादिष्ववरुद्धत्वान्नोच्यते ॥ ६

सुश्रुतसंहिता, सूत्रस्थानम्, २२ ।

lung. When it is of osseous origin, it often contains fat and small splinters of bone. If it takes origin in the glands of the skin, it produces a furuncle or a carbuncle--lesion, remarkable for the presence of sphacelated fragments of the cellular tissue, which constitutes the core.

Pyogenic agents : Pyogenic agents which can cause suppuration are numerous. (1) Bacteria habitually pyogenic : Staphylococcus aureus and albus, streptococcus, pneumococcus, colon bacillus and micrococcus tetragens are normally encountered upon our integuments and though in healthy condition of the tissues they usually live a harmless saprophatic or vegetative life, yet when the tissues are damaged or injured, and therefore are incapable of offering natural resistance to encroachment, they are particularly apt to provoke suppuration. Of them staphylococci are the most common pathologic agents, but take nearly 250,000,000 to 1,000,000,000 of them to provoke an abscess. (2) Specific pyogenic bacteria are yet recognized to be only three, namely : gonococcus, the bacillus of soft chancre and the bacillus glanders. (3) Bacteria accidentally pyogenic are those which cause specific and well differentiated lesions of their own, but may, also, cause suppuration under certain conditions, as the tubercle bacillus causes cold abscess, and typhoid bacillus pus in the bone. (4) Pyogenic fungi are the streptothrix, pergillus and odium. (5) The animal pyogenic parasites are the amœbas of dysentery which not only provoke ulcerations of the intestinal mucous membrane, but also abscesses in the liver, and the syphilitic spirocheta which may cause gumma and its ulceration. Gangrene is the morbid process charcterized by the mortification (*necrobiosis*) and the putrefaction of the tissues. The microbes causing gangrene act upon the altered tissues by interrupted circulation, by humoral changes or by the interference of the arterial circulation, especially in the extremities exactly as they would act upon the tissues of the cadavers. But between gangrene and the cadaveric putrefaction, there is this difference, that in the gangrene, the affected parts are still the seat of certain biotic reactions, as all the cells are not equally attacked by the bacteria and quite a few survive; and moreover, there is partial influx of serum, lymph, venous blood and blood pigments and the bacteria attacking the exudate produce new fermentations therein.

"The ingestion of heavy, unsuitable, dry, rotten, or disharmonious combinations of foods, venery, excessive exertion (fatigue), retention of the feces and the urine, and inflammatory beverage provoke bulbous abscess like an ant-hill, either by particular lesion or by their combined effects. In the anus, neck of the bladder, abdomen, axilla and the groin (*bubo*—an inflammatory swelling of the lymphatic gland, usually leading to suppuration), kidneys (*vṛkka*), spleen, liver and the lung abscesses are formed with the symptoms of superficial abscesses (*furuncles or boils*)" *Suśruta* II. 9. 13-14[150].

"In abortion or injurious delivery, a woman suffers with fever 'hyperæmia' from dangerous blood-abscess (*rakta-vidradhi* = *septico-pyemia* : if the entire organism is invaded by bacteria which are usually introduced through the septic handling of the genital puerperal wounds, it is

150. गुर्व्वसात्म्यविरुद्धान्न-शुष्कसंक्लिन्नभोजनात् ।
अतिव्यवायव्यायाम-वेगाघातविदाहिभिः ॥
पृथक् सम्भूय वा दोषाः कुपिता गुल्मरूपिणम् ।
वल्मीकवत् समुन्नद्धमन्तः कुर्व्वन्ति विद्रधिम् ॥ १३
गुदे वस्तिमुखे नाभ्यां कुक्षौ वङ्क्षणयोस्तथा ।
वृक्कयोः प्लीह्नि यकृति हृदये क्लोम्नि वा तथा ॥
तेषां लिङ्गानि जानीयाद्बाह्यविद्रधिलक्षणैः ॥ १४
सुश्रुतसंहिता निदानस्थानम्, ९ ॥

called *septicemia* ; but if the purulent foci are developed as the abscesses in the liver, kidney, lungs, heart etc. which are known as metastatic abscesses, it is called *pyemia.* In the transitory stage of both these morbid processes, it is often called *septico-pyemia.* However septicemia and pyemia are both usually attended by fever, diarrhœa and other symptoms of malaise according to the virulence of the infection and the bodily reaction)". *Suśruta* II. 9. 20[151].

"If any one neglects a suppurated abscess, it burrows through to an interior organ, and as it proceeds like a tube, it is called *'nāḍī-vraṇa'* (*fistular abscess*)." *Suśruta* II. 10. 9[152].

---

151. स्त्रीणामपप्रजातानां प्रजातानां तथाऽहितैः ।
दाहज्वरकरो घोरो जायते रक्तविद्रधिः ॥

सुश्रुतसंहिता, निदानस्थानम्, ९ ।

152. शोफं न पक्वमिति पक्वमुपेक्षते यो
यो वा व्रणं प्रचुरपूयमसाधुवृत्तः ।
अभ्यन्तरं प्रविशति प्रविदार्य्य तस्य
स्थानानि पूर्व्वविहितानि ततः स पूयः ॥
तस्यातिमात्रगमनाद्गतिरित्यतश्च
नाड़ीव यद्वहति तेन मता तु नाड़ी ॥ ९

सुश्रुतसंहिता, निदानस्थानम्, १० ।

"When a rounded and knotted swelling is developed by the corruption of the *'vāta, flesh, blood, serous fluid and the fat'*, it is called *'granthi'* (*cyst*).

In the *'vāta-granthi* (*aneurism*), pains are felt with the sensation that the cyst is being elongated by a gravitating force (expulsive pain), that it is being torn (terebrant p.), that it is being penetrated by needles (boring p.), as if dashed out (tensive p.), as if being lancinated (lancinating p.) or lacerated (lacerating pain) ; it is dark and shaped like the bladder, and if it bursts, pure blood comes out of it (*aneurism* is a blood-containing cyst formed by circumscribed enlargement of an artery through which the blood circulates. Such cysts are distinguished by their expansive pulsation with each systole of the heart, by a thrill to be felt on pulpation and by a *'bruit'* heard on auscultation. As they increase in size, they produce absorption of adjacent structures and give rise to distressing pain by their pressure on nerves, and their final tendency is to burst, and if a large artery is the seat of the cyst, to cause death).

In *'pitta-granthi'* (*hemangioma*), there is hyperemia, and the pain seems to be like that of the application of caustics and cautery : the cyst is of reddish or dark-yellowish color, and if it bursts, very hot blood comes out (*hemangioma* is a blood swelling or cyst due to the dilatation of the blood vessels).

The 'Kapha granthis' (*tubercles*) are cold, pale, slightly painful and are hard like stone, and take a long time for their growth (suppuration); when they burst, a thick whitish pus comes out of them); *tubercles* are ealled cold abscesses or they arouse no local or general reaction. Tubercles appear under three different aspects; gray granulation, Laenneck's tubercle and caseous mass. Gray granulation is a small, hard and non-nuclear nodule, surrounded by a reddish vascular zone and their dimensions vary from 0.5 millimeter to 2 or 3 millimeters. Laenneck's tubercle is more voluminous; it is a round, gray or yellow mass, having the volume of a pea, a hazelnut or a walnut. The caseous masses are greenish-yellow deposits and look like Roquefort cheese. The tubercular abscess may also arise from the breaking down of a tubercular lymphatic vessel).

The 'Meda-granthi' (*lipoma*) is bright, voluminous, slightly painful, but pruritic; it grows with the adiposity of the body, and declines with its decrease; if it bursts, fat like that of the kernel of the sesame or like clarified butter comes out (*lipoma* is a tumor of the fatty tissue, and grows in the subcutaneous tissues, especially in parts subjected to pressure—the shoulders and the buttocks, the abdominal wall and the breast, though it may be present in tissues containing very little fat as the dura matter, submucous tissue of the intestine, as a single or multiple flattened, rounded or pendiculated growth. When large it is always lobulated. The yellowish tissue of the lobules is usually softer and more plastic than the ordinary fatty tissue).

The 'Śirā-granthi' (*cirsoid aneurism*) is developed by the derangement of *'vāyu'* in a weak person through wrestling which causes arterial distension, distortion or contortion and elevates them (the arteries) like lotus stems, and makes of them roundish tumors ; if these tumors are painful and temporary, they can be cured with difficulty, but if they are painless, permanent, voluminous or developed in the vital organs, they are incurable (*cirsoid aneurism* is a tumor-like collection of dilated and elongated arteries. In the majority of cases, aneurisms are due to weakening of the arterial walls by arteriosclerosis. If the latter is diffuse, the dilatation is generally fusiform and irregular ; if circumscribed, the yielding is succular. Of the causes of the sclerotic changes, syphilis is the most important in producing aneurism. Prolonged high arterial tension as in laborious muscular work, cardiac hypertrophy, a great and sudden strain as in heavy lifting, violent coughing or straining may initiate the dilatation if, the coats are weakened by previous disease).

At the maxillary, clavicular, axillary, humero-ulnar (and radial, i. e. elbow), scapulo-clavicular (back-neck), and hyoid-thyroid-cartilaginous (front neck) joints, due to the accumution of fat, a solid and rounded tumor (*exostosis or osteoma*) or causes slightly painful fatty and serous inflammation ; if the tumor resembles the stone of myrobalan or the fish-roe, or any such similar substance and has the color of the skin, it is called *'apachi'* (*exostosis*) because of its swelling. Exostosis is pruritic and slightly painful ; some of them (exostosises) exudate when torn (or incised). It lasts for a long time, its nodules being destroyed and renewed. This disease develops from *'fat and kapha'* and is very hard to cure (*osteomas* and osteomatoid conditions, in which there is localized or general overgrowth of the bone, are of common occurrence. Both groups are found chiefly at the point of junction of a bone and its cartilage, fasciæ, periosteum, tendons and the ligaments, in the pia matter and the dura matter in the choroid and sclerotic coats of the eye at the apex of the lungs, in the skin and the mucous membrane, and sometimes even in the penis and in muscular tissues. They are usually divided into two groups, the exostosis, or those growing from the surface of the bone, and enostoses or those growing within the bone. And again they may be divided according to their structure, into eburnated exostosis intensely hard like that of the cement of the tooth and spongy or cauliflower exostosis).

Due to some lesion, the tissues become affected, and a rounded, solid neoplasm slightly painful, voluminous, and deep-seated but with slender base, grows without suppuration ; it is called *arvvuda* (*tumor, neoplasm or cancer*).

Due to contraction of the blood-vessels and the blood, owing to a papilliferous, slightly ulcerative and exudative meat-ball (*neoplasm*) is ferm which, grows rapidly ane causes incessant bleeding. This is called'*rakta-arvvuda*' (*papilloma*). Due to the complications (sequels) arising from the loss of blood, the papilloma victim becomes anemic. It is an incurable disease (*papilloma* is any abnormal excrescence having a villous structure, but more properly a tumor of the skin or of the mucous membrane, either sessile or pedunculated, consisting of hypertrophied or new-formed papillæ, covered by an envelope of the epithelial cells separately on each papillæ, so as to produce a villous or filiform appearance. Papilloma is usually benign but if neglected, it may form the starting point or be converted into benignant '*epithelioma*'. Also a destructive papilloma is known which is probably a carcinomatous form, and which is ulcerative and in which the papillary growth upon the surface extends into and destroys the subjacent tissues.

If any part of the body is lacerated by a blow, there is developed a painless, bright, skin-colored, non-suppurative, stone-hard and fixed tumor, due to the lesion of the tissues; and it is called *māṃsa arvvuda*, (*myxoma* usually occur in submucous, subcutaneous or other connective tissues in the intermuscular septa between the bundles of nerves, in periosteum and in sub-serous fat, and has the general character of tumors of this group).. If a myxoma victim partakes of meat. this tumor becomes thickened and incurable. And of the benign-symptomatic tumors those which are infiltrative (or malignant breast tumors) are incurable.

Of the above-mentioned tumors those which are exudative or develop in the vital organs or in the vessels (arterial, venous, lymphatic or nervous) or those which do not move (suppurate ?) are incurable. If a new tumor developes on another, it is called *'adhyarvvuda'* (secondary or proliferation tumors that develop adjacent to each other as pairs are called *'dvir-arvvuda'* (double tumors). It is also incurable".
"*Suśruta* II. 11. 2-15.[153]

---

153. वातादयो मांसमसृक् प्रदुष्टाः सन्दूष्य मेदश्च कफानुविद्धम् ।
वृत्तोन्नतं विग्रथितन्तु शोथं कुर्व्वन्त्यतो ग्रन्थिरिति प्रदिष्टः ॥ १५२
आयम्यते व्यथ्यत एति तोदं प्रत्यस्यते कृत्यत एति भेदम् ।
कृष्णोऽमृदुर्वस्तिरिवाततश्च भिन्नः स्रवेच्चानिलजोऽस्रमच्छम् ॥ ३
दन्दह्यते धूप्यति चातिमात्रं पापच्यते प्रज्वलतीव चापि ।
रक्तः सपीतोऽप्यथवापि पित्ताद्भिन्नः स्रवेदुष्णमतीव चास्रम् ॥ ४
शीतोऽविवर्णोऽल्परुजोऽतिकण्डूः पाषाणवत् संहननोपपन्नः ।
चिराभिवृद्धिश्च कफप्रकोपाद्भिन्नः स्रवेच्छुक्लघनञ्च पूयम् ॥ ५
शरीरवृद्धिक्षयवृद्धिहानिः स्निग्धो महानल्परुजोऽतिकण्डूः ।
मेदःकृतो गच्छति चातिभिन्ने पिण्याकसर्पिःप्रतिमन्तु मेदः ॥ ६
व्यायामजातैरबलस्य तैस्तैराक्षिप्य वायुर्हि शिराप्रतानम् ।
संपीड्य सङ्कोच्य विशोष्य वापि ग्रन्थिं करोत्युन्नतमाशु वृत्तम् ॥

"A neoplasm or tumor is a new formation of tissue, which is atypical in structnre, serves no useful purpose in the whole economy and the growth of which has no typical termination." According to Cohnheim there remains in the adult enough of unappropriated embryonic residues which if activated by any mechanical or microbic irritant outstrip the normal calculus growth and form a tumor possessing an unutilized and consequently an exaggerated power of proliferation. But the cells of the malignant neoplasms are themselves capable of starting new growths (*metastases*) if carried to

---

ग्रन्थिः शिराजः स तु कृच्छ्रसाध्यो भवेद्यदि स्यात् सरुजश्चलश्च ।
अरुक् स एवाप्यचलो महांश्च मर्म्मोत्थितश्चापि विवर्ज्जनीयः ॥ ७
हन्वस्थिकक्षाक्षकबाहुसन्धि-मन्यागलेषूपचितन्तु मेदः ।
ग्रन्थिं स्थिरं वृत्तमथायतं वा स्निग्धं कफश्चाल्परुजं करोति ॥ ८
तं ग्रन्थिभिश्चामलकास्थिमात्रैर्मत्स्याण्डजालप्रतिमैस्तथान्यैः ।
अनन्यवर्णैरुपचीयमानं चयप्रकर्षादपचीं वदन्ति ॥ ९
कण्डूयुतास्तेऽल्परुजः प्रभिन्नाः स्रवन्ति नश्यन्ति भवन्ति चान्ये ।
मेदःकफाभ्यां खलु रोग एष सुदुस्तरो वर्षगणानुबन्धी ॥ १०
गात्रप्रदेशे क्वचिदेव दोषाः संमूर्च्छिता मांसमसृक् प्रदूष्य ।
वृत्तं स्थिरं मन्दरुजं महान्तमनल्पमूलं चिरवृद्ध्यपाकम् ॥
कुर्व्वन्ति मांसोपचयञ्च शोफं तदर्ब्बुदं शास्त्रविदो वदन्ति ।

सुश्रुतसंहिता, निदानस्थानम्, ११ ।

distant parts by circulation, as a malignant tumor of the breast may start new cancers far removed from the original lesion into the lungs, ribs, brain and the abdomen through the lymphatic current. No microbic agent has yet been definitely identified with the tissues of the malignant tumor, though *'micrococcus neoforfans'* has been found in both benign and malignant neoplasms. However, the probability is that there is a specific pathogenic cancerous agent. Fortunately all neoplasms are not dangerous. The benign tumors are entirely harmless unless they are situated in a sensitive position, where by their growth they might cause pressure on the nerves or displace the vital organs. And they never reproduce themselves in distant parts by grafting like the malignant growths. And the fundamental difference between the two types, though the process of their growth has the same tendency of exxaggerated, abnormal proliferation and multiplication of their own cells, lies in the fact that the benign tumor does not eat its way into the surrounding tissues, but remains closed in its own fibrous capsule. While a malignant tumor infilters into the neighboring tissues, causes destruction of the healthy cells, creates an ulcerative zone and therein transplants a new colony.

But only sarcoma, endothelioma and carcinoma are malignant. However, between benign adenoma and malignant epithelioma there exist numerous transitions, and under certain circumstances, a benign tumor may turn into the malignant type as '*destructive papilloma*'. And though tumors may be observed in all ages, yet their frequency and nature vary considerably at different periods of life. In the defective development of the embryo, angiomata are frequently met. During early life sacromata are observed, located chiefly in the kidneys. At puberty exostoses are frequent. In women at a later period, ovarian cysts belonging to the group of adenomata and epitheliomata are encountered. From the age of fourteen onward, epithelioma becomes more and more common, reaching its maximum of frequency between the age of fifty and fifty-five years. Age exercises no less influence upon the localization than upon the nature of the tumors. In children, they affect, in order of frequency, the eye where melanotic sarcoma is met with, the kidney, testicles and spleen. In adults the part of the body most frequently attacked is the stomach, uterus, liver, mamma and the intestine in the order mentioned. It is certain that the irritation alone, microbic or mechanical,is not sufficient to develop tumor unless the organism is predisposed to it by heredity, or has aquired this characteristic through some morbid process of pathogenesis which is not yet understood.

The abscess (*Vraṇa*, *furuncle*, boil or carbuncle, differs from the furuncle or the boil in various points. (I) It generally occurs singly and usually appears at the back of the neck, the back or the buttocks. (2) It is very large in size like a hen's egg or even larger. (3) It contains more than one core (necrotic tissue or suppuration points as in furuncle), due to (corruption) of the '*vāyu*, '*pitta*, *kapha and the blood*', produces intense · burning, throbbing, tremulous and pricking pain, hyperæmia, suppuration, redness, swelling and hyperesthesia; and it causes various kinds of pain and exudation." *Suśruta* IV. I. 20[154].

"There are sixty treatments of '*vraṇa*' (suppurative tumor, especially furuncle) as follows: *fasting* (*apatarpaṇa*) to facilitate the elimination of the toxic and the effete matter circulating in

---

154. निर्द्दहननिर्म्मथनस्फुरणतोददाह-पाक-राग-कण्डू-स्वाप-वहुलो नाना-वर्णवेदनाश्रावविशेषोपेतः पवनपित्तकफशोणितेभ्यः ॥ २०

सुश्रुतसंहिता, चिकित्सास्थानम्, १ ।

the blood which predisposes the tissues to pyogenic infection), *epithem* (*ālepa*, to spread over the boil to releive pain, congestion, to focalize the inflammation and to bring out suppuration), *lotion* (*pariṣeka*, to wash the inflamed part for asepsis and to relieve pain), *salve* (*abhyaṅga* to smear over as an antiseptic and analgesic), *fomentation* (*śveda*, as an analgesic and suppurantia), *emollient* (*vimlāpana*, to soften and beat the boil), *cataplasm* (*upanāha*, as a suppurantia), *suppurantia* (*pāchana*, to cause early suppuration), *leeching* (*visrāvaṇa*, to apply sucking leeches to relieve congestion), *emulsion* (*sneha*, as a stimulating nourishment), *emetic* (*vamana*, to remove gastric irritants), *dissection* (*chhedana*, to remove the ulcerative parts of a non-suppurative tumor), *incision* (*vedana*= lancing to cause the drainage of the pus), *scarification* (*dāraṇa*, to soften the skin so as to cause spontaneous bursting of the abscess in the timid women and children who are afraid of lances and incision), *evacuation* (*lekhana*, to scratch and to wipe out the impacted caseous pus from the abscess cavity), *exploration* (*eṣaṇa* to find out the nature of the abscess cavity in a fistula), *extraction* (*āharaṇa*, to extract any foreign body from an abscess),*puncture* (*vyadhana*, exploratory puncture of a cavity or a tumor with a hollow needle to determine the presence or absence of fluid or gas, and its nature, if present), *suction* (*vidrāvaṇa*, to suck the liquid pus and exudation from an abscess cavity or serous fluid from hydrocele or ascites through a tube by exhausting the air in the front), *suture* (*sīvana*, to reunite by stitching a wide-gaping, non-suppurative wound with a silk-thread), *appositional reunion* (*sandhāna*, to put the wounded and operated parts in their proper place and to unite them together), *compressive epithem* (*pīḍana*, an epithem that draws the pus to the surface), *hemostatic* (*śoṇitāsthāpana*, to arrest bleeding of a wound), lenitive (*nirvvāpaṇa*, to soothe and to relieve irritation), medicinal *fomentation* (*utkārikā*, to provoke suppuration), *antiseptic astringent* (*kaṣāya*, to cleanse the wound-cavity), *collyrium* (*vartti*, as disinfectant),*mucilaginous paste* (*kalka*, as a disinfectant), *ointment* (*ghṛta*, as depurant), *oil* (*taila*, as depurant), *chemical action* [*rasa-kriyā*, of sesame decoction, thickened and made into paste with the mixture of iron sulphide (*surāṣṭrajāṃ sakāsīsāṃ*), *arsenic disulphide* (*manaḥśilā*) and arsenic *trisulphide* (*haritāla*)] to be applied to the abscess—*Suśruta* IV. I. 59], fine *bland powder* (*avachūrṇana*, as a deodorant), *fumigation* (*vraṇa-dhūpana*, to expose the abscess cavity to medicinal gases), *vulnerary* (*utsādana*, to promote healing and cicatrization), *inunction* (*avasādana*, to promote tissue formation and normal circulation in the cicatrized area), *emollient* (*mṛdu-karma*, to soften the skin), *tissue-hardener* (*dāruṇa karma*, to harden the tissues with tannic astringents), caustic (*kṣāra-karma* destroy a long standing ulcer, which is hard to cure), *cautery* (*agni-karma*, to scar the ulcerated tissues which do not easily cure, especially in the bladder and the joints), *pigmentary* (*kṛṣṇa-karma*, to promote pigment cells in the pale cicatrised area), *pigmento-lysin* (*pāṇḍu-karma*, to destroy the pigment, in order to bleach the darkened area), *pigment-normalizer* (*pratisāraṇa*, to normalise the skin-color of the affected area), hair-grower (*roma-sañjanana*, to promote the growth of hair, where the hair follicles have been destroyed), *depilatory* (*lomāpaharaṇa*, to cause the falling out of hair where it is not desirable, or by shaving), *clyster* (*vasti-karma*, as an antiseptic injection in a deep-seated abscess), *irrigation* (*uttara-vasti*, to wash out the purulent deep-seated abscess cavity), *bandage* (*vanda*, to protect the wound from microbic infection), *plaster* (*patra-dāna*, as a pepastic), *germicide* (*kṛmighna*, as a destructive agent of the microbes), detoxicants (*viṣaghna*), *stimulants* (*vṛṃhaṇa*, to activate the organism to fight against the disease, to throw off the toxins and to restore health) *sedatives* (*ṣiro-virechana*, to remove congestion from the upper parts of the body, in case of abscesses there), *snuff* (*nasya*, as a sedative), *mouth-wash* (*kavala-dhāraṇa*, as a disinfectant in stomatitis), *fumigation* (*dhūma*, exposure to the action of a disinfectant smoke), *analeptic* (*madhu-sarpi*, a restoration), *operation* (*yantra*, to operate where there is a foreign body in the wound and its mouth is narrow), *dietary* (*āhāra*, light and stimulating foods), and *hygiene* (*rakṣā-vidhāna*, as curative and preventive). "*Suśruta* IV. 1. 22. ; 59[155].

155. तस्य व्रणस्य षष्टिरुपक्रमा भवन्ति। तद्यथा—अपतर्पणमालेपः परिषेकोऽभ्यङ्गः स्वेदो विम्लापनमुपनाहः पाचनं विस्रावणं स्नेहो वमनं विरेचनं छेदनं भेदनं दारणं लेखनमेषणमाहरणं व्यधनं विद्रावणं सीवनं सन्धानं पीड़नं शोणितास्थापनं निर्व्वापणमुत्कारिका कषायो वर्त्तिः कल्कः सर्पिस्तैलं रसक्रियावचूर्णनं व्रणधूपनमुत्सादनमवसादनं मृदुकर्म्म दारुणकर्म्म क्षारकर्म्माग्निकर्म्म कृष्णकर्म्म पाण्डुकर्म्म प्रतिसारणं रोमसञ्जननं लोमापहरणं वस्तिकर्म्मोत्तरवस्तिकर्म्म वन्धः पत्रदानं कृमिघ्नं वृंहणं विषघ्नं शिरोविरेचनं नस्यं कवलधारणं धूमो मधुसर्पिर्यन्त्रमाहारो रक्षाविधानम् इति॥ २२

सुश्रुतसंहिता, चिकित्सितस्थानम्, १।

"After the above-mentioned treatment, if the inflammation is found to be of a suppurative kind, then by the application of a pustulant, it has to be made to suppurate, then lanced and disinfected." *Suśruta* IV. 16. 4[156].

Etiology : Furuncle or boil is not possible without the infection of staphylococcus pyogenes aureus which is invariably found in the pus. This gives rise to acute inflammation and exudation, leading to necrosis of the tissue. The infection of the staphylococcus pyogenes aureus is favored by the impairment of the tissue vitality, which is the natural consequence if the blood contains toxic, irritant or effete matters. In that case, the tissues are not only ill-nourished, and therefore incapable to offer natural resistance to microbic invasion, but

---

व्रणानां स्थिरमांसानां कुर्य्याद्‌द्रव्यैर्व्दीरितैः ।
कषायैर्विधिवत् तेषां कृते व्यामिश्रयेत् पुनः ॥
सुराष्ट्रजां सकासीसां दद्याच्चापि मनःशिलाम् ।
हरितालञ्च मतिमांस्ततस्तामवचारयेत् ॥ ५९

सुश्रुतसंहिता, चिकित्सितस्थानम्, १ ।

156. वेशवारैः सकृशरैः पयोभिः पायसैस्तथा ।
स्वेदयेत सततञ्चापि निर्हरेच्चापि शोणितम् ॥ ३

सुश्रुतसंहिता, चिकित्सितस्थानम्, १६ ।

especially when the kidney fails to eliminate the effete and the toxic substances in the blood, the burden falls on the skin as an emunctory organ. This naturally irritates the skin and predisposes it to the infection of staphylococcus which is ubiquitous causing furuncles, boils and carbuncles. And they are usually associated with the diseases, especially if the renal functions have been impaired, as in chronic dyspepsia, gout, rheumatism, scrofula, tuberculosis, diabetes and albuminuria. It is frequently met with in dyspepsia in which there is insufficiency or deficiency of the pepsin and the trypsin, especially the latter, leading to albuminous putrefaction, whose toxic products are absorbed into the blood, and are thrown over to the skin for elimination when the kidney alone is not equal to the task.

Therefore special attention should be paid to dietary and cleanliness. Fresh, healthy, wholesome light and easily digestible food should be taken in restricted quantity, especially of the albumins. All irritant foods, drinks and spices must be avoided. Whey or butter-milk which by its lactic acid producing content (*lactose*) counteracts putrefaction by changing the culture medium of the proteolytic bacteria is a very preferable addition to the diet, or an exclusive diet for a few days.

"A '*ślesma*' tumor which has not been remedied by any application, and which has not grown in any vital organ, should be dissected, extirpated, in its premature state. the wound cauterized and treated as any fresh wound. *Suśruta* IV. 18. 8[157].

"A tumor in its premature state (that is, it should be operated as early as possible) should be excised and cauterised. Or as according to the previous insrtuction, it should be scratched out, and the caustics should be applied to the wound. "*Suśruta* IV. 18. 16[158].

"If the neoplasm is not deep-rooted, then with a (wire) of tin (*trapu*), copper, lead or silk (cord) it should be surrounded, and carefully

---

157. असमर्म्मजातं श्लेष्मप्रजातमपक्वमेवापहरेद्विदार्य्य ।
दहेत् स्थिते वाप्यथ सिद्धकर्म्मा सद्यःक्षतोक्तञ्च विधिं विदध्यात् ॥ ८
सुश्रुतसंहिता, चिकित्सितस्थानम् , १८ ।

158. ग्रन्थीनमर्म्मप्रभवानपक्वानुद्धृत्य चाग्निं विदधीत पश्चात् ।
क्षारेण वापि प्रतिसारयेत्तु संलिख्य शस्त्रेण यथोपदेशम् ॥ १६
सुश्रुतसंहिता, चिकित्सास्थानम , १८ ।

the physician should use the knife, caustic or cautery, according to the strength of the patient. *Suśruta* IV. 18. 29[158a].

"If any part of the neoplasm remains and is not completely extirpated, then from the remnant the neoplasm reappears, as fire can grow from a small spark left-over; therefore all the growth (of the neoplasm) must be extirpated". *Suśruta* IV. 18. 33[159].

There is no question that the complete extirpation of either the benign or the malignant neoplasm is the best remedy, wherever possible, that is when they have not developed with a deep base in any vital organ.

VII —*Skin Disease.**

Prodromes of Leprosy :—"The thickening of

158a. यदल्पमूलं त्रपुताम्रसीस-पट्टैः समावेष्ट्य तदायसैर्वा ॥
क्षाराग्निशस्त्राण्यसकृद्विदध्यात् प्राणानहिंसन् भिषगप्रमत्तः ॥ २९
सुश्रुतसंहिता, चिकित्सितस्थानम्, १८।

159. सशेषदोषाणि हि योऽर्बुदानि करोति तान्याशु पुनर्भवन्ति।
तस्मादशेषाणि समुद्धरेत् तु हन्युः सशेषाणि यथा हि वह्निः ॥ ३३
सुश्रुतसंहिता, चिकित्सितस्थानम्, १८।

* The writer regrets that he lacks the clinical ex-

the skin, sudden horripilation, pruritus, hyperidrosis or anhydrosis, anesthesia of the skin, the extension of ulceration if any wound takes place, and the dark color of the blood are the prodromes of '*Kuṣṭha*' (*leprosy*)." *Suśruta* II. 5. 2[160].

"In the '*vāta*' leprosy, the lepromes are browny and slender with boring pain and anesthesia ; it is called '*aruṇa*' sun-colored '*lepra flava*' In the '*pitta*' leprosy, the nodosities are like the

---

perience of skin disease, especially the tropical dermatosis, and the diseases of the genital organs. His knowledge is limited to the studies of authorities on these subjects. And moreover as the cutaneous manifestations are hard to identify without the associated symptoms, and both Charaka and Sus ́ruta have given vague description of them, only those diseases will be mentioned which have a direct bearing on the history of syphilis in ancient India. It is very likely that the papulo-squamous syphilide, pustulo-crustaceous syphilide, tubercular syphilitic dactylitis, exostoses, osteo-periostitis, nodes, gummata and ulcerations have been classified as leprous manifestations or varieties of leprosy.

160. तस्य पूर्व्वरूपाणि त्वक्पारुष्यमकस्माद्रोमहर्षः कण्डूः स्वेदबाहुल्यमस्वेदनं व्यङ्गप्रदेशानां स्वापः क्षतविसर्पणमसृजः कृष्णता चेति ॥ २

सुश्रुतसंहिता, निदानस्थानम, ५ ।

ripe fruit of '*ficus glomarata*'; this is called '*auḍamvara*' leprosy (*lepra nodosities*, rounded, hemispherical, varying in size from a pin's head to a hazel-nut, hard and elastic to the touch, pale-red or brown in color, may appear from the beginning without any antecedent patches, scattered over the body, especially on the face, forehead, elbows, knees and legs). In the '*ṛṣya-jihva*' leprosy, it (*the lepra erythematous patch*) has the size and the roughness of antelope's tongue. Black scales appear in '*kapāla*' (*scabby leprosy : psoriasis*). Black-red patches like those of the fruit of '*abrus precatorius*' appear in '*kākaṇaka*' (*lepra nigricuns*, black in the centre and reddish at the edges as in the '*kākaṇaka*' fruit). Heat, tensive pain, hyperæmia and cloudy sensation (disturbances of the cutaneous nerves) are felt in these four kinds of leprosy. With microbes bullæ appear, burst and ulcerate.

'*Pauṇḍarika*' (*nodes*) are shaped like the lotus leaves; '*dadru*' is copper-colored or like that of the flower of '*linum usitaliosimum*' (dark) and the nodes continue to grow covered with herpes. The nodes of both '*pauṇḍarika* and *dadru*' are elevated, globular and pruritic and they take a long time for their growth. These are their general symptoms.

Minor *'kuṣṭha'*: Hard, broad-based, thick and dry nodules develop at the joints in *'sthūla-rukṣa'* (*dry leprosy*). There is contraction of the skin (the skin thickens by infiltration and forms deep sulci by folding on itself), boring pain and anesthesia in *'mahā-kuṣṭha'* (*anesthetic leprosy*). The disease in which the skin becomes dark-brown (bronzed) is called *'eka-kuṣṭha* (Addison's disease); this is incurable. In *'charmadala-kuṣṭha'* (tinea albigena ?) there are pruritus, tremor, tensive and burning pain in the palms of the hands and soles of the feet. The leprosy in which the skin, blood and the flesh become affected, and spread over the body, like erysipelas (*visarpa*), and which causes swooning, burning sensation, nervousness, pricking pain and ulceration, is called *'visarpa-kuṣṭha'* (cutaneous leprosy). The leprosy in which exudative bullæ repeatedly spread over the body is called *'parisarpa'* (*macular leprosy*). The skin lesion, in which there is pruritic, whitish, painless and scattered (*tanu=thin*) eruption in the upper part of the body, is called *'sidhma-kuṣṭha'*. The skin lesion in which very pruritic, painful and dry patches appear over the entire body, is called *'vicharchikā'* ; if this very pruritic and painful manifestation appears only on the foot, it is called '*vipādikā*' (*psoriasis*). The skin lesion which is exudative, globular, superficial, very pruritic, shiny and dark, is called '*kiṭima*' (acne *keloid*). If exudative, pruritic, inflammatory and tiny pustule appears over the entire body, it is called '*pāmā*' (*eczema*). If the '*pāmā*' becomes suppurative, it is called '*kachchhu*', '*pyosis tropica*'. Pruritic but non-exudative pustules that appear over the entire body, are called '*rakasā*' (dry eczema). *Suśruta* II. 5. 7-10[161].

---

161. तत्र वातेनारुणाभानि तनूनि विसर्पीणि तोदभेदस्वापयुक्तान्यरुणानि । पित्तेन पक्वोडुम्बरफलाकृतिवर्णान्यौडुम्बराणि ; ऋष्यजिह्वाप्रकाशखरत्वानि ऋष्यजिह्वानि ; कृष्णकपालिकाप्रकाशानि कपालकुष्ठानि ; काकणन्तिकाफलसदृशान्यतीव रक्तकृष्णानि काकणकानि । तेषां चतुर्णामप्योषचोषपरिदाहधूमायनानि क्षिप्रोत्थानप्रपाकभेदित्वानि क्रिमिजन्म च सामान्यानि लिङ्गानि ॥ ७

पुण्डरीकपत्रप्रकाशानि पौण्डरीकाणि ; अतसीपुष्पवर्णानि ताम्राणि वा विसर्पीणि पिड़कावन्ति च दद्रुकुष्ठानि । तयोर्द्वयोरप्युत्सन्नता परिमण्डलता कण्डूश्चिरोत्थानत्वञ्चेति सामान्यरूपाणि ॥ ८

क्षुद्रकुष्ठान्यत ऊर्द्ध्वं वक्ष्यामः ॥ ९

स्थूलानि सन्धिष्वतिदारुणानि स्थूलाकृति स्युः कठिनान्यरूंषि ।
त्वक्कोचभेदस्वपनाङ्गसादाः कुष्ठे महत्पूर्व्वयुते भवन्ति ॥
कृष्णारुणं येन भवेच्छरीरं तदेककुष्ठं प्रवदन्त्यसाध्यम् ।
स्युर्येन कण्डूव्यथनौषचोषास्तलेषु तच्चर्म्मदलं वदन्ति ॥
विसर्पवत् सर्पति सर्व्वतो यस्त्वग्रक्तमांसान्यभिभूय शीघ्रम् ।
मूर्च्छाविदाहारतितोदपाकान् कृत्वा विसर्पः स भवेद्विकारः ॥

"When the microbes begin to eat up the skin etc., various symptoms appear according to the nature of the lesion. Due to '*vāta*', (*lepromas*) become pale-white or sun-colored, rough and dry, and there are boring pain, emaciation, piercing pain, tremor, wrinkles of the skin, horripilation, lassitude, paralysis, anesthesia, gangrene and mutilations (of extremities). Due to '*pitta*' the following symptoms manifest, as burning sensation, sweating, effusion, decomposition (of the tissues), exudation, ulceration and bloody color (of the sores). From '*śleṣmā*' the following symptoms manifest as chilliness, whiteness (of the macular patches), pruritus, hardness (of the nodes), heaviness, elevation (of the nodes, thickening and folding of the skin), fattiness (fatty infiltration) and (ulcerous) crusts.

शनैः शरीरे पीड़काः स्रवन्त्यः सर्पन्ति यास्तं परिसर्पमाहुः ।
कण्ड्वन्वितं श्वेतमपायि सिध्म विद्यात् तनु प्रायश ऊर्द्ध्वकाये ॥
राज्योऽतिकण्ड्वर्त्तिरुजः सुरूक्षा भवन्ति गात्रेषु विचर्च्चिकायाम् ।
कण्डूमती दाहरुजोपपन्ना विपादिका पादगतेयमेव ॥
यत् स्रावि वृत्तं घनमुग्रकण्डू तत् स्निग्धकृष्णं किटिभं वदन्ति ।
सास्रावकण्डूपरिदाहवद्भिः पामाणुकाभिः पिड़काभिरुक्ता ॥
स्फोटैः सदाहैरति सैव कच्छुः स्फिक्पाणिपादप्रभवैर्निरुप्या ।
कण्ड्वन्विता या पिड़का शरीरे संस्रावहीना रकसोच्यते सा ॥ १०

चरकसंहिता, निदानस्थानम् ५ ।

"When the microbes eat up slowly the four (layers) of the skin (epidermis, corium, muesum and corneum), vessels and nerves (*śirā*), tendons and tender bones, then there are other complicating leprous symptoms as exudation, gangrene, deformations, polydipsia, fever, diarrhœa hyperæmia, debility, anorexia and indigestion, in which it becomes incurable". *Charaka* II. 5. 15-16[162].

Leprosy is caused by Hansen's '*bacillus lepræ*' which morphologically has a very striking resemblance to the tubercular bacillus, but according to Jamanito, the tubercular bacillus is stained black by the silver nitrate method, while the '*bacillus lepræ*' remain transparent. However, a large percentage of the lepers are found either tubercular or syphilitic. And these three diseases are very alike in their evolution and it is very hard often to diagnose one from the other without differential diagnosis. The '*lepra bacilli*' are found in all diseased tissues, in nasal, salivary, vaginal and urethral secretions, tears,

162. क्रिमयस्तु त्वगादींश्चतुरः सिराश्चाय चास्थीन्यपिच तरुणानि खादन्ति। अस्याञ्चैवावस्थायां कुष्ठिनमुपद्रवाः स्पृशन्ति। तद्यथा प्रस्रवणमङ्गभेदः पतनान्यङ्गाक्यवानां तृष्णाज्वरातिसारदाह-दौर्बल्यारोचकाविपाकाश्च तथाविधमसाध्यं विद्यादिति।

चरकसंहिता, निदानस्थानम्, ५।

sputum, semen, macular scales, exudation or discharges from the sores. It seems that the lepra bacillus takes a long period for the evolution of leprosy and incubation is very slow lasting from 2 to 20 years. The lepra bacillus is infectious, but its contagion is not of a virulent type, as is demonstrated by the fact that usually the attendants at the leper asylums with cleanliness of the body, hygienic living and nutritious dietary, escape from this loathsome malady. On the other hand it is undeniable that the segregation of the lepers in Norway, Hawaii and the Philippine Islands have shown a very promising result, in not only arresting the spread of leprosy, but also tending to uproot the disease entirely as it has been done in Europe. However, the mode of its infection is not yet known. It seems the lepra germs find a favorable medium for growth, like tubercular bacilli, in an organism devitalized by malnutrition, uncleanliness and unhygienic living. And that perhaps explains how with improved living and hygiene, it has practically died out of Europe. It is usually found in the East among the poorer classes who suffer from chronic malnutrition and live in unhygienic surroundings in the midst of filth and misery. The tissues therefore lack the resisting power against the invasion of the *'lepra bacilli'* though they possess but feeble virulence.

There are three froms of leprosy : (I) *'tubercular leprosy*, (2) *muculo-anesthetic leprosy* and (3) *mixed leprosy*. In the tubercular form, there are repeated attacks of fever as a reaction of the organism against the invasion of the lepra bacilli. There may be pruritus and hyperesthesia of the skin with neuralgic pain in all locations. In most cases there is a premonitory eruption of vesicles or bullæ, affecting the extremities chiefly. These bullæ appear rapidly, are usually painless, break spontaneously, and often heal as ulcers, leaving behind a pigmented spot, brown, black, or white. Spots gradually make thus their appearance in various parts of the body, and the macular eruption is more frequent as the disease progresses. This may continue for months or years according to the resisting power of the organism. The small tubercles appear, grow in size and become confluent. They may simply ulcerate, without marked destruction of tissue, leaving small superficial ulcers, covered with greenish or brown crusts, destroying by degrees the adjacent tissues, tendons, ligaments, and finally the bones. If treated, they cicatrize and produce deformities; but if neglected, they suppurate, and cause amyloidosis or gangrene. Almost from the beginning the senses are disturbed.

In the maculo-anesthetic or tropho-neurotic form of leprosy, the infiltration principally takes place into the nerves, causing their gradual irritation, inflammation, degeneration and destruction. In the first inflammatory stage, there is hyperesthesia, sensory, vaso-motor and motor disturbances manifested by burning numbness, formication (*sensory*), flushings of the face, glossy skin (*vaso-motor*), twitchings of the muscles (motor) particularly of the face, paroxysms of neuralgic pain and cutaneous manifestation. This is gradually succeeded by a period of nerve degeneration, marked clinically by anesthesia, paralysis, atrophies and distinct trophic disturbances. With the anesthesia, there appears a muscle-atrophy which first of all attacks the muscles of the hand (causing contraction), the extensors and flexors of the forearm, causing the charecteristic '*claw-hand*'. There is loss of power, sense of touch, of heat and cold, even of pain. The muscles of the feet are likewise affected. There is a variety of trophic disturbances at this stage —shedding of the nails, loss of pigment, loss of hair, loss of teeth, ulceration, followed by dry gangrene, necrosis and absorption of the bone with the resultant mutilation.

The '*mixed*' is really the typical form of leprosy, combining the tubercular and tropho-neurotic manifestations, and the symptoms of both types are present. Of course lepra bacillus is found in all cases in all leprous lesions, whether located in the skin, mucous membranes, nerves or internal organs. Malnutrition, uncleanliness, infections of tuberculosis or syphilis which are found among a large percentage of the lepers, not only predispose the organism to leprosy, but also accelerate the progress of this malignant disease and hasten death.

Treatment :—"For a pious leper who wishes to live and for whom the five methods of treatment have not been effective, the wise physician should treat him in the following manner :—Ripe fruits should be collected, in the rainy season of the '*tubara*' (*Faractogenos Kurzii:-chaulmugra*) tree which grows on the southern sea-coast (*Arakan*) and whose branches are agitated by the wind, raised by the ocean waves ; the kernel of the fruits is to be taken out, dried and made into fragments. And then they should be pressed in a mill like the sesame-oil press, or the oil extracted in a basin as with the saffron flower (*crocus sativus*). This should be put on fire (in a kettle) and when all the water has been evaporated from the oil, it ought to be taken out and placed (in a flask) in dried cow-dung for a fortnight. When the patient has been fattened by the treatment of oils, sweated by diaphoretics, cleansed (internally) by purgatives and emetics, then in a lunar auspicious evening, he should drink the oil, consecrated with the hymn that the essence of the kernel is the antidote of all poisons, etc. The '*tubara*' (*chaulmugra*) oil causes repeated evacuations of the toxin (of the leprous lesion) through the upper and lower channels (*chaulmugra oil* is very irritant, and causes vomiting and purgation. It should be given in a capsule, or better still, to be effective, ethyl ester preparations of the fatty acids of the '*chaulmugra oil*' can be administered intramuscularly with the hypodermic syringe with marvellous results). After this cold barley water should be drunk without any salt (which provokes vomiting) and fat (which stimulates peristalsis). Thus he shall drink for five days the oil, and for a fortnight giving up all injurious habits as anger etc., shall live on rice and the broth of '*mudga*' (phaseolus mungo, both of them are constipative). If thus for five days the patient drinks the oil, he gets cured of all kinds of leprosy. If this '*tubara*' oil is cooked together as before with three times the quantity of the decoction of *khadira* (*Mimosa ferruginacæ*) and he untiringly drinks it for a month, all leproma become destroyed, with the inunction and imbibition of the oil, together with proper dietary, and hoarseness of voice, red-eyes and ulcers eaten by bacteria are cured soon." *Suśruta* IV. 13. 8-9[163].

163. पञ्चकर्म्मगुणातीतं श्रद्धावन्तं जिजीविषुम् ।
योगेनानेन मतिमान् साधयेत् कुष्ठिनं नरम् ॥
वृक्षास्तुवरका ये स्युः पश्चिमार्णवभूमिषु ।
वीचीतरङ्गविक्षेप-मारुतोद्धतपल्लवाः ॥
तेषां फलानि गृह्णीयात् सुपक्वान्यम्बुदागमे ।
मज्ज तेभ्योऽपि संहृत्य शोषयित्वा विचूर्ण्य च ॥
तिलवत् पीड़येद्द्रोण्यां क्वाथयेद्वा कुसुम्भवत् ।
ततैलं संहृतं भूयः पचेदा तोयसंक्षयात् ॥
अवतार्य्य करीषे च पक्षमात्रं निधापयेत् ।
स्निग्धः स्विन्नो हृतमलः पश्चादूर्द्ध्वं प्रयत्नवान् ।
चतुर्थभक्तान्तरितः शुक्लादौ दिवसे शुभे ॥ ८
मन्त्रपूतस्य तैलस्य पिबेन्मात्रां यथाबलम् ।
तत्र मन्त्रं प्रवक्ष्यामि येनेदमभिमन्त्र्यते ॥

"If one eats the kernel of the '*tubara*' fruit, his body becomes cleansed of all impurities; it is very potent, and is the best medicine for leprosy." *Suśruta* IV. 13. 10[164].

Tubara or *chaulmugra* (*Taraktogenos kurzii*), by which name it is better known, is certainly the best medicine known yet in the treatment of leprosy. A few intramuscular injections of the ethyl esters or intravenous in-

---

मज्जसार महावीर्य्य सर्व्वान् धातून् विशोधय ।
शङ्खचक्रगदापाणिस्त्वामाज्ञापयतेऽच्युतः ॥
तेनास्योर्द्ध्वमधश्चापि दोषा यान्त्यसकृत् ततः ।
अस्नेहलवणां सायं यवागूं शीतलां पिवेत् ॥
पश्चाहं प्रपिवेत् तैलमनेन विधिना नरः ।
पक्षं परिहरेच्चापि मुद्गयूषौदनाशनः ।
पञ्चभिर्दिवसैरेवं सर्व्वकुष्ठैर्विमुच्यते ॥ ९
तदेव खदिरक्वाथे त्रिगुणे साधु साधितम् ।
निहन्ति पूर्व्ववत् पक्कं पिवेन्मासमतन्द्रितः ॥
तेनाभ्यक्तशरीरश्च कुर्व्वीताहारमीरितम् ।
भिन्नस्वरं रक्तनेत्रं विशीर्णं क्रिमिभक्षितम् ॥
अनेनाशु प्रयोगेण साधयेत् कुष्ठिनं नरम् ।

सुश्रुतसंहिता, चिकित्सितस्थानम्, १३ ।

164. शोधयन्ति नरं पीता मज्जानस्तस्य मात्रया ।
महावीर्य्यस्तुवरकः कुष्ठमेहापहः परः ॥ १०

सुश्रुतसंहिता, चिकित्सितस्थानम्, १३ ।

jection of the salts—chaulmoogric and hydnocarpic acids, result in the destruction of the lepra bacilli in the tissues, followed by the disappearance of the nodules and healing of the ulcers. The oral administration of the chaulmugra oil is not so successful, for the reason that it is nauseating and offensive to the stomach, and when injected intramuscularly, it is extremely painful and very slowly absorbed. Its fatty acids—chaulmoogric acid and hydnocarpic acid, being solids, are unsuited for hypodermic administration. But the ethyl esters of these acids, being thin fluid oils, are well suited for infection and are well absorbed. And they have given remarkable result within a short time. These ethyl ester derivatives have been in use at the United States Public Health Service leprosy investigation station at Kalihi in the Hawaiian Islands only for three years with a very limited supply of the oil, and within this short period 140 lepers have been paroled and return ed to their families, the disease apparently arrested, if not totally cured. From the joint report of J. T. Mc.Donald of the leprosy investigation, and A. L. Dean, President of the University of Hawaii, the following conclusion may be summarized : (1) The intramuscular injection of the ethyl esters of the fatty acids of the chaulmoogra oil usually leads to rapid improvement in the clinical symptoms of leprosy. In many cases the lesions disappear, except for scars and permanent injuries, and the leprosy bacillus can no longer be demonstrated. (2) When combined with iodine, the fatty acids of chaulmoogra oil and their esters give good result, but there is no adequate experimental proof that it causes any increase in the effectiveness of the materials used. (3) Although conclusive evidence is not at hand, it is probable that the oral administration of chaulmoogra oil derivatives is of minor importance compared with the injections. (4) In treating leprosy, it is important to make use of all auxiliary agencies to build up and maintain bodily vigor. (5) It has been sufficiently established that the chaulmoogra oil contains one or more agents which exert a marked therapeutic action in leprosy. We can not as yet say the disease is cured, since we have no test adequate to establish such a verdict. Whether or not the apparent cures are real and permanent, it is evident that we have a valuable agent at our disposal for the control of the disease.

In Burma and Assam, four varieties of

Chaulmugra trees (*Hydnocarpus castana, Hydnocarpus anthelmintica* in Siam where it is known as *Maikrabao* tree. *Gynocardia odoratta* and *Taraktogenos kurzii*, spoken of by the Burmese as '*kalaw*') are seen together, and they can not be easily distinguished one from the other without accurate botanical description. The trees, leaves, fruits and the oils are very similar. Only the genuine chaulmoogra *Taraktogenos kurzii* lacks the double testa on the fruit of the other varieties, and the oil derivatives of the '*Taraktogenos kurzii*' have the potent therapeutic value. Others only possess it to a lesser extent.*

VIII. *Diseases of the Genital Organs.*

"*Vṛddhi* (*oscheoncus*) is the vascular swelling of the sac (scrotum) containing the testes, due to various lesions. Pain in the bladder, groin, testes and the penis are its prodromal symptoms.

The scrotum is distended and rough like a bladder filled with gas, and without any apparent cause there is pain due to the gas, in

* The vivid description of the Chaulmoogra tree is given with illustrations in the March content of the *National Geographic Magazine,* Washington, 1922, by J. F. Rock who was sent by the U. S. A. Department of Agriculture to secure the seeds of Chaulmoogra.

vāta-vṛddhi (*emphysema* may be classified under two divisions : (1) benign, where the gas is introduced into the tissues through a local wound or where its source is from some distant wound which communicates with the air-passages or bowels ; and (2) malignant, where gas is generated in connection with bacterial fermentation. The benign form gets well spontaneously. For the malignant form, incision, drainage and thorough disinfection are necessary).

The scrotum has the color of the ripe fruit of '*ficus glomerata*' and it (inflammation) grows and suppurates rapidly, in '*pitta-vṛddhi*' (*epididymo-orchitis*' in which the symptoms somewhat differ according to whether the epididymis or the testis is more affected. On the whole the symptoms are more severe with the latter than with the former, though suppuration is more frequent in epididymitis. Premonitory symptoms are fever, headache and general malaise, followed by tenderness and pain in the affected parts. This disease might arise from the extension of the chronic gonorrheal inflammatory process or secondary manifestation of syphilis in interstitial or gummatous forms. The patient must be put to bed and have the scrotum raised and supported with a pillow and ice-bag. The bowels are to be opened with a purgative to remove internal congestion and light liquid food should be given as milk. After the inflammation has subsided, hot lead-lotion dressings or hot fomentations can be used advantageously to increase the vascularity of the part, thus aiding in the removal and absorption of the inflammatory products. If suppuration takes place, the abscess must be incised, drained off and the abscess cavity disinfected. If the lesion is of syphilitic origin, antisyphilic treatment is very beneficial).

It is tense, slightly painful, cold and pruritic in '*śleṣma-vṛddhi*' (*edema* is common as the scrotum being elastic and distensible, is especially liable to be invaded by general dropsical effusions).

The scrotum encloses a dark tumor and has all the symptoms of epididymo-orchitis in '*rakta-vṛddhi*' (*hematocele* which is a tumor caused by collection of blood in the cavity of the tunica vaginalis. It differs from hydrocele in that it is not transparent. It is usually associated with some traumatism, and is accompanied by inflammatory symptoms. Any variety of hydrocele or spermatocele may rapidly refill with blood, after being tapped, thus forming hematocele or by filaria. Hemorrhage also may take place into the loose tissues about the cord, forming a tumor, sometimes called, diffused hematocele of the cord. For treatment, the sac should be incised antiseptically, the clot removed, the cavity irrigated, and drainage established and continued until such time as the obliteration of the sac by granulations has been accomplished).

It is boggy, glistening, pruritic, slightly painful and looks like the fruit of the palmyra tree (Borassus flabelliformis) in *'medo-vṛddhi'* (*elephantiasis*, the Scrotum is a favorite seat of this affection. The growth is slow, painless and progressive and may reach the weight of 150 pounds or more, and is caused by the blocking of the afferent lymph ducts by the adult worms and the eggs of Filaria bancrofti. The disease is confined to high temperature region and the egg of the Filaria bancrofti is introduced into the body by the bite of the mosquito, belonging to different species which are known to be its carrier as Culex fatigans, Mansonia uniformis, Mansonia pseudotitillans, Pyretophorus costalis, Myzomia rossii, Myzorhynchus nigerrimus, Cellia albimana. The only effective treatment of the disease is operative removal which is very easy and successful, if special attention is paid to antisepsis, so that there can be no septic absorption from the stump. To keep the skin clean and aseptic, and to choose the parts of the skin as flaps are rather important factors of a successful operation. The pedicle is clamped and the scrotal tissue removed, care being taken to leave the testicles and penis and ligaturing the vessels as they are exposed. The exposed testicles become covered by granulation and cicatrization).

Due to the retention of urine, the scrotum palpitates like a leather-bag filled with water ; it is boggy and in this disease, there are strangury, pain in the testes and edema of the scrotum ; it is called *'mūtra-vṛddhi'* [urinary extravasation or *hydrocele*, possibly the latter. Urinary extravasation invades the scrotal tissues, causing a tumefaction as in simple edema (*śleṣma-vṛddhi* hydrosscheocele). The urine however excites greater irritation than serous effusion, and consequently the scrotal tissues speedily become infiltrated by inflammatory exudates. If it be not relieved with a puncture-needle, trocar or incision, it usually results in abscess formation. Vaginal hydrocele on the other hand, consists of a collection of fluid, more or less serous, in the cavity of the tunica vaginalis. Perhaps by *'śleṣma-vṛddhi'* (oschedema) hydrocele was meant. But according to the tradition, '*mūtra-vṛddhi*' is taken for hydrocele. The etiology of vaginal hydrocele is yet obscure. In the tertiary stage of syphilis, there is diffuse gummatous infiltration or the formation of localized gumma in the testes accompanied usually by a small hydrocele. In infancy the hydrocele is generally connected with gastro-intestinal fermentation ; in childhood and early adult life, it is very often associated with some abnormal condition of the testicle or spermatic cord ; later in life it is perhaps concerned with the vascular changes that take place with the degenerative involution of the testes]. "*Suśruta* II. 12. 2-5[165].

---

165. वातपित्तश्लेष्मशोणितमेदोमूत्रान्त्रनिमित्ताः सप्त वृद्धयः। तासां मूत्रान्त्र-निमित्ते वृद्धी वातसमुत्थे केवलमुत्पत्तिहेतुरन्यतमः ॥ २

अधःप्रकुपितोऽन्यतमो हि दोषः फलकोषवाहिनीरभिप्रपद्य धमनीः फलकोषयोर्वृद्धिं जनयति, तां वृद्धिमित्याचक्षते ॥ ३

तासां भविष्यन्तीनां पूर्वरूपाणि वस्तिकटीमुष्कमेढ्रेषु वेदना मारुतनिग्रहः फल-कोषशोफश्चेति ॥ ४

ततानिलपरिपूर्णां वस्तिमिवाततां परुषामनिमित्तानिलरुजं वातवृद्धिमाचक्षते। पक्वोडूम्बरसङ्काशां ज्वरदाहोष्मवतीञ्चाशु समुत्थानपाकां पित्तवृद्धिम्। कठिनाल्प-वेदनां शीतां कण्डूमतीं श्लेष्मवृद्धिम्। कृष्णस्फोटावृतां पित्तवृद्धिलिङ्गां रक्तवृद्धिम्। मृदुस्निग्धां कण्डूमतीमल्पवेदनां तालफलप्रकाशां मेदोवृद्धिम्। मूत्रसन्धारणशीलस्य मूत्रवृद्धिर्भवति, सा गच्छतोऽम्बुपूर्णा दृतिरिव क्षुभ्यति मूत्रकृच्छ्रं वेदनां वृषणयोः श्वयथुं कोशयोश्चापादयति, तां मूत्रवृद्धिं विद्यात् ॥ ५

सुश्रुतसंहिता, निदानस्थानम, १२।

Treatment : "'In '*vāta-vṛddhi*' (*emphysema*) apply soothing salve and emplasterum (*anilāpahāna*=relief of '*vāyu*' =soothing) ; in case it is of a suppurative type (malignant emphysema), use a pustulant and after it has suppurated, incise (and drain) it without hurting the raphe, and treat it according to the prescribed rules in these cases.

In '*pitta-vṛddhi*' (*epididymo-orchitis*), the treatment of aneurism is beneficial ; if it suppurates, incise it and disinfect it with (antiseptic) ointment (*kṣaudra-sarpi* = honied fat) and then apply vulnerary oil and mucilaginous paste.

In '*rakta-vṛddhi*' (*hematocele*), apply leeches for withdrawal of blood, or give as a sedative (diuretic) honey and sugar ; in suppurative or non suppurative form, hematocele should be attended to.

In '*śleṣma-vṛddhi*' (hydroscheocele or vaginal hydrocele), apply emplasterum of calorific substances as (cow) dung and urine, drink the infusion of Circuma aromatica (or pinus longifolia) mixed with urine ; except compression, all other treatments of '*śleṣma-granthi*' are beneficial. If it suppurates, incise it, and as a vulnerary of the wound, the restorative oil concocted with Tritico estivo, Semicarpo anacardia, Alangio hexapetalo and Echite scholari, should be applied.

In '*medovṛddhi*' (*elephantiasis*), use an emplasterum of a gum-resinous substance as myrrha or any other sedative, warmed with cow's urine to soften the scrotum, and when it is done, it should be bandaged (as antisepsis). Then with encouraging words to the patient, it should be incised with a leaf-shaped instrument, sparing the testes and the raphe, and all the fats removed (Filaria bancrofti and the larva which block the lymph-channels and cause the inflammation of the scrotal tissue), then green vitriol (*kāsīsa* = sulphate of iron) and rock salt (as disinfectant) should be applied and the wound sutured properly. As vulnerary, oil cooked with arsenic disulphide, arsenic sulphide, sodium chloride and semicarpus anacarda is to be applied.

In '*mūtrā-vṛddhi*' (*urinary extravasation or vaginal hydrocele*), fomentation should be applied to the scrotum (to make it tense) and then have it bandaged (as antisepsis). By the raphe downward, an instrument like the sharp point of a grain (trocar) should be introduced, and thereby a double-barrelled cannula

(through the one cannula air is passed to cause pressure so that through the other the fluid content may be completely drained off), the urine (fluid) is evacuated. Then the cannula is to be withdrawn and ligature applied. If the wound remains clean (non-suppurated or granulated), the vulnerary is to be applied. (The only difference in the modern method of tapping in hydrocele, is that after the fluid is evacuated, the cannula is not withdrawn usually, but a syringe which fits it, is filled with half a drachm of a solution of ten parts of carbolic acid to one of glycerine, and is injected into the cavity. This causes but slight pain. However the sac refills partially due to the inflammatory reaction caused by the carbolic acid, but the inflammatory exudate is gradually reabsorbed after the inflammatory process giving rise to it has subsided. However, tapping is but a palliative measure. It has to be done once or twice a year. But perhaps because it causes so little inconvenience and discomfort, it is preferred to operation by excision of a portion of the sac especially in old hydroceles with thickened walls due to sclerous and calcerous changes in the subserous tissues, which gives a more satisfactory result. However, whether in tapping or in operation, care has to be taken to avoid wounding the testes or scrotal vessels). *Suśruta* IV. 19. 3-8[166].

---

166. स्नेहापनाहौ कुर्य्याच्च प्रदेहांश्चानिलापहान् ॥
विदग्धां पाचयित्वा वा सेवनीं परिवर्ज्जयेत् ।
भिन्द्यात् ततः प्रभिन्नायां यथोक्तं क्रममाचरेत् ॥ ७
पित्तजायामपक्वायां पित्तग्रन्थिक्रमो हितः ।
पक्वां वा भेदयेद्भिन्नां शोधयेद् क्षौद्रसर्पिषा ।
शुद्धायाश्च भिषग्दद्यात् तैलं कल्कञ्च रोपणम् ॥ ४
रक्तजायां जलौकाभिः शोणितं निर्हरेद्भिषक् ।
पिबेद्विरेचनं वापि शर्कराक्षौद्रसंयुतम् ।
पित्तग्रन्थिक्रमं कुर्य्यादामे पक्वे च सर्व्वदा ॥ ५
वृद्धिं कफात्मिकामुष्णैर्मूत्रपिष्टैः प्रलेपयेत् ।
पीतदारुकषायञ्च पिबेन्मूत्रेण संयुतम् ॥
विम्लापनादृते वापि श्लेष्मग्रन्थिक्रमो हितः ॥
पक्वायाश्च विभिन्नायां तैलं शोधनमिष्यते ।
सुमनारुष्कराङ्कोट-सप्तपर्णेषु साधितम् ॥ ६
मेदःसमुत्थां संस्वेद्य लेपयेत् सुरसादिना ।
शिरोविरेकद्रव्यैर्वा सुखोष्णैर्मूत्रसंयुतैः ॥
स्विन्नाञ्चावेष्ट्य पट्टेन समाश्वास्य तु मानवम् ।
रक्षेत् फले सेवनीञ्च वृद्धिपत्रेण दारयेत् ॥
मेदस्ततः समुद्धृत्य दद्यात् कासीससैन्धवे ।
बध्नीयाच्च यथोद्दिष्टं शुद्धे तैलञ्च दापयेत् ॥
मनःशिलालवणैः सिद्धमारुष्करेषु च ॥ ७
मूत्रजां स्वेदयित्वा तु वस्त्रपट्टेन वेष्टयेत् ।
सेवन्याः पार्श्वतोऽधस्ताद्विध्येद्व्रीहिमुखेण च ॥

"Carriage of a heavy burden, wrestling with a strong man, fall from a tree—all these strains increase *'vāyu'* which enlarges the viscera and which in its downward course makes a tumor-like formation in the groin (*inguinal hernia*). If it be not attended to, it descends to the scrotum (osceocele) and causes the inflammation of the testes. This causes the distension of the scrotum like that of the bladder, and if it be pressed, gas ascends with noise, but descends again when left. This is called *'antra-vṛddhi'* (inguinal hernia). It is an incurable disease. "*Suśruta* II. 12. 6[167].

"The hernia that has reached the groin, to

अथात ह्विमुखां नाड़ीं दत्त्वा विस्रावयेद् भिषक्।
मूत्रं नाड़ीमथोद्धृत्य स्थगिकाबन्धमाचरेत्॥
गुह्वायां रोपणं दद्याद्वर्ज्जयेदन्त्रवृद्धिकीम्॥ ८

सुश्रुतसंहिता, चिकित्सितस्थानम, २१।

167. भारहरणवलवद्विग्रह-वृक्षप्रपतनादिभिरायासविशेषैर्वायुरतिप्रवृद्धः प्रकुपितस्य स्थूलान्त्रस्येतरस्य चैकदेशं द्विगुणमादायाधो गत्वा वङ्क्षणसन्धिमुपेत्य ग्रन्थिरूपेण स्थित्वा प्रतिक्रियमाणे च कालान्तरेण फलकोशं प्रविश्य मुष्कशोफमापादयत्याध्मातो बस्तिरिवाततः प्रदीर्घः शोफो भवति सशब्दमवपीड़ितश्चोर्द्ध्वमुपैति, विमुक्तश्च पुनराध्मति, तामन्त्रवृद्धिमसाध्यामित्याचक्षते॥ ६

सुश्रुतसंहिता, निदानस्थानम् १२।

obstruct its passage, should be cauterized by a semilunar-shaped cautery. *Suśruta* IV. 19. 10[168].

Hernia is the protrusion of the abdominal viscera through weak spots in the abdominal wall, which develop either due to congenital deficieney of muscular or tendonous development or due to their degenerative changes. It is met with in two extremes of life. In infancy when the inguinal rings are as yet imperfectly formed, uncontrolled crying, coughing or any other form of severe strain may subject the tissues to give way. In old age tissues begin to degenerate, while the weight of the viscera is heavier, and under severe straining as in asthmatic paroxysm, the weak spots in the parietes are easily apt to yield.

"If the prepuce has been forcibly drawn back (over the glans, and its return ia prevented by the arrest of the narrow opening behind the corona), during coitus with narrow vagina, masturbation, accident, play or detumescence, it is called '*avapātikā*' (*paraphimosis* ; if this condition is left unrelieved, the circulation in the parts beyond may be interfered with sufficiently to

168. तव या वङ्क्षणस्था तां दहेदर्द्धेन्दूवक्रया ।
सम्यङ्मार्गावरोधार्थं कोषप्राप्तान्तु वर्ज्जयेत् ।
सुश्रुतसंहिता, चिकित्सितस्थानम, २१ ।

make them swell, as to render retraction very difficult even when the preputual orifice is not very tight).

In '*niruddha-prakaśa*' (*phimosis*) the prepuce adheres to the glans penis, and therefore also contracts the meatus. But if it be not complete, the urine flows drop by drop with pain, ballooning the prepuce but without rupturing the glans penis. (The best remedy of phimosis is circumcision with lateral incision as the dilatation of the preputial opening by any method is only a half measure, involving as much pain as cutting or operating. Phimosis should be corrected as early as possible, as the abdominal pressure exerted in the straining to evacuate the urine and in the crying which often accompanies the effort in such children, is sufficient to prevent the firm closure of the natural hernial openings and to cause yielding of those which have already closed. Another consequence of the mechanical obstruction is the obstacle which it offers to cleanliness, resulting in a balano-posthitis induced by the retention of the smegma which consists of the secretion of the glands of the lining membrane of the prepuce together with the dead epithelial cells from those surfaces, the decomposition of which is hastened by the admixture of urine. This inflammation reacts on the nervous system and causes its irritability which is expressed in the peevishness of the child, and urinary disturbances such as frequent micturition, involuntary micturition especially at night, and spasmodic and painful micturition. The acrid and irritable decomposition product also provokes priapism in children and for the relief of this they learn and gradually habituate themselves to the pernicious practice of masturbation. In the adult the sexual erethism causes self-abuse, venery, spermatorrhea, premature ejaculation, backache and their various reactions. Circumcision is a great hygienic measure, especially in a tropical country). *Suśruta* II. 13. 40-41[169].

---

169. अल्पीयःखां यदा हर्षाद्बालां गच्छेत् स्त्रियं नरः ।
हस्ताभिघातादथ वा चर्मण्युद्वर्त्तिते बलात् ॥
मर्द्दनात् पीड़नाद्वापि शुक्रवेगविघाततः ।
यस्यावपाट्यते चर्म्म तां विद्यादवपाटिकाम् ॥ ४०
वातोपसृष्टमेवन्तु चर्म्म संश्रयते मणिम् ।
मणिश्चर्म्मोपनद्धस्तु मूत्रस्रोतो रुणद्धि च ॥
निरुद्धप्रकशे तस्मिन् मन्दधारमवेदनम् ।
मूत्रं प्रवर्त्तते जन्तोर्मणिर्न च विदीर्य्यते ॥
निरुद्धप्रकशं विद्यात् सरुजं वातसम्भवम् ॥ ४१

सुश्रुतसंहिता, निदानस्थानम्, १३

"Application of '*śūka*' for the enlargement of the penis, causes eighteen kinds of diseases. *Suśruta* II. 14. 2[170].

Traditionally '*śūka*' is taken as a pruritic water insect and used externally as an aphrodisiac. As '*śūka*' is used in the plural, it is possible that it includes some species of the insects, belonging to the 'Coleoptera' order as 'Lytta or Cantharus corulea' (blue blistering fly of Bengal) or 'Lytta nepalensis' (Nepal blistering fly, a black species having filiform attenæ and elytra broadened toward the apex), having its active irritating principle '*cantharidin*' and which is used as an aphrodisiac. When dried powder or its active principle is applied to the skin, it causes burning sensation and hyperemia, to which in the course of a few hours, succeeds the formation of vesicles. If the application is continued, it forms a blister, and if it goes on like that for a long time, sloughing and ulcerating result. If it is applied to the penis, it causes a voluminous swelling and engorgement of corpus cavernosum, and violent erection.

---

170. लिङ्गवृद्धिमिच्छतामक्रमप्रवृत्तानां शूकदोषनिमित्ता दश चाष्टौ च व्याधयो जायन्ते ।

सुश्रुतसंहिता, निदानस्थानम्., १४ ।

"Due to the undue application of '*śūka*', vesicles develop like the mustard seed, and are called '*sarṣapikā*' (*cantharidal vesicles*).

Due to the application of poisonous '*śūka*', a stone-hard unsymmetrical tumor develops which is called '*aṣṭhīlikā*', *osteoma or chondroma* of the penis : ossification and calcification of the penis have been reported in many cases. The parts involved are the sheaths of the corpora cavernosa and the septum pectiniform. Ossification which is partial takes place usually in the plates very insiduously and without pain, and the patient first becomes aware of its existence by the impediment it offers to coitus or the curvature which it causes to the organ. Tuffier reports a case in which he found a bean-sized chondroma growing on the external surface of one of the corpora cavernosa, near the middle of the organ and which he removed by operation).

If the penis is repeatedly engorged by the '*śūka*', the vesicles that are developed like neoplasm, are called 'grathita' (*soft vegetations* of succulent warts of the mucous membranes and muco-cutaneous junctions, especially found in the coronal sulcus and near frenum).

Darkish vegetation that develops like the seed of '*Eugenæ jambu*' is called '*kumbhīkā*

(*corneous vegetations*, consisting of brown or dirty-brown, sessile, rounded growths, quite firm in structure, growing in the penis, scrotum, crural fields and anus in the male, on the labia majora, perineum and anus in woman).

Ophthalmia (*alajī*) is similar to that of gonorrhea (*prameha*; it is probable that by *alajī* is here either meant the gonorrheal conjunctivitis of the eye, or syphilitic gumma of the conjuctiva or sclera or parenchymatous keratitis).

If through derangement of '*vāyu*' the penis is pressed and beaten (lacking the power of erection and is pendulous) and on it appears vesicles with edema, it is called '*mṛdita*' (*syphilitic edema of the penis*).

The vesicles that develop, in masturbation, are called *sammūḍha* (*herpes progenitalis* which is very pruritic appears about the glans and the foreskin, accompanied with a little moisture. When the parts are inspected in the early stages, small pin-head vesicles will be seen at the edge of the foreskin, in the neighborhood of the corona or near the meatus. When the vesicles have broken, they leave superficial erosions surrounded by minute circular or crescentric areola).

Numerous elongated growths appear, breaking

in the middle, causing pain, and horripilation, and are called '*avamantha*' (*horns of penis*, which are usually dark-brown or green in color, in texture resembling the nails, but rough on the surface, arising from the coronal sulcus, especially near the frenum, and may attain a length of three inches. They possibly are papillomatous growths, and when protected from the air, remain moist, soft and pinkish, and when exposed become dry, hard and dark-brownish in color. On removal, usually a wart is found at their bases, and they are found in persons of careless habits and advanced life).

Due to the (corruption of) '*blood and pitta*' the sore that develops in the shape of the petal of lotus, surrounded by pustules, is called '*puṣkarikā*' (*chancroid* : it is very hard sometimes to distinguish from syphilitic initial lesion-chancre and the pyogenic ulcer-chancroid. Chancroid is contagious, its secretions being always auto-inoculable, but it is essentially a local lesion, in contradistinction to chancre which is an expression of syphilitic constitutional affection. Chancroid is due to Ducrey's streptobacillus and does not usually appear single, is not sharply circumscribed and is not indurated like the syphilitic sore. The ulcer is surrounded by minute pustules on the rugged edge, which is slightly inflamed, and from which if pressed, appears a thin brownish pus, for the streptobacillus is pyogenic, while the spirochete pallida is not. Differential diagnosis is very important before treatment is given, for if the chancroid is treated with mercury or iodoform ointment, it may seriously complicate the case, while with thorough cleansing and antisepsis, it can be easily cured).

If due to the lesion of '*śūka*', the (corrupt) blood causes anesthesia, it is called '*sparśa-hāni*' (*syphilitic anesthesia* of the penis and impotence).

Due to the indigestion, caused by '*sūka*' (taken internally as an aphrodisiac), '*the blood and pitta*' become deranged, and the growths that appear thereby like Phaseolus mungo and Phaseolus radiatum are called '*uttamā*' (milia, resembling millet seeds, usually benign growths, are not infrequently found in the cutaneous investment of the penis).

If due to the (corruption of) '*vāyu and blood*', the penis is covered with perforating tissues like a sieve, it is called '*śata-ponaka*' (*tuberculosis of penis* occurs in two forms. The majority of cases are examples of chronic tuberculous ulceration of the skin or the mucous membrane, the ulcers having the same irregular worm-eaten shape, blue undermined edges and slowly sloughing or granulating cases. The other form which is rarer, appears to begin in the depth of the erectile tissue, producing a necrotic mass, closely resembling the tuberculous sequestra seen in a spongy bone. The latter form is perhaps indicated by '*śata-ponaka*').

If due to '*pitta and blood*', the skin of the penis ulcerates, with burning and fever, it is called '*tvak-pāka*' (*erysipelas* or *cantharidal ulceration*, due to its excessive and concentrated application).

The dark, blood-tumor covered with very pruritic vesicles, is called *śoṇitārvvuda*' (*angioma*: though angima is more frequent than other benign tumors, it does not attack the penis so commonly as the female organs of generation. Angioma is generally seen in children, forming a superficial flat tumor, giving rarely any symptoms, unless a considerable part of the organ is involved and in that case troublesome priapism has been observed.

Due to the lesion of the tissues, develops a neoplasm, called '*māṃsārvuda*' (*epithelioma or cancer of the penis* : cancer almost invariably originates on the prepuce, glans or both combined and is a disease of advanced life. The most common mode of origin of epithelioma of the penis is in warty growths, which may promptly or after the lapse of months or years, degenerate into a malignant type. The etiology of the disease is obscure. Beside the unknown factor— tissue susceptibility, chronic irritation caused by phimosis, balanitis, venereal ulcer, especially a chronic ulcer of syphilitic origin seems to be the chief cause of cancer of the penis. It may be grafted from the cancer of the uterus where it is commoner than in man, during coitus. If the diagnosis is correct, amputation or extirpation according to the severity of the lesion, is the only safe remedy. For in many cases, destruction of tissue is marked as well as growth, and the malignant growth consists of an ulcer which may be very deep in the center with greatly thickened and indurated borders, the induration preceding the spread of the ulcer on all sides, and often the urethra is perforated so that the urine can only pass through the soft sloughing tissues, thus producing extensive ulceration).

When ulceration takes place (of the epithelioma), it is called malignant '*māṃsa-pāka*' (ulceration of the cancer).

All the symptoms of complicated tumor,

mentioned before (*Suśruta* II. 9) are the same in the case of the *'vidradhi'* (*sarcoma* of the penis, like the sarcoma of the other parts of the body, may be found at any time of life from childhood to old age, and is chiefly found in the tissues of the corpora cavernosa, running a rapid and insidious course, forming a tumor without any painful sensation, but enlarging and distorting the penis. If the tumor is extirpated, there is always great danger of the return of the morbid process).

If the poisonous black or multicolored *'śūka'* is used, then the tissues ulcerate with dark pigmentation and fall off ; this disease originates from the (corruption) of the three humors and is called *'tila-kālaka'* (*gangrene* : Gangrene of the penis is observed in young, but more commonly in elderly, subjects. In some cases balanitis, phimosis, paraphimosis, chancre, or chancroid has been the starting point. Cases have been reported in which gangrene of the penis was said to be due to ingestion of ergot and cantharides). *

(Of these diseases), *epithelioma* (*māṃsārvvuda*), *ulceration of the cancer* (*māṃsa-pāka*), *sarcoma*

* R. W. Taylor : *Genito-urinary and Venereal Diseases*, p. 270.

(*vidradhi*) and *gangrene* (*tilakālaka*) of the penis are incurable." *Suśruta* II. 14. 3-32[171].

"Masturbation, manipulation or traumatism of the penis causes the derangement of the '*vāyu*', which corrupts the (mucous membrane of) prepuce and causes intumescence, of the glans ; it is called '*pari-vartikā*' (*balanitis*) and being of '*vāyu*' and infectious origin, it is

171 गौरसर्षपतुल्या तु शूकदुष्टनिमित्तका ।
पिड़का कफरक्ताभ्यां ज्ञेया सर्षपिका बुधैः ॥ ७
कठिना विषमैरन्तैर्मारुतस्य प्रकोपतः ।
शूकैस्तु विषसंयुक्तैः पिड़काष्ठीलिका भवेत् ॥ ४
शूकैर्यत् पूरितं शश्वद्ग्रथितं तत् कफोत्थितम् ॥ ५
कुम्भीका रक्तपित्तोत्था जाम्बवास्थिनिभा शुभा ॥ ६
अलजीलक्षणैर्युक्तामलजीञ्च वितर्कयेत् ॥ ७
मृदितं पीड़ितं यत् तु संरब्धं वायुकोपतः ॥ ८
पाणिभ्यां भृशसंमूढ़े संमूढ़पिड़का भवेत् ॥ ९
दीर्घा बह्वाश्च पीड़का दीर्यन्ते मध्यतस्तु याः ।
सोऽवमन्थः कफासृग्भ्यां वेदनारोमहर्षकृत ॥ १०
पित्तशोणितसम्भूता पीड़का पिड़काचिता ।
पद्मपुष्करसंस्थाना ज्ञेया पुष्करिकेति सा ॥ ११
जनयेत् स्पर्शहानिन्तु शोणितं शूकदूषितम् ॥ १२
मुद्गमाषोपमा रक्ता पीड़का रक्तपित्तजा ।
उत्तमैषा तु विज्ञेया शूकाजीर्णनिमित्तजा ॥ १३
छिद्रैरणुमुखैर्यत् तु चितं मेढ्रं समन्ततः ।
वातशोणितजो व्याधिर्विज्ञेयः शतपोनकः ॥ १४

painful, causes burning and occasionally suppurates. If it originates from '*śleṣmā*', it is hard and pruritic (papilloma or any other vegetation." *Suśruta* II. 13. 39[172].

पित्तरक्तकृतो ज्ञेयस्त्वक्पाको ज्वरदाहवान् ॥ १५

कृष्णस्फोटैः सरक्ताभिः पिड़काभिश्च पीड़ितम् ।

यस्य वस्तिरुजश्चोग्रा ज्ञेयं तच्छोणितार्व्वुदम् ॥ १६

मांसदोषेण जानीयादर्व्वुदं मांससम्भवम् ॥ १७

शीर्य्यन्ते यस्य मांसानि यस्य सर्व्वाश्च वेदनाः ।

विद्यात् तं मांसपाकन्तु सर्व्वदोषकृतं भिषक् ॥ १८

विद्रधिं सन्निपातेन यथोक्तमभिनिर्द्दिशेत् ॥१९

कृष्णानि चित्राण्यथवा शूकानि सविषाणि च ।

पातितानि पचन्त्याशु मेढ्रं निरवशेषतः ॥ २०

कालानि भूत्वा मांसानि शीर्य्यन्ते यस्य देहिनः ॥

सन्निपातसमुत्थानं तं विद्यात् तिलकालकम् ॥ २१

तत्र मांसार्व्वुदं यच्च मांसपाकश्च यः स्मृतः ।

विद्रधिश्च न सिध्यन्ति ये च स्युस्तिलकालकाः ॥ २२

सुश्रुतसंहिता, निदानस्थानम्, १४ ।

172. मर्द्दनात् पीड़नाच्चापि तथैवाप्यभिघाततः ।

मेढ्रचर्म्म यदा वायुर्भजते सर्व्वतश्चरः ॥

तदा वातोपसृष्टन्तु चर्म्म प्रतिनिवर्त्तते ।

मणेरधस्तात् कोषश्च ग्रन्थिरूपेण लम्बते ॥

सवेदनः सदाहश्च पाकञ्च व्रजति क्वचित् ।

मारुतागन्तुसम्भूतां विद्यात् तां परिवर्त्तिकाम् ॥

सकण्डुः कठिना चैव सैव श्लेष्मसमुत्थिता ॥ ३९

सुश्रुतसंहिता, निदानस्थानम्, १३ ।

Balanitis is the inflammation of the mucous membrane of the glans, or of the prepuce (posthitis), or to both conditions combined. The two surfaces are generally attacked simultaneously, except in chronic processes which are limited to small areas. The predisposing cause to inflammation of these parts is the difficulty or impossibility of cleansing them, especially when the foreskin is long and narrow. The active cause may be the retained pus or irritating substances of gonorrhea, chancroid, secretions of primary or secondary syphilitic lesions, or the decomposition of the accumulated smegma mixed with urine and perhaps leucorrheal discharge added to it in coitus. The existence of vegetations under the prepuce provokes balanitis especially when the lodgment of the gonorrheal pus excites the inflammation. Balanitis may occur also in diabetic patients, on account of the ready decomposition of their sugar-laden urine, and a certain fungus, for it is found in the smegma under the prepuce. The treatment of balanitis consists chiefly in the establishment of cleanliness, and if the prepuce can be retracted, this will usually suffice to cure. Parts may be washed with warm water of mild boric acid solution, but strong antiseptics are not desirable as before they can exert their germicidal effect, they are apt to provoke further irritation of already inflamed surfaces and cause the necrosis of the delicate cells, thus postponing their recuperative power.

"Excess in coitus (*simple urethritis* may be provoked, especially in gouty diathesis), continence (herpes progentitalis and reflex nervous irritability), coitus with a nun or one who has had no sexual intercourse for a long time (urethritis if the vagina is not kept clean), with a menstruating woman (menstrual blood has been regarded as an etiological factor of urethritis from remote antiquity in diverse lands. The menstrual fluid, unless decomposed or mixed with the products of bacterial evolution of one kind or another, whether the germs be autogenetic or heterogenetic, is inconsequential—can not possibly produce urethritis. Apparent contradictions are due to the autogenesis of urethritis in a previously damaged urethra, or to the washing down of the products of an old infection from the upper portion of the female sexual tract by the out-flowing menstrual secretion) or coitus with a woman whose vulva is long-haired, coarse-haired, thick-haired or there is hair in the vulvar orifice(abrasions, excoriations, fissure or fine cuts made by sharp edges of the hair at certain angles by the copulative paroxysmal movements when the genital organs are in intumescent state, are the necessary and favorable conditions for the venereal germs when deposited there, to grow and multiply. Chancroidal, syphilitic or gonorrheal germs can not cause a lesion unless they can find a lodgment and form a colony, otherwise they will be washed away by the mucous and the urinal discharges. It is only when there is an abrasion, cut, wound, tear, rent or solution of any kind of the mucous membrane, that they can find an entrance, and in the delicate epithelium, with its warmth and moisture, they find it very favorable to multiply to destroy the cells, and invade the economy in syphilis), with a woman of narrow or large vulvar orifice (strain and injuries may be caused by narrow orifice and a flabby large vaginal passage is indicative of some disease or the reaction of the diseased condition of the genitals, as otherwise in the normal state there should be vaginal muscular contraction by the sexual stimuli and the passage of the penis), with an unpleasant or repulsive woman (venereal diseases, especially syphilis causes many disfigurements of the body), with a woman who makes lavation of her vagina with contaminated water, or one who does not make any lavation of her vagina at all, or a woman who has a genital disease, or who has a chronic lesion in her genitals, or unnatural intercourse (sodomy does not necessarily cause any lesion unless there is an infection in either party, or venery ; excess might cause enervation and its reflex reactions on the organism, thus predisposing to any infection), injury to the penis by nails, teeth, toxic cantharides, compression, masturbation or bestiality (no infection can take place unless there is contact with some venereal pathogenic virus, except it might cause local injuries and pyogenic infection), ablution of the penis with contaminated water, or its strangulation, or retention of urine or semen, or non-lavation (uncleansing) of the penis after coitus—all these causes produce the derangement of the *'vāyu'*, and provoke the inflammation of the penis, whether it has been wounded or not ; this is called *'upadaṃśa'*

There are five kinds of *'upadaṃśa'*, each infection originating from five different kinds of contagions of women.

Scaliness (roughness), ulceration of the skin, torpor of the penis and inflammation with induration takes place in *'vāta-upadaṃśa'*(*syphilitic chancre*: The initial lesion is first seen as a papule, varying in size from a pea to a bean, pinkish-brown in color, dry and scaling, imparting a slight resistance to the touch, which appears after an incubation of two to four weeks in syphilis, three to seven days in chancroid (which is of diagnostic value in distinguishing chancre frem chancroid) after suspicious coitus or contact, and which slowly ulcerates with slightly inflamed and indurated, circumscribed or oval edges, leaving a superficial or eroded depression, having a thin serous or sero-purulent secretion, or it may be covered with a thin grayish pellicle).

Fever (as a reaction of the organism against the invasion of syphilitic '*Spirocheta pallida*') and intumescence like the color of '*Ficus glomerata*' (which is pinkish-brown, the color of chancre) develop, and which rapidly ulcerates with '*pitta*' pain in '*pitta-upadaṃśa*' (ulcerating chancre).

Intumescence is pruritic, hard and shiny with slight (*śleṣma*) pain, in *ślemṣa-upadṃśa*) (chancre in the first stage).

A dark tumor which bleeds excessively with fever, burning, and emaciation with all '*pitta*' symptoms, and which sometimes (spontaneously) cures, is called *'rakta upadaṃśa'* (angioma of the penis on a large artery).

The intumescence ulcerates with the development of germs, which might bring about death, with all the symptoms of the corruption of the three humors in *'sarvva-upadaṃśa'* (syphilitic sore)." *Suśruta* II. 12. 7-13 [173]

"The contagion (syphilitic *'Spirocheta pallida'*) infecting the tissues and the blood, causes their

---

173. तत्रातिमैथुनादतिब्रह्मचर्य्याद्वा तथा ब्रह्मचारिणीं चिरोत्सृष्टां रजस्वलां दीर्घरोमां कर्कशरोमां सङ्कीर्णरोमां निगूढ़रोमामल्पद्वारां महाद्वाराममप्रियामकामामचौक्षसलिलप्रक्षालितयोनिमक्षालितयोनिं योनिरोगोपसृष्टां स्वभावतो वा दुष्टयोनिं वियोनिं वा नारीमत्यर्थमुपसेवमानस्य तथा करजदशनविषशूकनिपातनादङ्गनाद्हस्ताभिघातात्चतुष्पदीगमनादचौक्ष - सलिलप्रक्षालनादवपीड़नाच्छुक्रमूत्रवेगविधारणान्मैथुनान्ते वाप्रक्षालनादिभिर्मेढ्रभागस्य प्रकुपिता दोषाः क्षतेऽक्षते वा श्वयथुमुपजनयन्ति तमुपदंशमित्याचक्षते ॥ ७

स पञ्चविधस्त्रिभिर्दोषैः पृथक् समस्तैरसृजा चैकः ॥ ८

तत्र वातिके पारुष्यं त्वक्परिपुटनं स्तब्धमेढ्रता परुष-शोफता विविधाश्च वातवेदनाः ॥ ९

पैत्तिके ज्वरः श्वयथुः पक्वोडुम्बरसङ्काशस्तीव्रदाहः क्षिप्रपाकः पित्तवेदनाश्च ॥ १०

श्लैष्मिके श्वयथुः कण्डूमान् कठिनः स्निग्धः श्लेष्मवेदनश्च ॥ ११

रक्तजे कृष्णस्फोटप्रादुर्भावोऽत्यर्थमसृक्प्रवृत्तिः पित्तलिङ्गान्यत्यर्थं ज्वरदाहौ शोषश्च याप्यश्चैव कदाचित् ॥ १२

सर्व्वजे सर्व्वलिङ्गदर्शनमवदरणं शेफसः क्रिमिप्रादुर्भावो मरणञ्चेति ॥ १३

सुश्रुतसंहिता, निदानस्थानम्, १२।

pruritis; from pruritis develops sore; in the sore malignant nodules are formed, enveloped in a film-like membrane, and from it exudates a viscous serous fluid (when the syphilitic process dips down into the subcutaneous tissue, and is complicated with indurating edema, the chancrous erosion becomes covered with '*indurated nodules*', while if the sore remains superficial and compact, the induration is spread out into a disk-like mass and is called *parchment-like chancre.* Parchment-like chancres are mostly found on the integument of the penis and sometimes on the vulva. '*Indurated chancres*' are mostly found in the sulcus coronarius, particularly near the frenum. When, owing to excessive cell-increase, the chancrous erosion becomes salient above the level of the parts, it is called '*ulcus elevatum*'. Ulcus elevatum becomes covered with a film-like membrane, having a color which is a mixture of cream with a light-green tint which degenerates into brownish black, if the membrane is not shod and exists for a long period. But if an antiseptic or iodoform is used, it melts away, leaving an erosive chancrous surface. This is known as 'chancre with the cream and the green-colored membrane). This (chancrous nodule) kills virility and destroys the penis (*phagedenic chancre*); the lesion infecting the vulva of woman produces soft, foul-smelling, umbrella-like (circumscribed) nodular chancre from which a viscid serous fluid exudates; and this contagion ascending upward, produces gummata in the ear, eye, nose and throat. The *gummata* of the ear cause deafness, otalgia and suppuration of the ear (gumma of the auricle leads at times to deep ulceration and destruction of cartilage; gummata on the membrane tympani occasionally cause the destruction of the membrane with ulceration; condylomata of the meatus causes severe pain with tension and fullness and deafness may be produced merely by the mechanical closure of the meatus, but the drum membrane occasionally becomes inflamed and may suppurate. Suppurative inflammation (Otitis media suppurativa) occurs in syphilitic subjects as the direct result of the syphilitic manifestations in the naso-pharynx, and also from other causes, but the syphilitic dyscrasia is a serious complication). In the (gummatous syphilitic) affection of the eye there is obstruction of the palpabra (Tarsitis syphilitica = gummatous infiltration of the tarsus; ulcerated syphilitic mucous patches on the free margin of the lower eyelid is commoner), ofthalmag..., lippitude (in Iritis gummosa, the exudation is gelatinous, made up of fine filaments which may be absorbed without alterations in appearance or may be changed into a bluish-white homogenous mass), and blindness (amblyopia = partial loss of vision, amaurosis = complete loss of vision in syphilis of the optic nerve, which is marked by visible changes in the papilla through : (1) choked disk or papillitis as a symptom of various intracranial processes ; (2) neuro-retinitis descendens, accompanying the various changes in the brain and its meninges which have extended along the sheath of the optic nerve, or due to gumma ; (3) atrophy of the optic nerve may take place either as a result of choked disk, neuritis descendens or inflammatory degeneration). Nasal (syphilitic) affection causes catarrh (the pituary membrane may be the seat of erythema, superficial ulcerations and mucous patches which give rise to symptoms of ordinary catarrh), excessive sneezing (as a reflex excited by the irritation of the nasal mucous membrane by syphilitic erythema, mucous patches, condylomata, gummata or ulcerations), dyspnea (difficulty in breathing results from mechanical obstruction, caused by the swollen folds or in the development of adenoids stopping up the nasal passages as may be seen in congenital syphilis), ulcer of the septum (if a gumma on the septum breaks down and ulcerates, plugs or casts of inspissated mucous, mixed with blood and pus of a very disagreeable appearance and an almost intolerable odor are discharged, especially if the necrosis of the bone has occurred. Should the lesion involve the vomer extensively, characteristically syphilitic flattening of the nose may be produced by the falling in of the bridge. The sense of smell is impaired by the failure of the odorous particles to reach the olfactory tract, owing to the obstruction of crusts and plugs of putrefying inspissated mucous), nasal voice (owing to the obstruction of the eustachian tube and nasal passages by swollen folds, gummata or condylomata) and headache (syphilitic neuralgia, the headaches being due to the lesion of the meninges which are supplied by the ramification of the trigeminal nerve : it is a very characteristic symptom of syphilis). Affections in the pharynx, larynx and palate, cause hoarseness of voice (huskiness of the voice is found in the syphilitic erythema of the larynx, and the phonation is interfered with, ranging from slight hoarseness to complete aphonia according to the extent of ulceration), ageusia (loss of taste occurs with the ulceration and destruction of the gustatory nerve or the nerve endings on the tongue), and the ulceration of buccal cavity (mucous patches, gummata, etc.)" *Suśruta* II. 2. 15 [174]

"In '*udāvarta*' (*dysmenorrhea*) foamy (menstrual) blood is discharged with colicky spasm (*colicky dysmenorrhea* results from the attempt of the uterus to expel foreign bodies as squamous pellicles, epithelial cells, blood clots, mucous membrane and exudations, originating either from neoplasms or inflammation, which is prevented from freely flowing out with the menstrual

---

174. प्रकुपितास्तु दोषा मेढ्रमभिप्रपन्ना मांसशोणिते प्रदूष्य कण्डूं जनयन्ति, ततः कण्डूयनात् क्षतं समुपजायते, तस्मिंश्च क्षते दुष्टमांसजाः प्ररोहाः पिच्छिलरुधिरस्राविणो जायन्ते कूर्च्चिनोऽभ्यन्तरमुपरिष्टाद्वा। ते तु शेफो विनाशयन्त्युपघ्नन्ति च पुंस्त्वम्, योनिमभिप्रपन्नाः सुकुमारान् दुर्गन्धान् पिच्छिलरुधिरस्राविणश्छत्राकारान् करीरान् जनयन्ति त एवोर्ध्वमागताः श्रोत्राक्षिघ्राणवदनेष्वर्शांस्युपनिर्व्वर्त्तयन्ति। तत्र कर्णजेषु बाधिर्य्यं शूलं पूतिकर्णता च। नेत्रजेषु वर्त्मावरोधो वेदनास्रावो दर्शननाशश्च। घ्राणजेषु प्रतिश्यायोऽतिमात्रं क्षवथुः कृच्छ्रोच्छ्वासता पूतिनस्यं सानुनासिकवाक्यत्वं शिरोदुःखञ्च। वक्त्रजेषु कण्ठौष्ठतालूनामन्यतमस्मिंश्च गद्गदवाक्यता रसाज्ञानं मुखरोगाश्च भवन्ति। व्यानस्तु प्रकुपितः श्लेष्माणं परिगृह्य बहिःस्थिराणि कीलवदर्शांसि निर्व्वर्त्तयन्ति तानि चर्म्मकीलान्यर्शांसीत्याचक्षते॥ १५

सुश्रुतसंहिता, निदानस्थानम्, २।

blood, by some obstruction as a tumor of the cervix or an atresia, caused by inflammation, following child-birth). '*Naṣṭārtava*'(ovarian *lesion*) causes sterility. In '*viplutā*' (*hysteralgia*), the (female) genital region is always painful. In '*pariplutā*' (*dyspareunia*), coitus is very painful (coitus may be painful to a woman due to (1) vaginismus ; (2) tender carunculæ myrtiformes, or soreness from the laceration of the hymen in a newly married woman ; (3) inflammation of the vagina or the vulva ; (4) disproportion in size of the penis and the vaginal orifice, especially osteum vaginæ ; (5) prolapsed ovaries or uterus ; (6) pelvic peritonitis, even in multiparous women). In '*vātalā*' (*vaginitis dissecans*, in which the vaginal mucous membrane becomes dry in most instances and the superficial squamous epithelium undergoes '*cornification*' and if the venereal vaginitis persists, a formation of '*acuminated condylomata*' may take place in the vagina). In *raktaksārā* (*inflammatory ulceration* of the internal genital organs), the menstruation flows with burning sensation (burning sensation is felt as the blood flows over the inflammatory ulcerated surfaces, due generally to gonorrhea or syphilis). In '*vāminī*' (*carcinoma uteri*) sanious mucous discharge appears with gas (leucorrhea or flour albus, a whitish discharge of a more or less viscid fluid, mucous or pus cells, is due to, '*chronic cervicitis*' and known by another name '*śveta-pradara*'). In *prasraṃsinī*' (*colpitis emphysematosa*) the vagina is tremulous and tumorous (colpitis emphysematosa is distinguished by small-celled infiltration and hyperemia in the vicinity of numerous bubbles in and beneath the epithelium of the vaginal mucosa, formed perhaps by a gas-forming anærobic bacterium). In '*putraghnī*' (*endometritis*), though there are conceptions, abortion takes place with hemorrhage (recurrent abortion is usually either syphilitic in origin, or due to endometritis from any cause or retroflexion of the uterus). In '*pittalā*' (*gonorrheal acute salpangitis*) there are intense burning pain, suppuration and fever (gonorrheal inflammation and the degenerative changes of the oviducts—salpingitis, is responsible for the frequent cases in which pregnancy, happening shortly after marriage, terminates by an abortion or so called '*one-child-strerility*'). In '*atyānandā*' (*senile vaginitis*) coitus is not enjoyed (due to gonorrheal degenerative changes, the mucosa, especially in the upper part of the canal, sheds its epithelium in patches, becomes here and there studded with papillary granulations, shows a tendency to cicatrical contractions, and during coitus turgescence and voluptuous sensations are missing). In *karṇinī (neoplasms)*, due to *'śleṣma and the blood'* growths are formed (in vagina myomata, fibromata, sarcomata, carcinomata, and cystomata are seen ; in the uterus diffuse adenomata, polypoid adenomata, fibromata, fibroid polypuses, carcomata and carcinomata are more common). In *'acharaṇā'* (*vaginismus*), there is a repulsion against coitus (vaginismus is an abnormal sensitiveness of the external genitalia which may occasionally develop to spasmodic contraction of the constrictor, cunni, the levator ani and the muscles of the entire pelvic floor ; nervous virgins on the wedding night might be its subjects if brutal attacks are made by inconsiderate husbands, if they have got leathery hymen or especially in women in whom the vulva extends far forward, so that the urethral and hymenial orifices lie upon the symphysis or the ligamentum and arquatium and such women are mostly sterile, even if cohabitation in spite of the pain is enforced). *'Aticharaṇā yoni'* (female sexual apparatus habituated to excessive copulation) due to excesstve coitus, is neither capable of conception (it is well known that courtesans and prostitutes who have not contracted venereal diseases are also usually sterile). In '*śleṣmalā*' (*pruritus vulvæ*), the vulva is gummy, pruritic and chilly (vulvar pruritis may originate from various causes, as acne, eczema, acrid gonorrheal discharges from the vagina, or the high uric acid containing or sugar-laden urine may exercise a cotinuous irritation, the decomposed and stagnated secretion makes the genital apparatus sticky, and it should be removed as in all other local lesion by frequent irrigations with weak antiseptic solutions as lysole one per cent, thymol one-tenth of a per cent, or sublimate one-twentieth of a per cent). In '*śaṇḍī*' a woman does not menstruate, her breasts are very little developed and during coitus, the vagina appears rough (*infantilismus genitalium* in which the uterus and the ovaries are incompletely developed, or androgynous masculine *pseudohermaphroditism* in which the penis is rudimentary and perforate, the scrotum fused and empty, and the central resembling the labia majora, together with the absence of testicles and the development of large breasts all conspire to convey the impression of the female sex). If a maiden with a narrow vaginal orifice has copulation with a man of very large penis, and a fruit-like tumor is formed, it is called '*phalinī*' (cervicitis ; it may be also provoked by the repeated use of nodular condom)". *Suśruta* VI. 38. 5-8[175].

It has been often questioned whether the '*upadaṃśa*' of Charaka and Suśruta is really

---

175. सा फेनिलमुदावर्त्ता रजः कृच्छ्रेण मुञ्चति ॥
वन्ध्यां नष्टार्त्तवां विद्याद्विप्लुतां नित्यवेदनाम् ॥
परिप्लुतायां भवति ग्राम्यधर्म्मे रुजा भृशम् ॥
वातला कर्कशा स्तब्धा शूलनिस्तोदपीड़िता ॥
सदाहं प्रकिरत्यस्रं यस्याः सा लोहितक्षरा ॥
सवातमुद्गिरेद्वीजं वामिनी रजसा युतम् ॥
प्रस्रंसिनी स्पन्दते तु क्षोभिता दुःप्रसूश्च या ॥
स्थितं स्थितं हन्ति गर्भं पुत्रघ्नी रक्तसंस्रवात् ॥
अत्यर्थं पित्तला योनिर्दाहपाकज्वरान्विता ।
चतसृष्वपि चाद्यासु पित्तलिङ्गोच्छ्रयो भवेत् ॥ ६
अत्यानन्दा न सन्तोषं ग्राम्यधर्म्मेण गच्छति ॥
कर्णिन्यां कर्णिका योनौ श्लेष्मासृग्भ्यान्तु जायते ॥
मैथुनाचरणात् पूर्व्वा पुरुषादतिरिच्यते ॥
वहुशश्चातिचरणादन्या वीजं न विन्दति ॥
श्लेष्मला पिच्छिला योनिः कण्डुयुक्तातिशीतला ॥
चतसृष्वपि चाद्यासु श्लेष्मलिङ्गोच्छ्रितिर्भवेत् ॥ ७
अनार्त्तवस्तना षण्डी खरस्पर्शा च मैथुने ॥
अतिकायगृहीतायास्तरुण्याः फलिनी भवेत् ॥

सुश्रुतसंहिता, उत्तरतन्त्रम्, ३८

syphilis and whether the disease was known in ancient India before it was introduced into India by the Portuguese in the sixteenth century and is described graphically in *Bhāva-Prakāśa*, a work of the same age, as '*phiraṅga-roga*', the disease of the Franks, by which name Europeans were known in India, identical with the '*mal Francais or morbus gallicus*' by which it was known all over Europe.

It is well known that during the return voyage of Cristoval Colon (Cristopher Columbus) from West Indies to Spain, many of the sailors who had intercourse with the Indian women of the Islands, developed specific lesions of syphilis, and they were treated on landing by Ruy Diaz de Isla who has left clinical pictures of the lesions, typical of syphilis as known to-day. In the year 1492 Cristoval Colon sailed across the Atlantic and discovered some of the outlying islands of Central America. On the fourth of January, 1493, he sailed from the West Indies on his return to Spain which was reached in the following March. Many of the sailors were treated on landing for a new disease, which is now identified with syphilis, and the symptoms of which appeared on the shipboard before their landing. On the fourteenth of June of the year following, Nicholas Scyllatius reported an epidemic of syphilis. Soon after this Gonzalez Fernandez de Cordova, left Spain for Italy, where in a second campaign, his troops were brought into contact with those of the French. The French army numbering about 8 to 10 thousand soldiers, recruited from all parts of Europe, crossed into Piedmont on the eighth of December, in an expedition against Naples. According to the fashion of the day both the Spanish and the French army were accompanied by numerous courtesans and prostitutes for the entertainment of the soldiery. Nor was this enough. It is said that when the French soldiers reached Naples, in the intoxication of victory and unrestrained license of the age, they pillaged the convents and the homes of the rich, and spared neither the nuns nor the virgins. The army quartered in many important Italian and French cities on its return journey, left behind always in its track the *'fearful scourge of God,'* as it was called by the Church, and with the dispersal of the army, as the soldiers returned to their homes in all parts of Europe, the disease began to spread like a plague, sparing neither the cardinals, royalties nor the laity. It was known by different names, as the *'malady of* *the Neapolitans, Portuguesse, or Spainards,*' but it was '*par excellence*' known as the disease of the French (*morbus gallicus*). And one thing is clear that the history of modern syphilis can be traced step by step to the Neapolitan expedition of the French monarch Charles VIII. Bones have been exhumed of the ancient Indians, in scattered parts of America, as Colorado and Lima, exhibiting syphilitic exostosis and the results of periositis, osteitis, sclerosis, caries and other morbid processes.*

All this definitely proves that syphilis was endemic in America, and the sailors of Columbus contracted the disease in their sexual intercourse with the Indian women, and on their return home, from their contact, it spread gradually to the rest of Europe and the modern world. But this can not warrant the assumption that syphilis in some other modified or attenuated form was not known to the ancient world. The Old Testament, the ancient Chinese medical works, and especially Charaka and Suśruta have left incontestable testimonials of the pathogenesis, evolution and the malignant course of this fateful disease. The initial lesion with chancre,

* Peabody Museum of American Archeology and Ethnology, Cambridge, Mass.

cutaneous manifestations, laryngeal symptoms, caving in of the nasal bridge, condylomata, gummata in the nose, ears and eyes, exostoses of the bones (*apachi*), all these make a complete picture of syphilis (*Suśruta* II. 11. 15). But it may be said that if '*lingārśa* or *upadaṃśa*' were really syphilis, there would have been no need of writing a chapter on '*phiraṅga*' malady (morbus gallicus) with clear and systematic clinical picture of typical syphilis, by Bhāva-Miśra in his well-known '*Bhāva-Prakāśa*' after the Portuguese had introduced it in India, in addition to that of '*upadaṃśa*', thus artificially adding a disease without reason, if both were indeed identical. Strangely, '*Mādhava-Nidāna*', a work of pathology, composed between the seventh and eighth centuries, gives its seventy-seventh chapter to '*phiraṅga roga*' and the language of both '*Mādhava-Nidāna*' and '*Bhāva-Prakāśa*' is the same. It seems clear that this must have been a later interpolation, for in Mādhavakara's time, the word '*phiraṅga*' was not known. Whatever may be the case, whether the passages are spurious or '*Mādhava-nidāna*' is a much later work than it is generally believed, it must not be forgotten that the pathogenic micro-organisms do not possess the same virulence under all circumstances. As the seeds of a plant sown in different soils—marshy, sandy, fertile, rocky or desert wastes, and according to the mineral contents of the soil, sunshine, humidity and temperature—will vary in their folliage, growth, size of the plant and the fruit, and in course of time would evolve into sub-species, so a disease germ in the history of its evolution passes through an eventful career of exuberant growth and vitality or arrested development, its life being conditioned by the nourishment it receives and the environmental influences it is subjected to. Disease is the expression of the reactions of the organism in the struggle that ensues between the invading pathogenic germs and the host at whose expense the specific germs want to live and multiply. Two organisms are never the same. The American Indians were virtually nomads who lived by hunting. Their civilization was crude and primitive. They lacked personal and communal hygiene. They knew not the comforts of advanced '*social organizations*'—progressive and well-ordered States and Empires—in which life was settled, peaceful and regulated, and there was plenty of nutrition, medical attention and hospital facilities for all. So there is no wonder that syphilis ran a very virulent course with them. While in Asia, it became controlled and its virulence was attenuated. Moreover, in course of time a disease becomes milder as the race becomes partially immunized by the antibodies that are elaborated by the organism as a reaction of the disease and those characteristics are transmitted from generation to generation, thus developing a partial or complete racial immunity against a specific disease. A new disease is always virulent, for the body has not yet developed antibodies as a defensive mechanism against its attack. In the fifteenth century, after its introduction by the sailors of Columbus, syphilis overran Europe as a terrible epidemic. Now the European races have been partially immunized against it, and it usually runs a very mild course, even milder than what it was fifty years ago, as descriptions left by reliable medical writers unmistakably show the horrible syphilitic ravages which are almost unknown to-day. Possibly better nutrition and hygiene have been not unimportant factors. When syphilis was first introduced in the Sandwich Islands, more than half the population was exterminated by it within a short time as by a plague. So it is very likely that when the Portuguese introduced the virulent type of

European syphilis, it appeared almost like a new disease in the severity of the symptoms and malignant sequela. The etiology of the disease became more definite and certain, and therefore all the primary and tertiary manifestations of the lesion became united and related together, and not as described before as separate diseases.

"Because in the land of the Frank(European), this disease (syphilis) is very prevalent, it is called by the pathologists, '*phiraṅga*' (Frank's or European) disease. This disease is developed by the physical contact of a Frank or coitus with a Frankish woman. Its another name is '*gandha-roga*' (the disease that smells). It is contagious. After the incubation of the disease, the '*vāta*' becomes affected, and according to the symptom, the lesion of the '*vāta*' is to be determined.

"Syphilis manifests itself in three ways, externally, internally, or both combined. External syphilis manifests as a slightly painful papule which ulcerates like a tumor, but is easily curable. Internally gumma appears like tumescence at the joints with pain and inflammation and is very difficult to cure.

"Emaciation, loss of strength, caving in of the nasal bridge, anorexia, osteitis and osteocampsia are the symptoms of (tertiary) syphilis.

External syphilitic eruption and uncomplicated condylomata are curable. Internal manifestation (*gummata*) of syphilis is very hard to cure. But the internal complications of syphilis in a debilitated person are incurable.

Treatment : The ancient therapeutists have said that the application of (calcinated and incinerated) mercury (*karpūrarasa*) positively controls (the progress of) syphilis. And if the mercury is given in the following manner, it does not cause ulceration of the mouth : Press wheat flour with water and make a cup (out of the paste); place into the cup four *'guñjas'* (the berries of Abrus precatorius, weighing about a grain and a half each) of mercury and make such a capsule of it that no mercury can be seen on the surface. Then rolling the capsule (enclosing mercury) on clove-powder, swallow it carefully with water, so that it does not come in contact with the teeth. Later, betel-nut should be chewed, and vegetables (consisting of leaves), acids and sodium chloride should not be indulged in. Especially fatigue, exposure to the sun, exertion and coitus must be avoided. About one-fourth of an ounce of mercury, one-fourth of an ounce of Acacia catechu, half an ounce of *'ākāra-karabha'* (Echinopea echinatus ?) and three-fourths of an ounce of honey pounded together in a mortar should be made into seven pills. Syphilis is destroyed by taking each of the pills every morning with water. After taking the pill, acids and sea-salt should be avoided.

Fumigation : Mercury one ounce, sulphur one ounce and Embelia ribes one ounce should be pounded together and made into a paste, and seven pastils are to be made out of it. If the syphilitic is subjected to the fumigation for seven days, by putting a ball into fire each day, then syphilis is certainly cured.

Inunction : One-fourth of an ounce of mercury is to be rubbed over the body with the juice of Michelia champaka and Barleria pubiflora by hand, as long as mercury does not entirely disappear. The fomentation is to be applied (to facilitate absorption) and if thus avoiding acids and sea-salt, inunction is applied for seven days, syphilis is cured." *Bhāva-prakāśa* IV. 50. 1-20[176].

---

176. फिरङ्गसंज्ञके देशे बाहुल्येनैव यद्भवेत्।
तस्मात् फिरङ्ग इत्युक्तो व्याधिर्व्याधिविशारदैः॥ १

विप्रकृष्टनिदानमाह—गन्धरोगः फिरङ्गोऽयं जायते देहिनां ध्रुवम्। फिरङ्गिनोऽङ्गसंसर्गात् फिरङ्गिण्याः प्रसङ्गतः॥ व्याधिरागन्तुजो ह्येष दोषाणामव संक्रमः। भवेत्तं लक्षयेत्तेषां लक्षणैर्भिषजां वरः॥ २।३

रूपमाह—फिरङ्गस्त्रिविधो ज्ञेयो वाह्य आभ्यन्तरस्तथा। वहिरन्तर्भवश्चापि तेषां लिङ्गानि च ब्रुवे॥ तत्र वाह्यः फिरङ्गः स्याद्विस्फोटसदृशोऽल्परुक्। स्फुटितो व्रणवद्वैद्यः सुखसाध्योऽपि स स्मृतः॥ सन्धिष्वाभ्यन्तरः स स्यादामवात इव व्यथाम्। शोथञ्च जनयेदेष कष्टसाध्यो बुधैः स्मृतः॥ ४—६

उपद्रवानाह—कार्श्यं वलक्षयो नासाभङ्गो वह्नेश्च मन्दता। अस्थिशोषोऽस्थिवक्रत्वं फिरङ्गोपद्रवा अमी॥ ७

साध्यत्वादिकमाह—वहिर्भवो भवेत् साध्यो नवीनो निरुपद्रवः। आभ्यन्तरस्तु कष्टेन साध्यः स्यादयमामयः॥ वहिरन्तर्भवो जीर्णः क्षीणस्योपद्रवैर्युतः। व्याप्तो व्याधिरसाध्योऽयमित्याहुर्मुनयः पुरा॥ ८।९ इति फिरङ्गनिदानम्।

अथ फिरङ्गस्य चिकित्सा (कर्पूररसः)—फिरङ्गसंज्ञकं रोगं रसकर्पूरसंज्ञकः। अवश्यं नाशयेदेतदूचुः पूर्व्वचिकित्सकाः॥ लिख्यते रसकर्पूरप्राशने विधिरुत्तमः। अनेन विधिना खादेन्मुखे शोथं न विन्दति॥ गोधूमचूर्णं सन्नीय विदध्यात् सूक्ष्मकूपिकाम्। तन्मध्ये निःक्षिपेत् सूतं चतुर्गुञ्जामितं भिषक्॥ ततस्तु गुटिकां कुर्य्याद् यथा न दृश्यते वहिः। सूक्ष्मचूर्णं लवङ्गस्य तां वटीमवधूलयेत्॥ दन्तस्पर्शो यथा न स्यात् तथा ताम्भसा गिलेत्। ताम्बूलं भक्षयेत् पश्चाच्छाकाम्ललवणान् त्यजेत्॥ श्रममातपमध्वानं विशेषात् स्त्रीनिषेवणम्॥ १०—१४

सप्तसालिवटी—पारदष्टङ्कमानः स्यात् खदिरष्टङ्कसंमितः। आकारकरभश्चापि ग्राह्यष्टङ्कद्वयोन्मितः॥ टङ्कद्वयोन्मितं क्षौद्रं खल्वे सर्व्वं विनिःक्षिपेत्। संमर्द्य तस्य सर्व्वस्य कुर्य्यात् सप्तवटीर्भिषक्। स रोगी भक्षयेत् प्रातरेकैकामम्बुना वटीम्। वर्ज्जयेदम्ललवणं फिरङ्गस्तस्य नश्यति॥ १५—१७

धूमप्रयोगः—पारदः कर्षमात्रः स्यात्तावानेव हि गन्धकः। तण्डुलाश्चाक्षमात्राः स्युरेषां कुर्व्वीत कज्जलीम्॥ तस्याः सप्तवटीः कुर्य्यात्ताभिर्धूमं प्रयोजयेत्। दिनानि सप्त तेन स्यात् फिरङ्गान्तो न संशयः॥ १८—१९ इति धूमप्रयोगः।

पीतपुष्पवलापत्ररसैष्टङ्कमितं रसम्। हस्ताभ्यां मर्द्दयेत्तावद् यावत् सूतो न दृश्यते॥ ततः संस्वेदयेद्धस्ताविवं वासरसप्तकम्। त्यजेल्लवणमम्लञ्च फिरङ्गस्तस्य नश्यति॥

भावप्रकाशः, मध्यखण्ड, ४।

VI.—THERAPEUTICS.

"The agent that normalises a diseased function is called '*therapeutics*' and the application of it is the duty of the physician. That the principles of the body remain normal and do not become abnormal, is the object of '*therapeutics*.'" *Charaka* I. 16. 18[177]

Disease is frequently caused directly and by certain states of the blood. If certain principles in the blood are diminished, due either to faulty dietary or pathogenesis, as iron or thyroid secretion which are necessary for metabolic processes, morbid conditions of health result from these causes, known as anemia (*oligochromemia*, lacking sufficient iron for the formation of hemoglobin), or myxedema (due to deficiency of thyroid secretion). They can be easily remedied by giving iron in an assimilable form as milk, meat or spinach, or thyroid glands or sea-weeds contain-

---

177. याभिः क्रियाभिर्जायन्ते शरीरे धातवः समाः ।
सा चिकित्सा विकाराणां कर्म्म तद्भिषजां मतम ॥
कथं शरीरे धातूनां वैषम्यं न भवेदिति ।
समानाञ्चानुबन्धः स्यादित्यर्थं क्रियते क्रिया ॥
चरकसंहिता, सूत्रस्थानम्, १६ ।

ing iodine as *Durvillae utilis, Lamianria sacarina* etc., so that the thyroid glands may manufacture the necessary colloids from them. The blood being faulty, the tissues are ill-nourished and lack the necessary resisting power against the invasion of pathogenic micro-organisms. (2) There may be also disorders due to the excess of substances in the blood as '*glucose*' in glycosuria, or uric acid in gouty diathesis. If diabetes is due to defective carbohydrate metabolism, it can be cured by withholding carbohydrates from the diet, if begun when the case is not too advanced. Colchicum seems to remove the pain symptoms of gout. (3) There may be foreign bodies in the blood and their abnormal secretions, as the germs of malaria (*Plasmodium malariæ*), leprosy (*Bacillus lepræ*) or syphilis (*Spirocheta pallida*). Quinine kills the malarial spores of plasmodia, chaulmoogra and its derivatives the lepra bacilli, and mercury the syphilitic spirocheta.

It is very likely that a majority of the drugs that have found place in the '*Materia Medica*' of various countries, have very little positive value. They are more or less empirical. If they cure at all, it is but symptomatic, if not psycho-therapeutic, and can not be radical.

Many people subconsciously, as in various other superstitions, feel assured against a disease, if they have taken some kind of medicine. Lacking faith in religion, they confide in pseudo-science, for the word '*science*' has a magic charm and the people are swayed by it, as by religion in the past, and the medicine-man is but a successor of the priest. That is why, the list of drugs has swelled in volume and a new drug is being added every day. The fact is that a medicine can not destroy the pathogenic germs lodged in the tissues or blood-corpuscles without destroying the tissues, or, the corpuscles. If the chemical is strong enough to kill the pathogenic micro-organisms, it might cure the disease, but it is apt to kill the patient. Of all medicines in all '*Materia Medicas*', only quinine, chaulmoogra and mercury have proved to be of some value in the treatment of malaria, leprosy and syphilis. Yet the sequela of their treatment are many and are injurious to the organism. If the organism needs iron or phosphorus, it is not only useless, but harmful, to give inorganic ferric or phoshoric salts or compounds, for the body is incapable of assimilating them and they throw additional burden upon the over-worked kidney to eliminate them.

However, from this, it will be unjust to conclude that therapeutics is a failure. As far as medication is concerned, it is certainly getting obsolete, as the people are growing in intelligence, and learning reactions of drugs. But the disease is being controlled and conquered by hygiene, prophylaxis, dietary, serum therapy, opo therapy, surgery and antisepsis,

Ancient Hindu Medicine was justified in emphasizing the cardinal value of hygiene and dietary in the treatment of disease, by promoting the resisting power of the organism, to enable it to cure itself of the pathogenesis, Charaka severely warns against the prescription of drugs whose action is not well-known and thoroughly tested :—

"The organism suffers if drugs are given whose names, description and actions are not well-known, or if known, has not been properly given (chemical incompatibility or over-dose). By proper chemical combination and application, even a deadly poison can become a good medicine, while a good drug by improper combination (chemical incompatibility) and application can be venomously injurious. Therefore any intelligent person who wishes cure and long life, should not take an improper medicine. *Charaka* I. 1. 48 [178].

"Medicines are derived from three sources—animals, minerals and vegetables." *Charaka* I. 1. 35[179].

"Of animals, honey, milk and milk-products, bile, fat, bone-marrow, blood, flesh, excreta, urine, skin (including membrane), semen, bone, tendon, horn, claw, hoof, hair, down and gall-stone are used in medicine.

Gold, five metals (silver, copper, tin, lead and iron) and their oxides, sand, carbonate of lime, arsenous disulphide, arsenous sulphide, precious stone (diamond), sea-salt, ferric carbonate of calcium and antimony (are used in medicine of the minerals).

Vegetable drugs are from four sources : '*vanas-*

---

178. औषधं ह्यनभिज्ञातं नामरूपगुणैस्त्रिभिः ।
विज्ञातमपिदुर्युक्तमनर्थायोपपद्यते ॥
योगादपि विषं तीक्ष्णं उत्तमं भेषजं भवेत् ।
भेषजं वापि दुर्युक्तं तीक्ष्णं सम्पद्यते विषम् ॥
तस्मान्न भिषजा युक्तं युक्तिबाह्येन भेषजम् ।
धीमता किञ्चिदादेयं जीवितारोग्यकाङ्क्षिणा ॥

चरकसंहिता, सूत्रस्थानम्, १ ।

179. तत्पुनस्त्रिविधं ज्ञेयं जाङ्गमौद्भिदपार्थिवम् ।

pati' (*gymnosperms*), '*vānaspatya*' (*angiosperms*), '*oṣadhi*' (*herbs*) and '*vīrudh*' (*archegoniates*). Those who have fruits without flowers are called '*vanaspati*' (*gymnosperms*). Those whose fruits develop from flowers, are called *vānaspatya* (*angiosperms*). Those who only persist for the development of seeds are called '*oṣadhi*' (*herbs*). Those which expand (*pratāna*, by climbing, as the fern Lygodium palmatum) are called, '*vīrudh*' (*archegoniates*.)." *Charaka* I. 1. 36-38[180].

"Root (*mūla*), bark (*tvak*), pith (*sāra*), gum-resin (*niryyāsa*), culm (*nāḍa*), juice (*svarasa*), leaves and flowering top (*pallava*), vegetable alkali (*kṣāra*), milky exudation (*kṣīra*), fruit (*phala*), flower (*puṣpa*), ash (*bhasma*), oil (*taila*),

---

180. मधूनि गोरसाः पित्तं वसा मज्जासृगामिषम् ॥
विन्मूत्रचर्म्मरेतोऽस्थिस्नायुशृङ्गनखाः खुरा ।
जङ्गमेभ्यः प्रयुज्यन्ते केशलोमानि रोचनाः ॥
सुवर्णं समलाः पञ्चलोहाः ससिकता सुधा ।
मनःशिलाले मणयो लवणं गैरिकाञ्जने ॥
भौममौषधमुद्दिष्टमौद्भिदन्तु चतुर्व्विधम् ।
वनस्पतिस्तथा वीरुद्वानस्पत्यस्तथौषधिः ॥
फलैर्व्वनस्पतिः पुष्पैर्व्वानस्पत्यः फलैरपि ।
ओषध्यः फलपाकान्ताः प्रतानैर्वीरुधः स्मृताः ॥
चरक-संहिता, सूत्र-स्थानम्, १ ।

thorn (*kaṇṭaka*, for opening superficial cutaneous abscess), leaf (*patra*), flower-bud (*śūṅga*), rhizome and bulb (*kanda*), and bud (*praroha* = undeveloped shoot) of plants are used as medicines." *Charaka* I. 1. 38[181].

"The fluid that is extracted by pressing any (vegetable or animal) substance in a machine, is called juice (*svarasa*). Anything that is beaten into semi-solid consistency in a mortar, is called *paste* (*kalka*). The liquid preparation of any (vegetable) drug, obtained by boiling with water, is called by the therapeutists, *Decoction* (*śṛta*). The preparation that comes out by steeping a (crude) drug in cold water, and passing it through a sieve after exposing it to the dew-drops of the night (that is the crude drug is to be kept soaked in water at least for 12 hours), is called *Infusion* (*śīta*). If any ground drug is poured into boiling water, and the preparation is passed through a sieve, it is called, *Tea* (*phāṇṭa*)." *Charaka* I. 4. 8[182].

---

181. मूलत्वक् सारनिर्य्यास-नाड़-स्वरसपल्लवाः ।
क्षाराः क्षीरं फलं पुष्पं भस्म तैलानि कण्टकाः ।
पत्राणि शुङ्गाः कन्दाश्च प्ररोहाश्चौद्भिदो गणः ॥
चरक-संहिता, सूत्र-स्थानम्, १ ।

182. यन्त्रप्रपीड़नाद्द्रव्याद्रसः स्वरस उच्यते ।
यत् पिण्डं रसपिष्टानां तत् कल्कं परिकीर्त्तितम् ॥

Cerebral Sedatives : "Fructus Achyranthes aspera (*apāmārga*), Piper longum (*pippalī*), Piper nigrum (*maricha*), Embelia ribes (*viḍaṅga*), Moringa pterygosperma (*śigra*), Sinapis alba (*saṣarpa*), Xanthoxylon alatum (*tumburu*), Nigella sativa (*ajāji*), Ocymum gratissimum (*ajagandhā*), Salvadora persica (*pīlu*), Elletaria major (*elā*),Piper aurantiacum (*hareṇukā*), cardamomi semina (*pṛthvīkā*), Ocimum basilicum (*surasā*) Clitoria ternatea (*śvetā*), Ocimum sanctum (*kuṭheraka*) Ocimum villosum (*phaṇijjhaka*), fructus Albizzia lebbek (*śirīṣa*), Allium sativum (*laśuna*), Curcuma longa and Berberis asiatica (*haridrā* and *dāru-haridrā*), sodium chloride and rock-salt (*lavaṇa-dvaya*), Cardiospermum halicacabum (*jyotiṣmatī*),and zingiber officinale (*nāgara*) these are *Cerebral Sedatives*. These are also used in migraine, cephalalgia, catarrh, helmet-headache, syphilitic gumma (*krimivyādhi*-bacterial lesion ?), apoplexy, anosmia and epilepsy.

Emetics : Randia dumetorum (*madana*), Gly-

वह्नौतु क्वथितं द्रव्यं शृतमाहुश्चिकित्सकाः ।
द्रव्यादापोत्थितात्तोये तत् पुनर्निशि संस्थितात् ॥
कषायो योऽभिनिर्याति स शीतः समुदाहृतः ।
क्षिप्त्वोष्णतोये मृदितं तत् फाण्टं परिकीर्तितम् ॥

चरक-संहिता, सूत्रस्थानम्, ४ ।

cyrrhiza glabra (*madhuka*), Azadirachta indica (*nimba*), Achyranthes aspera (*jīmūta*), Achyranthes fruticosa (*kṛta-vedana*), Piper longum (*pippalī*), Mallotus philippinensis (*kūṭaja*), Citrullus colocynthis (*ikṣvāku*), Elletaria major (*elā*) and Achyranthes obtusifolia (*dhāmārgava*) are to be used as Emetics in proper doses, in intestinal, '*pitta*' and '*ślesma*' diseases without causing any injury to the organism.

Purgatives : Ipomoea (Convolvulus), turpethum (*trivṛt*), Terminalia chebula, Terminalia belerica (Myrobalan) and Emblica (Phyllanthus) officinalis (*tri-phalā*), Baliospermum montanum (*dantī*), Ipomoea caerulea (*nīlinī*, Abrus precatorius (*saptalā*), Acorus calamus (*vacha*), Mallotus philippinensis (*kampillaka*), Clitoria ternatea (*gavākṣi*), Mimusops kauki (*kṣīriṇi*), Luffa amara (*udakīryyka*), Salvadora persica (*pilu*), Cassia fistula (*āragvadha*), Uvae passæ (*drākṣā*), Baliospermum indicum (*dravantī*) and Barringtonia acutangula (*nichula*) are to be used as *Purgatives* in intestinal diseases, Sterospermum suaveolens (*pāṭali*), Premna serratifolia (*agnimantha*), Aegle marmelos (*vilva*), Oroxylum (Calosanthus), indicum (*śyoṇāka*), Gmelina arborea (*kāśmaryya*), Desmodium triflorum (*śālaparṇī*), Uraria logopodioides (*pṛśniparṇī*), solanum xanthocarpum (*nidigdhikā*),

Sida cordifolia (*valā*), Tribulus lanuginosus (*asvadaṃṣṭrā*) Solanum indicum (*vṛhatī*), Ricinus communis (*eraṇḍa*), Boerhaavia procumbens (*punarnavā*), Hordeum hexastichum (*yava*), Dolichos uniflorus (*kulattha*), Zizyphus jujuba (*kola*), Tinospora cordifolia (*guḍuchī*), Randia dumentorum (*madana*), Butea frondosa (*palāśa*), Andropogon citratum (*karttṛṇa*), oils and salts are to be used (as purgatives) in constipation and in the formation of the feces." *Charaka* I. 2. 2-5[183].

183. अपामार्गस्य बीजानि पिप्पली मरिचानि च ।
विडङ्गान्यथ शिग्रूनि सर्षपास्तुम्बुरूणि च ॥
अजाजीञ्चाजगन्धाञ्च पीलून्येलां हरेणुकाम् ।
पृथ्वीकां सुरसां श्वेतां कुठेरकफणिज्झकौ ॥
शिरीषबीजं लशुनं हरिद्रे लवणद्वयम् ।
ज्योतिष्मतीं नागरञ्च दद्याच्छीर्षविरेचने ॥
गौरवे शिरसः शूले पीनसेऽर्द्धावभेदके ।
क्रिमिव्याधावपस्मारे घ्राणनाशे प्रमोहके ॥
मदनं मधुकं निम्बं जीमूतं कृतवेधनम् ।
पिप्पलीकुटजेक्ष्वाकुण्येलां धामार्गवाणि च ॥
उपस्थिते श्लेष्मपित्ते व्याधावामाशयाश्रये ।
वमनार्थं प्रयुञ्जीत भिषग् देहमदूषयन् ॥
त्रिवृतां त्रिफलां दन्तीं नीलिनीं सप्तलां वचाम् ।
कम्पिल्लकं गवाक्षीञ्च क्षीरिणीमुदकीर्य्यकाम् ॥

Antiparasitics : Cassia fistula (*āragvadha*), Cassia tora (*aiḍagaja*), Luffa amara, Justicia adhatoda (*vāsā*), Tinospora cordifolia, Randia dumentorum, Curuma longa, Berberis asiatica, Acacia gummifera (*śryāhva*), Cedrus deodara (*surāhva*), Acacia catechu (*khadira*), Tomentosa latifolia (*dhava*), Azadirachta indica, Embelia indica, Nerium odoratum (*karavīraka*), Betula bhojpattra (*bhūrjja*), Allium sativum, Albizzia lebbek, Laurus cassia (*lomaśa*), Balsamodendron pubescens (*guggulu*), Moringa (*zeylanica*) pterygosperma (*kriśṇagandhā*), Ocimum villosum, Mallotus philippinensis, Alstonia scholaris, Salvadora persica, Saussurea lappa (*kuṣṭha*), Jasminum grandiflorum (*sumana*), Acorus calamus, Piper angustifolium (*reṇukā*), Ipomoe turpethum, Baliospermum montanum, Acaju officinalis

---

पीलून्यारग्वधं द्राक्षां द्रवन्तीं निचुलानि च ।
पक्वाशयगते दोषे विरेकार्थं प्रयोजयेत् ॥
पाटलिञ्चाग्निमन्थञ्च विल्वं श्योणाकमेव च ।
काश्मर्य्यं शालपर्णीञ्च पृश्निपर्णीं निदिग्धिकाम् ॥
वलां श्वदंष्ट्रां वृहतीमैरण्डं सपुनर्नवम् ।
यवान् कुलत्थान् कोलानि गुडूचीं मदनानि च ॥
पलाशं कत्तृणञ्चैव स्नेहांश्च लवणानि च ।
उदावर्त्ते विवन्धेषु युञ्ज्यादास्थापनेषु च ॥

चरकसंहिता, सूत्र-स्थानम् २

(*bhallātaka*), ferric calcium carbonate (*gairika*), antimonious sulphide (*añjana*), arsenous sulphide (*āla*), arsenous disulphide (*manaḥśilā*), fuliginis alcalina (*gṛha-dhūma* = a complex empyreumatic substance, deposited from smoke, made up chiefly of a resinous substance combined with lactic acid, carbonous matters and creasote, besides various mineral salts), Elletaria major (*elā*), ferric sulphide (*kāśīsa*), Symplocos racemosa (*lodhra*), Terminalia arjuna (*arjjuna*), Achyranthes aspera (*musta*) and Shorea robusta (*sarjja*) are kept together with the bovine gallstone for seven days, and then having crushed the gallstone, the linimenta is mixed with oleum sinapis, and applied over the body as an unguent, then obstinate psoriasis, leucoderma, alopecia, keloid, tinea imbricata, scrofulide, fistula-in-ano and eczema are cured within a short time.

Saussurea lappa, Curcuma longa, Berberis asiatica, Ocimum basilicum, Trichosanthes dioica, Azadirachta indica, Withania somnifera (*aśvagandhā*), Cedrus deodara, Moringa pterygosperma, Sinapis alba, Xanthoxylon budrunga (*tumvurū*), Coriandri fructus, Scrupus capsularis (*vanya*) and Andropogon acicularis (*chaṇḍā*) are to be ground in equal proportion and mixed with whey, and if then it be rubbed over the body as an unguent, pruritus, eruption, urticaria and tumescence become cured.

Saussurea auriculata, Cocculus cordifolius (*amṛta*), Hydrocarpus kurzii or copper-sulphide (*asanga*), Berberis asiatica, ferric sulphide, gummi Rotleria tinctoria (*kampillaka*), Achyranthes aspera, Symplocos racemosa, Andropogon shoenanthus (*saugandhika*), Shorea robusta, gummi Vateria indica (*sarja-rasa*), Embelia indica, arsenous disulphide, arsenous sulphide, and Nerium odorum—relieve tinea imbricata, pruritus, keloid, eczema and scrofulide, if these are ground and rubbed over the body, smeared with unguents." *Charaka* I. 3. 2-4 [184].

---

184. आरग्वधः सैड़गजः करञ्जो वासा गुड़ुची मदनं हरिद्रे ।
श्र्याह्वः सुराह्वः खदिरो धवश्च निम्बो विड़ङ्गं करवीरकत्वक् ॥
ग्रन्थिश्च भौर्ज्जो लशुनः शिरीषः सलोमशो गुग्गुलुकृष्णगन्धे ।
फणिज्झको वत्सकसप्तपर्णौ पीलूनि कुष्ठं सुमनःप्रवालाः ॥
वचाहरेणुस्त्रिवृता निकुम्भो भल्लातकं गैरिकमञ्जनञ्च ।
मनःशिलाले गृहधूम एलाकाशीशलोध्रार्ज्जुनमुस्तसर्ज्जाः ॥
इत्यर्द्धरूपैर्विहिताः षड़ेते गोपित्तपीताः पुनरेव पिष्टाः ।
सिद्धाः परं सर्षपतैलयुक्ताश्चूर्णप्रदेहा भिषजा प्रयोज्याः ॥
कुष्ठानि कृच्छ्राणि नवं किलासं सुरेन्द्रलुप्तं किटिभं सदद्रु ।
भगन्दरार्शांस्यपचीं सपामां हन्युः प्रयुक्तास्त्वचिरान्नराणाम् ॥
कुष्ठं हरिद्रे सुरसं पटोलं निम्बाश्वगन्धे सुरदारु शिग्रु ।
ससर्षपं तुम्बुरुधान्यवन्यं चण्डाञ्च चूर्णानि समानि कुर्य्यात् ॥

Anodynes : "Radix Nymphaea lotus, Cedrus deodara, Saussurea lappa, Glycyrrhiza glabra, Elletaria major, Nelumbium speciosum (*kamala*) Nyphaea stellata (*utpala*), Aquilaria agallocha (*loha*), Typha angustifolia (*erakā*), Nymphaea lotus (*padmaka*), Andropogon acicularis—if these are used as a liniment, headache is relieved. Aerides tessalatum (*rāsnā*), Curcuma longa, Berberis asiatica, Valeriana dioica, Fœniculum vulgare and Anisi fructus, Cedrus deodara, Saccharum officinarum andCælogyne ovalis(*jīvantī* = *cæla*) if compounded and mixed with clarified butter and oleum sesami, and applied as a liniment after warming it, pain is relieved.

Demulcents : Musci (*śaivāla*), Nymphæa lotus, Nymphæa stellata, Calamus rotang (*vetra*), Calophyllum inophyllum (*tuṅga*), radix Nymphæa lotus, Andropogon muricatum, Symplocos racemosa, Aglaia edulis, Pterocarpus

---

तैलक्कपिष्टैः प्रथमं शरीरं तैलाक्तमुद्वर्त्तयितुं यतेत।
तेनास्य कण्डूः पिड़काः सकोठाः कुष्ठानि शोफाश्च शमं व्रजन्ति॥
कुष्ठामृतासङ्गकटङ्कटेरी काशीशकम्पिल्लकमुस्तलोध्रम्।
सौगन्धिकं सर्जरसो विड़ङ्गं मनःशिलाले करवीरकत्वक्॥
तैलाक्तगात्रस्य कृतानि चूर्णान्येतानि दद्यादवचूर्णनार्थम्।
दद्रुः सकण्डूः किटिमानि पामा विचर्च्चिका चैव तथैति शान्तिम्॥

चरकसंहिता, सूत्र-स्थानम्, ३।

santalinus, if applied as a liniment, after pasting and mixing them with clarified butter, the irritation of a burn is relieved. Ipomoea digitata (*sitā*), Rubia cordifolia, Calamus rotang, radix Nymphæa lotus, Glycyrrhiza glabra, Citrullus colocynthis (*aindrī*), Nymphæa lotus, Panicum frumentaceum (*durvvā*), radix Hedysarum alhagi (*yavāsa-mūla*), Poa cynosuroides, Saccharum spontaneum (*kāśa*), and Typha angustifolia, if applied as a liniment, irritation of the skin is relieved. Lichen (*śaileyam*), Elletaria major, Aquilaria agallocha, Saussurea lappa, Andropogon acicularis, Tabernæmontana coronaria (*nata*) Cinnamonum zeilanicum (*tvak*), Cedrus deodara, Aerides tessellatum, Albizzia lebbek and Mimosa indica, if applied as a plaster on a venous bite, the burning irritation is relieved.

Diaphoretics : Albizzia lebbek, Mimosa indica, Mesua speciosa (*hema*), and Symplocos racemosa, if rubbed upon the skin in the powder form, it relieves skin-lesion and causes perspiration." *Charaka* I. 3. 16-21[185].

---

185. प्रपौण्डरीकं सुरदारु कुष्ठं यष्ट्याह्वमेला कमलोत्पले च ।
शिरोरुजायां सघृतः प्रदेहो लोहैरकापद्मक-चोरकैश्च ॥
रास्नाहरिद्रे नलदं शताह्वे द्वे देवदारूणि सितोपलाश्च ।
जीवन्तिमूलं सघृतं सतैलमालेपनं पार्श्वरुजासु कोष्णम् ॥

Analeptics : "Celtis orientalis minor (*jïvaka*), Vitis vinifera (*ṛṣavaka*), Leptadenia reticulata (*medā*), Leptadenia spartium (*mahamedā*), Gymnema balsamicum (*kākolï*), Gymnema lactiferum (*kṣïra-kākolï*), Phaseolus trilobus (*mudga-parṇï*), Teramnua labialis (*māṣaparṇï*), Cælogyne ovalis and Glycyrrhiza glabra—these ten are vitalizing astringent drugs.

Tonics : Mimusops kauki (*kṣïriṇï*), Oxystelma esculentum (*rājakṣavaka*), Cordia latifolia (*valā*), Gymnema balsamicum, Gymnema lactiferum, Cordia officinalis, Cordia myxa, Hibiscus vitifolius, Batatas paniculata and Ipomoæ batatas—these ten are tonic astringents.

Epispastics : Cyperus rotundus, Saussurea lappa, Curcuma longa, Berberis asiatica, Acorus calamus, Aconytum heterophyllum, Picrorrhiza

---

शैवालपद्मोत्पलवेत्रतुङ्गं प्रपौण्डरीकाण्यमृणाललोध्रम् ।
प्रियङ्गु कालीयकचन्दनानि निर्व्वापणः स्यात् सघृतः प्रदेहः ।
सितालतावेतसपद्मकानि यष्ट्याह्वमैन्द्री नलिनानि दूर्व्वा ।
यवासमूलं कुशकाशयश्च निर्व्वापणः स्यात् जलमेरका च ॥
शैलेयमेलागुरुणी सकुष्ठे चण्डा नतं त्वक् सुरदारुरास्ना ।
शीतं निहन्यादचिरात् प्रदेहो विषं शिरीषस्तु ससिन्धुवारः ॥
शिरीषलामज्जकहेमलोध्रै स्त्वग्दोषसंस्वेदहरः प्रघर्षः ।

चरक-संहिता, सूत्र-स्थानम्, ३ ।

kurroa, Plumbago zeylanica, Pongamia glabra and Ipomoæ indica—these ten are reductive.

Pustulants : Convolvulus turpethum, Asclepias gigantea, Ricinus communis, Gloriosa superba, Rubia cordifolia, Plumbago zeylanica, Pongamia glabra, Andropogon acicularis, Picrorrhiza kurroa and Cleome felina—these ten cause suppuration.

Vulneraries : Glycyrrhiza glabra, Tinospora cordifolia, Uraria logopodioides, Stephania herandifolia, Mimosa pudica, Bombex malabarcum, Grislea tomentosa, Symplocos racemosa, Aglaia edulis, and Myrica sapida—these ten promote the healing of wounds..

Irritants : Piper longum, radix Piper longum, Piper chava, Plumbago zeylanica, Zingiber officinale, Rumex vesicarius, Piper nigrum, Pimpinella saxifraga, Semecarpus anacardium and Ferula asafœtida—these ten are rubefacient.

Tonics : Citrullus colocynthis, Carpopogon pruriens, Asparagus sarmentosus, Phaseolus trilobus, Convolvulus paniculatus, Withania somnifera, Desmodium triflorum, Picrorrhizza kurroa, Sida cordifolia, and Sida rhombifolia—these ten are tonics (strengthening).

Rubefacients: Pterocarpus santalinus, Calphyllum inophyllum, Nymphæa lotus, Andropogon muriculatum, Glycyrrhiza glabra, Rubia cordifolia, Hemidesmus indicus, Convolvulus paniculatus, Panicum frumentaceum and Panicum dactylon—these ten bring redness to the complexion.

Expectorants: Hemidesmus indicus, radix Saccharum officinarum, Glycyrrhiza glabra, Piper longum, Uvæ passae, Convolvulus paniculatus, Myrica sapida, Hydroctyle asiatica, Solanum indicum, and Solanum xanthocarpum—these ten stimulate bronchial (mucous membrane).

Heart-Stimulants: Mangifera indica, Spondias mangifera, Artocarpus lakoocha, Carissa carandas, Tamarindus indica, Rumex vesicarius, Prunus acida, Prunus acacia, Punica granatium, and Citrus medica—these ten stimulate the heart.

Refrigerants: Zingiber officiniale, Plumbago zeylanica, Piper chaba, Embelia ribes, Saussurea zeylanica, Tinospora cordifolia, Acorus calamus, Cyperus rotundus, Piper longum and Trichosanthes—these ten allay thirst.

Hemostatics: Holarrhena antidysenterica, Aegle marmelos, Plumbago zeylanica, Aconitum heterophyllum, Terminalia chebula, Alhagi maurorum, Berberis asiatica, Acorus calamus, and Piper chava—these ten cure piles.

Antiparasitics: Acacia catechu, Terminalia chebula, Phyllanthus emblica, Curcuma longa, Semescarpum anacardium, Alstonia scholaris, Cassia fistula, Nerium odorum, Embelia ribes, and Jasminum grandiflorum, Pterocarpus santalinus, Nardostachys jatamansi, Cassia fistula, Pongamia glabra, Azadirachta indica, Holarrhena antidysenterica, Sinapis alba, Glycyrrhiza glabra, Berberis asiatica and cyperus rotandus cure the skin diseases.

Counter-irritants: Pterocarpus santalinus, Nardostachys Jatamansi, Cassia fistula, Pongamia glabra, Azadirachta indica, Holarrhena antidysenterica, Sinapis alba, Glycyrrhiza glabra, Berberis asiatica and cyperus rotundus relieve pruritus (by dilating the superficial vessels).

Anthelmintics: Moringa pterigosperma, Piper nigrum, Tithymalus antiquorum, Colocasia antiquorum, Vitex negundo, Embelia ribes, Achyranthes aspera, Tribulus terrestris, Clerodendron serratifolium and Salvadora persica are vermifuge (cause the destruction or expulsion of the intestinal worms).

Antidotes: Curcuma longa, Rubia cordifolia, Aerides tessallatum, Ichnocarpus frutescens, Pterocarpus santalinus, Strychnos potatorum, Albizzia, lebbek, Vitex negundo and

Cordia myxa—these ten destroy (neutralize) poisons.

Galactogogues: Andropogon muricatum, Oryza sativa, a sub-species of Oryza sativa, Saccharum officinarum, Saccharum cylindricum, Poa cynosuroides, Saccharum spontaneum, Tinospora cordifolia, Abelmoschus moschatus, and Hemionetis esculenta—these ten increase milk.

Anti galactogogues: Stephania hernandifolia, Zingiber officinale, Cedrus deodara, Cyperus rotundus, Saussurea zeylanica, Tinospora cordifolia, Holarrhena antidysenterica, Agathotes cherayta, Picrorrhiza kurroa, and hemidesmus—these ten reduce the production of milk.

Aphrodisiacs: Celtis orientalis, Vitis vinifera, Gymnema balsamicum, Gymnema lactiferum, Phaseolus trilobus, Teramnus labialis, Leptademia spartium, Asparagus racemosus, Nardostachys jatamansi and Rhus succedania—these ten increase semen.

Anaphrodisiacs: Saussurea auriculata, Feronia elephantum, Myrica sapida, os sapiæ, Nauclea cadamba, saccharum purificatum, Hygrophila spinosa, Ruellia longifolia, Sesbania grandiflora and Andropogon muricatum—these ten reduce semen (diminish sexual desire and power).

Adipogenous agents :—Uvae passœ, Glycyrrhiza glabra, Tinospora cordifolia, Leptademia spartium, Convolvulus paniculata, Gymnema balsamicum, Gymnema lactiferum, Celtis orientalis, Caelogyne ovalis and Desmodium triflorum —these ten cause the formation of fat (in the body.)

Diaphoretics :—Moringa pterigosperma, Ricinus communis, Asclepias gigantea, Boerhaava diffusa, Boerhaava procubens, Hordium hexastichum, Sesamum indicum, Dolichos biflorus, Phaseolus trilobus, and Zizyphus jujuba—these ten increase perspiration (by stimulating the sudoriparous glands).

Emetics :—Mel, Glycyrrhiza glabra, Bauhinia variegata, Bauhinia acuminata, Nauclea cadamba, Calamus fasciculatus, Cephalandra indica, Crotalaria verrucosa, Asclepias gigantica and Achyranthus aspera—these ten cause vomiting.

Purgatives :—Uvae passae, Gmelina arborea, Grewia asiatica, Terminalia chebula, Phyllanthus emblica, Terminalia belerica, Zizyphus laccifera, Zizyphys jujuba, Zizyphus napeca and Salvadora persica—these ten are purgatives.

Enemata :—Ipomœa turpethum, Aegle marmelos, Piper longum, Holarrhena antidysenterica, Sinapis alba, Acorus calamus, fructi Holarrhena antidysenterica, Peucedanum graveolens, Glycyrrhiza glabra, and fructus Randia dumetorum—these ten are (suited) for enema.

Oily-enemata :—Vanda roxburghii, Cedrus deodara, Aegle marmelos, Randia dumetorum, Peucedanun graveolens, Boerhavia diffusa alba, Boerhavia diffusa rubra, Tribulus terrestris, Premna serratifolia and Oroxylum indicum—these ten are (fitted) for oily-enemata.

Cerebral sedatives :—Cardiospermum halicacabum, Sinapis nigra, Piper nigrum, Piper longum, Embelia ribes, Achyranthes aspera, Sinapis alba, Moringa pterogospermum, Clitorea ternatea, and Clitorea mariana—these ten are Cerebral sedatives (possibly an errhine is meant).

Anti-emetics :—Eugenia jambolana, Mangifera indica, Citrus medica, Zizyphus jujuba, Punicum granatum, Hordeum hexastichum, Andropogon muricatum, diatomacious earth, and pop corn—these ten are anti-emetics (by allaying the irritablity of the gastric nerves or the vomitting centers or neutralizing the toxins which irritate those centers).

Refrigerants:—Cyperus pertenuis, Alhagi maurorum, Cyperus rotundus, Oldenlandia herbacea, Pterocarpus santalinus, Agathotes chirayata, Tinospora cordifolia, Pavonia odorata, corandrum sativum and Trichosanthes dioica—these ten allay thirst.

Pulmonary sedatives: Curcuma zerumbet Costus speciosus, Zizyphus jujuba, Solanum xanthocarpum, Solanum indicum, Cymbidium tessaloides, Terminalia chebula, Piper longum, Alhagi maurorum and Rhus succedania—these ten relieve hiccup (by allaying irritability of the respiratory center or the terminal fibers of the nerves distributed to the bronchi and lungs).

Laxatives: Aglaia roxburghiana, Hemidesmus indicus, fructus Mangifera indica, Colosanthus indicus, Symplocus racemosa, gummi Bombax malabaricum, Mimosa pudica, Grislea tomentosa, Clerodendrum indicum, and fructus Nymphaea lotus—these ten cause the formation (evacuation) of feces.

Cholagogues:—Eugenia jambolana, Boswellia serrata, Mucuna pruriens, Glycyrrhiza glabra, Bombax malabaricum, Pinus longifolia, edible diatomacious earth (containing oxide of iron which gives it a red-yellowish color), Balatas paniculatus, Nymphaea stellata, and fructus Sesamum indicum—these ten give color to the feces (by causing the increased secretion of the bile).

Urinary diluents :—Eugenia jambolana, Mangifera indica, Ficus infectoria, Ficus Bengalensis, Spondias mangifera, Ficus glomerata, Ficus religiosa, Semecarpus anacardium, Oxalis acetosella and Acacia catechu—these ten increase the quantity of urine.

Urinary-antacids or anticeptics :—Nelumbian speciosum, Nymphæa stellata, Nymphæa alba, Nymphæa rubra, Nymphæa odorata, Nymphæa lotus, Nymphæa pubescens, Glycyrrhiza rubra, Aglaia roxburghiana and Grislea tomentosa—these ten purify the urine.

Diuretics :—Costus speciosum, Tribulus terrestris, Sesbania grandiflora, Cleome viscosa, Colcus amboinicus, Imperata cylindrica, Poa cynosuroides, Saccharum spontaneum, Panicum frumentaceum and Saccharum sara—these ten increase the excretion of urine.

Pulmonary sedatives :—Uvae passae, Terminalia chebula, Phyllanthus emblica, Piper longum, Alhagi maurorum, Rhus succedania, Solanum xanthocarpum, Boerhavia diffusa rubra, Boerhavia diffusa alba, and Phyllanthus nirury—these ten relieve coughing (expectorants ?).

Respiratory stimulants :—Curcuma zerumbet, Costus speciosum, Rumex vesicularis, Elletaria cardiamomum, Ferula assafoetida, Ocimum sanctum, Phyllanthus niruri, Caelogne ovalis, and Andropogon—these ten relieve dyspnea.

Styptics :—Stereospermum suaveolens, Premna serratifolia, Aegle marmelos, Colosanthes indica, Gmelina arborea, Solanum xanthocarpum, Solanum indicum, Desmosium trilobum, Uraria logopodioides, and Tribulus terrestris—these ten reduce inflammation.

Antipyretics : Hemidesmus indicus, rock candy, Stephania rotunda, Rubia cordifolia, Uvæ passæ, Salvadora persica, Grewia asiatica, Terminalia chebula, Phyllanthus emblica and Terminalia bellerica—these ten relieve fever.

Spinal stimulants : Uvæ passæ, Phœnix sylvetris, Buchanania latifolia, Zizyphus jujuba, Punica granatum, Ficus glomerata, Grewia asiatica, Saccharum officianarum, Hordeum hexastichum and a variety of Oryza sativa—these ten remove fatigue.

Vascular sedatives : Pop corn, Santalnum album, fructus Gmelina arborea, Glycyrhiza glabra, rock-candy, Nymphæa stellata, Andropogon muricatum, Hemidesmus indicum, Tinospora cordifolia and pavonia odorata—these ten relieve 'æstus' (internal congestion), by moderating the cardiac excitement, and rendering the heart's action more slow or less forcible.

Vascular stimulants : Cassia auriculata (Tabernaemontana coronaria ?), Aquilaria agallocha, Coriandrum sativum, Zingiber officinale, Carum ajowan, Acarus calamus, Solanum xanthocarpum, Paemna serratifolia, Colosanthus indica, and Piper longum—these ten relieve the chilly sensation (by accelerating the circulation, acting on the heart and the blood-vessels).

Emollients : Diospyros glutinosa, Buchanania latifolia, Zizyphus jujuba, Acacia catechu, Acacia bombolah, Alstonia scholaris, Shorea robusta, Terminalia arjuna, Terminalia tomentosa, and Acacia farmensiana—these ten relieve (the burning sensation) of erysipelas.

Antirheumatics : Desmodium trilobum, Uraria logopodioides, Solanum indicum, Solanum xanthocarpum, Ricinus communis, Gymnema balsimicum, Santalanum album, Andropogon muricatum, Eleteria cardamamum, and Glycyrrhiza glabra—these ten relieve rheumatic (gouty) pain (by dissolving uric acid deposits),

Counter-irritants : Piper longum, radix Piper longum, Piper chaba, Plumbago zeylanica, Zingiber officianale, Piper nigrum, Pimpinella involucrata, Seseli ubanotis, Cuminum cyminum, and Achyranthes repens—these ten relieve pain,

Styptics : Mel, Glycyrhiza glabra, Crocus sativus, Bombax malabaricum, diatomacious earth (containing oxide of iron), ferric calcium carbonate, Symplocos racemosa, Aglaia roxburghiana, rock candy, and pop corn—these ten arrest the flow of blood (by vascular contraction).

Anodynes :—Shorea robusta, Myrica sapida, Nauclea cadamba. radix Nymphaea lotus, Calophyllum, inophyllum, Bombax malabaricum, Albizzia lebbek, Calamus rotung, Feronia elephantum and Saraca indica—these ten relieve pain.

Anaesthetics : Ferula assafœtida, Melia azedarach, Acacia farnesiana, Acorus calamus, Andropogon acicularis, Herpestis monieria, Corydalis cava, Nardostachys jatamansi, Saraca indica, and Picrorrhizah kurroa—these ten abolish consciousness (by inhibiting the functions of the higher cerebral centers).

Aphrodisiacs : Citrullus colocynthis, Herpestis monieria, Panicum dactylon, Panicum frumentaceum, Steriospermum suaveolens, Terminalia chebula, Picrorrhiza kurroa, Sida cordifolia, and Aglaia roxburghiana—these ten increase the reproductive powers.

Analeptics : Tinospora cordifolia, Terminalia chebula, Phyllanthus emblica, Vanda roxburghii, Panicum dactylon, Caelogyne ovalis, Hemidesmus indica, Hydrocotyle asiatica, Desmodium trilobum, and Bœrhaavia asiatica—these ten prolong life." *Charaka* I. 4. 12-62[186].

---

186. जीवकर्षभकौ मेदा महामेदा काकोली क्षीरकाकोली मुद्गमाषपर्ण्यौ जीवन्ती मधुकमिति दशेमानि जीवनीयानि भवन्ति ।

क्षीरिणी राजक्षवकं बला काकोली क्षीरकाकोली वाट्यायनी भद्रौदनी भारद्वाजी पयस्यर्षगन्धा इति दशेमानि बृंहणीयानि भवन्ति ।

मुस्तकुष्ठहरिद्रा दारुहरिद्रा वचातिविषा कटुरोहिणी चित्रक
चिरबिल्वहैमवत्य इति दशेमानि लेखनीयानि भवन्ति ।

सुवहार्करुबुकाग्निमुखी चित्रा चित्रक चिरबिल्वशङ्खिनी
शकुलादनीस्वर्णक्षीरिण्य इति दशेमानि भेदनीयानि भवन्ति ।

मधुक मधुपर्णी पृश्निपर्ण्यम्बष्ठकी समङ्गा मोचरस धातकी
लोध्र प्रियङ्गु कट्फलानीति दशेमानि सन्धानीयानि भवन्ति ।

पिप्पलीपिप्पलीमूलचव्यचित्रकशृङ्गवेराम्लवेतस मरिचाजमोदा
भल्लातकास्थि हिङ्गु निर्य्यासा इति दशेमानि दीपनीयानि भवन्ति ।

ऐन्द्र्यृषभ्यतिरसर्ष्य प्रोक्ता पयस्याश्वगन्धास्थिरा रोहिणी
बलातिबला इति दशेमानि बल्यानि भवन्ति ।

चन्दनतुङ्गपद्मकोशीर मधुकमञ्जिष्ठासारिवापयस्या सितालता
इति दशेमानि वर्ण्यानि भवन्ति ।

सारिवेक्षुमूलमधुक पिप्पली द्राक्षाविदारीकैटर्य्यहंसपादी-
बृहती कण्टकारिका इति दशेमानि कण्ठ्यानि भवन्ति ।

आम्राम्रातकनिकुचकरमर्द्द वृक्षाम्लाम्लवेतसकुवलबदरदाडिम-
मातुलुङ्गानीति दशेमानि हृद्यानि भवन्ति ।

1. *Pectorals :* "Desmodium trilobum, Batatas paniculata, Sida cordifolia, Sida spinosa, Tribulus terrestris, Uraria logopodiodes, Aspara-

---

नागर चित्रकचव्यविड़ङ्गमूर्व्वागुडूचीवचामुस्त पिप्पली
पटोलानीति दशेमानि तृप्तिघ्नानि भवन्ति।
कूटज विल्व चित्रक नागरातिविषाभया धन्वयासक-दारु-
हरिद्रा-वचाचव्यानीति दशेमानि अर्शोघ्नानि भवन्ति।
खदिराभयामलक हरिद्रारुष्कर सप्तपर्णारग्वध करवीर-
विड़ङ्गजातिप्रवाला इति दशेमानि कुष्ठघ्नानि भवन्ति।
चन्दननलदकृतमालनक्तमाल निम्बकूटज सर्षपमधुकदारु-
हरिद्रामुस्तानीति दशेमानि कण्डूघ्नानि भवन्ति।
अक्षीवमरीचगण्डीरकेबूक विड़ङ्ग निर्गुण्डी-किणिह्नीश्वदंष्ट्रा-
वृषपर्णिकाखुपर्णिका इति दशेमानि क्रिमिघ्नानि भवन्ति।
हरिद्रामञ्जिष्ठासुवहासूक्ष्मैलापालिन्दीचन्दन कतक शिरीष
सिन्धुवार श्लेष्मातका इति दशेमानि विषघ्नानि भवन्ति।
वीरण-शालीषष्टिकेक्षुवालिका दर्भकुश-काशगुन्द्रेत्कट
कर्त्तृणमूलानीति दशेमानि स्तन्यजननानि भवन्ति।
पाठामहौषध सुरदारुमुस्तमूर्व्वा गुडूचीवत्सक-फलकिराततिक्त-
कटुरोहिणीसारिवा इति दशेमानि स्तन्यशोधनानि भवन्ति।
जीवकर्षभककाकोलीक्षीरकाकोलीमुद्गपर्णी माषपर्णीमेदावृद्ध-
रुहाजटिलाकुलीङ्गा इति दशेमानि शुक्र-जननानि भवन्ति।
कुष्ठैलवालुककट्फलसमुद्रफेण कदम्बनिर्य्यासेक्षुकाण्डेक्षु-
क्षुरकवसुकोशीराणीति दशेमानि शुक्रशोधनानि भवन्ति।
मृद्वीकामधुकमधुपर्णीमेदाविदारी काकोलीक्षीर-काकोली
जीवकजीवन्ती-शालपर्ण्य इति दशेमानि स्नेहोपगानि भवन्ति।

gus racemosus, Ichnocarpus frutescens, Hemidismus indicus nigra, Celtis orientalis minor,

---

शोभाञ्जनकैरण्डार्कवृश्चीर पुनर्नवायवतिलकुलत्थमाषबद-
राणीति दशेमानि स्वेदोपगानि भवन्ति।
मधुमधुक कोविदार कर्व्वुदारकनीप-विदुलविम्बीशणपुष्पी-
सदापुष्पी प्रत्यक्पुष्पा इति दशेमानि वमनोपगानि भवन्ति।
द्राक्षाकाश्मर्य्य परूषकाभयामलक-विभीतक कुवलवदर-
कर्कन्धुपीलुनीति दशेमानि विरेचनोपगानि भवन्ति।
त्रिवृद्विल्व पिप्पली कुष्ठ सर्षपवचा वत्सकफल शतपुष्पा-
मधुकमदनफलानीति दशेमान्यास्थापनोपगानि भवन्ति।
रास्नासुरदारुविल्वमदन शतपुष्पा-वृश्चीरपुनर्नवा श्वदंष्ट्रा-
ग्निमन्थ श्योनाका इति दशेमान्यनुवासनोपगानि भवन्ति।
ज्योतिष्मतीक्षवक मरिचपिप्पलीविड़ङ्ग शिग्रु सर्षपापामार्गतण्डुल-
श्वेता महाश्वेता इति दशेमानि शिरोविरेचनोपगानि भवन्ति।
जम्बाम्रपल्लवमातुलुङ्गाम्लवदरदाड़िमयव यष्टिकोशीर-
मृल्लाजा इति दशेमानि छर्द्दि निग्रहणानि भवन्ति।
नागरधन्व यासकमुस्तपर्पटक-चन्दनकिराततिक्तकगुड़ूचीह्रीवेर
धान्यक पटोलानीति दशेमानि तृष्णा-निग्रहणानि भवन्ति।
शटीपुष्करमूलवदरवीज कण्टकारिका वृहतीवृक्षरुहाभयापिप्पली-
दुरालभाकुलीरशृङ्ग्य इति दशेमानि हिक्कानिग्रहणानि भवन्ति।
प्रियङ्ग्वनन्तामास्थि कट्वङ्ग-लोध्र मोचरस समङ्गा धातकीपुष्प
पद्मा पद्मकेशरानीति दशेमानि पुरीषसंग्रहणीयानि भवन्ति।
जम्बुशल्लकीत्वक् कच्छुरा मधुक शाल्मली श्रीवेष्टक भृष्ट
मृत्पयस्योत्पलतिलकणा इति दशेमानि पुरीष-
विरजनीयानि भवन्ति।

Vitis vinifera, Teramnus labialis, Phaseolus trilobus, Solanum indicum, Solanum xanthocarpum, Bœrhaavia diffusa, Ricinus communis,

---

अम्बाम्रप्लक्ष वट कपीतनोडुम्बराश्वत्थ-भल्लातकाश्मन्तकसोम
वल्का इति दशेमानि मूत्रसंग्रहणानि भवन्ति ।
पद्मोत्पल नलिनकुमुदसौगन्धिक पुण्डरीक शतपत्रमधुक-
प्रियङ्गुधातकीपुष्पाणीति दशेमानि मूत्रविरजनीयानि भवन्ति ।
वृक्षादनीश्वदंष्ट्रावसुकवशिर पाषाणभेद दर्भकुशकाशगुन्द्रेत्
कटमूलानीति दशेमानि मूत्रविरेचनीयानि भवन्ति ।
द्राक्षाभयामलक-पिप्पलीदुरालभा शृङ्गीकण्टकारिका वृश्चीर
पुनर्नवा तामलक्य इति दशेमानि कासहराणि भवन्ति ।
शठी पुष्करमूलाम्लवेतसैलाहिङ्गुगुरु सुरसा तामलकी
जीवन्ती चण्डा इति दशेमानि श्वासहराणि भवन्ति ।
पाटलाग्निमन्थ विल्वश्योणाक-काश्मर्य्यकण्टकारिका वृहती शालपर्णी
पृश्निपर्णी-गोक्षुरका इति दशेमानि शोथहराणि भवन्ति ।
शारिवाशर्करा पाठा मञ्जिष्ठा द्राक्षा पीलु परूषकाभया-
मलकविभीतकानीति दशेमानि ज्वरहराणि भवन्ति ।
द्राक्षाखर्ज्जुर पियाल वदर दाड़िम फल्गु परूषकेक्षुयव-
यष्टिका इति दशेमानि श्रमहराणि भवन्ति ।
लाजाचन्दनकाश्मर्य्यफलमधुक शर्करा नीलोत्पलोशीर शारिवा
गुड़ूचीह्रीवेराणीति दशेमानि दाहप्रशमनानि भवन्ति ।
तगरागुरु-धान्यक-शृङ्गवेरभूतीकवचा कण्टकारिकाग्निमन्थ
श्योनाकपिप्पल्य इति दशेमानि शीतप्रशमनानि भवन्ति ।
तिन्दुकपियालवदर खदिरकदर सप्तपर्णाश्वकर्णार्ज्जुनासना-
रिमेदा इति दशेमान्युदर्द्द प्रशमनानि भवन्ति ।

Clitoræ ternata, Tragia involucrata, and Mucuna (Carpopogon) pruriens. These are called '*vidārī*' and they relieve the derangements of '*vāyu*' and '*pitta*', consumption, tubercles, gouty pains, dyspnea and other bronchial troubles.

II. *Antiseptics* : Cassia fistula, Randia dumentorum, Flacourtia ramontchi, Holarrhena antidysenterica, Stephania capilata, Acacia catechu, Stereospermum suaveolens, Sanseviera zeylanica, Holarrhena antidysenterica, Alstonia scholaris, Azadirachta indica, Barleria prionitis, Barleria buxifolia, Tinospora cordifolia, Plum-

---

विदारिगन्धापृश्निपर्णीबृहती कण्टकारिकैरण्डकाकोलीचन्द-
नोशीरैलामधुकानीति दशेमान्यङ्गमर्द्दप्रशमनानि भवन्ति ।
पिप्पली पिप्पलीमूल चव्य-चित्रक शृङ्गवेर मरिचाजमोदाज-
गन्धाजाजी गण्डीराणीति दशेमानि शूलप्रशमनानि भवन्ति ।
मधुमधुकरुधिर मोचरस मृत्कपाललोध्रगैरिक प्रियङ्गु-
शर्कराखाजा इति दशेमानि शोणितस्थापनानि भवन्ति ।
शाल कट्फल कदम्बपद्मक तुङ्ग मोचरस शिरीषवञ्जुलैलवालु-
काशोका इति दशेमानि वेदनास्थापनानि भवन्ति ।
हिङ्गुकैटर्य्यारिमेदा वचा चोरक वयःस्थागोलोमी जटिलाप
लङ्कषाशोकरोहिण्य इति दशेमानि संज्ञास्थापनानि भवन्ति ।
ऐन्द्रीब्राह्मीशतवीर्य्यासहस्रवीर्य्यामोघाव्यथा शिवारिष्टा वाट्यपुष्पी-
विश्वक्सेनकान्ता इति दशेमानि प्रजास्थापनानि भवन्ति ।
अमृताभया धात्री मुक्ताश्वेता जीवन्त्यतिरसा मण्डूकपर्णी
स्थिरा पुनर्नवा इति दशेमानि वयःस्थापनानि भवन्ति ।

चरक-संहिता, सूत्र-स्थानम्, ४।

bago zeylanica, Pongamia glabra, Carissa caranda, Trichosanthes dioica, Ophelia chirayta, and Momordica charantia are called *'āragdhādi'*, and they are disinfectants in catarrh, toxemia, gonorrhea, skin disease, and abscess-cavities and relieve fever, vomiting and pruritus (as symptomatic expressions of the former lesions).

III. *Hæmatinics* : Cratæva religiosa ; Barleria cærulea, Morunga plerygosperma, Hyperanthera morunga, Sesbania aculeata, Gymnema sylvestris, Guilandina bonducella, Pongamia glabra, Sanseviera zeylanica, Premna serratifolia, Barleria cristata, Momordica monadelpha, Coccinea indica, Calotropis gigantica, Pothos officinalis, Plumbago zeylanica, Asparagus racemosus, Aegle marmelos, Gymnema sylvestris, Imperata cylindrica, Solanum indicum and Solanum xanthocarpum are called *'varuṇādi'*, and they relieve (the derangements of) *'kapha'* and adiposis, headache, adenoncosis and adenitis.

IV. *Lithontriptics* : Pentaptera arjuna, Barleria caerulea, Barleria cristata, Imperata cylindrica. Vanda roxburghii, Cyperus pertinens, Arundo indica latifolia, Poa cynosuroides, Saccharum spontaneum, Coleus aromaticum, Premna serratifolia, Sanseviera zeylanica,

Calotropis gigantea, Scindapsus officinalis, Calosanthes indica, Barleria prionitis, Nymphæa stellata, Herpestis monieria, and Tribulus terrestris are called *'vïratarvvādi'* and they relieve stranguary, gravel and urinary calculus.

V. *Oxidizer* : Resina Shorea robusta, Terminalia alata tomentosa, Acacia catechu, Acacia arabica, Diospyros embryosteris, Areca catechu, Betula bhojapatra, Gymnema sylvestris, Ougenia dalbergisides, Santalum album, Pterocarpus santalinus, Dalbergia sissoo, Albizzia lebbek, Terminalia tomentosa, Anogeissus latifolia, Terminalia arjuna, Borassus flabelliformis, Tectona grandis, Pongamia glabra, Guilandina bonducella, Shorea robusta, Aquilaria agallocha, and Santalaum xanthocarpum are called *'sāla-sārādi'*, and these relieve phlegma, ediposis, and skin-diseases, gonorrhea and anemia.

VI. *Astringent disinfectants* : Symplocos racemosa, Symplocos alstonia, Butea frondosa, Calosanthes indica, Clerodendron siphoanthus, Myrica sapida, Myrica rubra, Boswellia serrata, Rubia cordifolia, Shorea robusta and Musa sapientum are called *'rodhrādi'*, and they relieve phlegmatic disposition and adiposis, and vaginal diseases, arrest diarrhœa, disinfect abscess cavity and neutralize toxins.

VII. *Disinfectants* : Calotropis gigantica, Calotropis gigantica alba, Pongamia glabra, Guilandenia bonducella, Heliotropium indicum, Achyranthes aspera, Clerodendrum, (siphonanthus, Vandra roxburghii, Gloriosa superba, Batatas paniculata Batatas epulis, Tragia involucrata, rock salt, Balanites roxburghii are called '*arkādi*' and they relieve phlegmatic disposition, adiposis, intestina, worms, skin diseases, neutralize toxins and disinfect abscess cavity.

VIII. *Pectorals* :—Ocimum sanctum, Ocimum hirsitum, Ocimum frutescens, Andropogon shœnanthus, Andropogon martiny, Andropogon muricatum, Andropogon iwaraneusa, Cassia esculenta, Achyranthes aspera ; Hygrophylla spinosa, Embelia ribes, Myrica sapida, surasi, Vitez negundo, Celsia caromandeliana, Salvinia cucullata, Clerodendron siphonanthus, Ruta graveolens, Solanum nigrum and Strychnos nux-vomica are called '*surasādi*' and they relieve phlegmatic disposition, bacterial flora, catarrh, anorexia, dyspnea and cough and disinfect abscess cavity.

IX. *Lithontriptics* :—Bignonia indica, Butea frondosa, Grislea tomentosa, Plumbago zeylanica, Randia dumetorum, Dalbergia sissoo, Euphorbia neriifolia, Terminalia, chebula, Terminalia belerica and Phyllanthus embelica are called *'muskādi'* and they relieve adiposis, urethral diseases, gonorrhea, chancre, anemia (symptomatic of the other lesions), gravel and urinary calculus.

X. *Stomachics* : Piper longum, radix Piper longum, Piper chaba, Plumbago zeylanica, Zingiber officinale, Piper nigrum, Scindapsus officinales, Piper auranticum, Elettaria cardamomum, Pimpinella involucrata, fructus Holarrhena antidysenterica, Stephania hernandifolia. Cuminum Cyminum, Sinapis alba, fructus Melia azadaroch, Ferula assafœtida, Clerodendron siphonanthus, Sanseviera zeylanica, Aconitum heterophyllum, Acorus calamus, Embelia ribes and Picrorrhiza kurroa are called *pippalyādi'* and they are appetizing, stomachic and dessicant, and they relieve catarrh, flatulence, anorexia, glandular swelling and pain.

XI. *Carminatives*: Elettaria cardamomum, Tabernæmontana coronaria, Saussurea auraticulata, Nardostachys jatamansi, Andropogon shœnan thus, Cinnamomum zeylanicum, Cinnamomum tamala, Mesua ferrea, Agraia roxburgiana, Piper aurantiacum, operculum of Purpura. Tamirindus indica,(*śukti*=pearl-oyster), *'sthauneyaka'* (a yellowish fragrant plant), Canscora decussata, Pinus longifolia, Cinnamomum pauciflorum, Andropogon acicularis, Sida cordifolia, Balsamodendron mukula, Shorea robusta, Liquidambar orientalis, Boswellia seratta, Aquilaria agallocha, Trigonella corniculata, Andropogon muricatum, Cedrus deodara, Crocus sativus, and Calophyllum inophyllum are called *'elādi'* and they relieve flatulence, phlegmatic disposition, pruritus and urticaria.

XII-XIII. *Stomachics*: Acorus calamus, Cyperus rotundus, Aconitum heterophyllum Terminalia chebula, Cedrus deodara, Mesua ferrea, Curcuma longa, Berberis asiatica, Uraria logopodioides, Holarrhena antidysenterica, and Glycyrrhiza glabra are called *vachādi* and *haridrādi* and they are galactogogue, antidysenteric and particularly stomachic.

XIV. *Laxatives*: Hemidesmus indicus, Ichnocarpus-frutescens, Ipomœa turpethum, Baliospermum montamum, Canscora decussata, Symplocos racemosa, Mallotus philippenensis, Trichosanthes dioica, Areca catechu, Salvinia cucullata, Citrullus colocynthis, Cassia fistula, Pongamia glabra, Guilandina bonducella, Tinospora cordifolia, Stereospermum suaveolens, Argyreia speciosa, Eupholia neriifolia and Cleome felina are called *śyāmādi* and they relieve tympanites and ascites.

XV. *Diureties*: Solanum indicum, Solanum xanthocarpum, Holarrhena antidysenterica, Stephania hernandifolia, and Glycyrrhiza glabra are called *'vṛhatyādi'* and they relieve the excess of the humors, anorexia, eructation and strangury.

XVI. *Disinfectants*: Trichosanthes dioica, Santalum album, Pterocarpus santalinus, Sanseviera zeylanica, Tinospora cordifolia, Stephania hernandifolia, and Picrorrhiza curroa are called *paṭalâdi* and they are beneficial in anorexia, fever, pruritus, and particularly in the asepsis of the abscesses.

XVII. *Analeptics*: Gymnema balsamicum, Gymnema lactiferum, Celtis orientalis, Vitis vinifera, Phaseolus trilobus, Teramnus labialis, Leptadenia spartinum, Leptadenia reticulata, Tinospora cordifolia, Rhus succedama, manna Bambucæ, Prunus padus (?), Nymphæa lotus, Nymphæa odorata, Nymphæa pubescens, Mimusops kauki and Glycyrrhiza glabra are restorative, stimulant, tonic galactogogue and phlegmatic.

XVIII. *Lithontriptics*: Alkalies, rock salt, Bitumen, iron sulphide, Assafœtida and copper sulphide are called *uṣakâdi* and they relieve phlegmatic disposition and adiposis, and urinary calculus, gravel and strangury.

XIX. *Vascular Sedatives :* Ichnocarpus frutescens, Glycyrrhiza glabra, Santalum album, Pterocarpus santalinus, Prunus padus, Gmelina arborea, Bassia latifolia, and Andropogon muricatum are called *sārivādi* and they relieve polydipsia, hemorrhage, bilious fever and especially hyperemia.

XX. *Hemostatics* : Sulphate of antimony, incinerated antimony, Mesua ferrea, Aglaia roxburghiana, Nymphaea stellata, Andropogon muricatum radix, Nelumbium speciosum, and Glycyrrhiza glabra are called *añjanādi* and they relieve hemorrhage, toxemia and internal congestion.

XXI. *Carminatives* : Grewia asiatica, Uvae passae, Myrica sapida, Punica granatum, Mimusops indica, Strychnos potatorum, Tectonia grandis, Terminalia chebula, Terminalia belerica, and Phyllanthus emblica are called *paruṣkādi* and they relieve flatulence, urinary troubles, polydipsia, and are appetizing and cardiac stimulants.

XXII. *Antiseptics* : Aglaia roxburghina, Mimosa pudica, Woodfordia floribunda, Calophyllum inophillum, Pterocarpus santalinus, Cæsalpinia sappan, Bombax malabaricum, antimony sulphide, diatomacious mixture of antimony (?), Nelumbium speciaosum, Rubia cordifolia, and Ichnocarpus frutescens are called '*priyangvādi*' and they are beneficial in ulcerative dysentery, for rejoining the fractured bones and as pustulants for the tumors.

XXIII. *Pustulants* : Stephania hernandifolia, Woodfordia floribunda, Mimosa pudica, Calosanthes indica, Glycyrrhiza glabra, Aegle marmelos, Symplocos racemosa, Symplocos alstonia, Butæ frondosa, Nerium coronarium, and Nelumbium speciosum are called *ambaṣṭhādi* and they are pustulant, and are beneficial in fractured bones.

XXIV. *Pustulants* : Ficus bengalensis, Ficus gloremata, Ficus religiosa, Ficus infectoria, Bassia latifolia, Spondias mangifera, Terminalia arjuna, Mangifera indica, Mangifera sylvatica, Andropogon acicularis, Cinnamomum tamala, Eugenia corymbosa, Buchanania latifolia, Glycyrrhiza glabra, Picrorrhiza kurroa, Mimusops elengi, Nauclea cadamba, Zizyphus jujuba, Diospyros embryosterus, Boswellia serrata, Symplocos racemosa, Symplocos alstonia, Semicarpus anacardium, Butea frondosa, and Cedrela toona are called '*nyagrodhādi*' and they are pustulants and beneficial in the reunion of the fractured bones and are vaginal disinfectants.

XXV. *Antipyretics* : Tinospora cordifolia,

Azadirachta indica, Coriandrum sativum, Santanum album and Prunus padus are called '*guḍuchyâdi*' and they are febrifuge, stomachic and relieve eructation, anorexia, polydipsia and *hyperemia*.

XXVI. *Refrigerants* : Nymphæa stellata, Nymphæa rubra, Nymphæa alba, Nymphæa odorata, Nymphæa cærulea, Nelumbium speciosum and Glycyrrhiza glabra are called '*utpalâdi*' and are refrigerant, antitoxic, hematinic, antiemetic, and relieve heart diseases and epilepsy.

XXVII. *Oxidizers*: Cyperus rotundus, Curcuma longa, Terminalia chebula, Phyllanthus emblica, Terminalia belerica, Saussurea auriculata, Acorus calamus, Stephania hermanifolia, Picrorrhiza kurroa, Pongamia glabra, Aconitum heterophyllum, Elettaria cardamomum, Semicarpus anacardium and Plumbago zeylanica are called '*mustâdi*' and they are oxidizing agents (reducing phlegma) stimulating digestion,increasing the secretion of milk (in woman) and act as disinfectants in vaginal diseases.

XXVIII. *Astringent antiseptics* : Terminalia chebula, Terminalia belerica, and Phyllanthus embelica are known as *triphalā* and they are beneficial in gonorrhea, skin-diseases, in some eye-troubles and they are stomachic.

XXIX. *Stomachics* : Piper longum, Piper nigrum and Zingiber zerumbet are called *trikaṭu* and they are oxidizing agents and are beneficial in phlegmatic disposition, adiposis, diabetes, skin-diseases, glandular swelling, and anorexia.

XXX. *Stomachics* : Phyllanthus emblica, Terminalia chebula, Piper longum and Plumbago zeylancia are called *āmalakyādi'* and they are tonic, stimulating, febrifuge and beneficial to the eyes.

XXXI. *Metallic salts* : Tin, lead, silver, iron and gold (salts), and iron-oxide are called *trapādi* and they are bacteri-cidal, antitoxic and beneficial in anemia and gonorrhea. (*Tin* compounds are no more used in modern medicine except as filings though in former times stannum oxidatum and butyrum stanni, were popular. *Lead* oxide, unguentum plumbi iodidi, and various other salts and preparations of lead are in use, usually for external application. *Copper* likewise has various external therapeutic uses. The oleate of copper is an admirable astringent, antiseptic and anti-parasitic prepartion, especially valuable in various forms of tinea trichophytesis ; copper sulphate in solid stick is effectively used as a surperficial caustic in indolent ulcers, exuberant granulations, and in syphilitic and other sores in the mouth and the throat. *Silver nitrate* in weak solutions has been used externally as an astringent caustic and internally in nervous disorders with marked benefit. But as it leaves a dark stain on the skin, *argentum Crede* is preferred by many, as the lactate and citrate of silver is claimed to possess the power of penetrating the entire organism and effecting a general disinfection of the entire organism. Argonin, an organic combination of silver with casein, soluble in water, but non-irritant, has been lately introduced in the market and is claimed to be antidotal to the gonococcus. Argyrol, another non-irritant combination, is used in 2 p. c. solution in gonorrheal eye-diseases. Various *iron preparations* are still in vogue and administered internally to supply iron to hemoglobin in its deficiency as in anemia. *Gold* and sodium chloride has marked bactericidal powers, resembling mercuric chloride and internally in very small doses it acts upon the glandular structures of the stomach and the liver, stimulating nutrition and assimilation; but in larger doses it produces violent gastro-enteritis without salivation or ulceration).

XXXII. *Antiparasitics* : Lac, Cassia fistula, **Holarrhena antidysenterica, Nerium odorum, Myrica sapida, Curcuma longa, Berberis asiatica,**

Azardirachta indica Alstonia, scholaris,Jasminum grandiflorum and Ficus heterophylla are called '*lākṣādi*' and they are of astringent, bitterish sweetish taste and are antiparasitical.

XXXIII. *Tonics* : The roots of Trilobus terrestris, Solanum indica, Solanum xanthocarpum, Uraria logopodiodes, Desmodium trilobus, are known as '*pañcha-mūla*' and they are of astringent sweet-bitterish taste and are restorative tonics.

XXXIV. *Stomachics* : The roots of Aegle marmelos, Premna serratifolia, Calosanthes indica, Stereospermum suaveolens and Gmelina arborea are called large '*pañcha-mūla*' and they are stomachics of slightly bitter-sweetish taste.

XXXV. *Oxidizers* : The five small roots and the five large roots, are called together '*daśa-mūla*' and they are stomachic and febri-fuge.

XXXVI. *Antiseptics* : The roots of Batatas paniculata, Ichnocarpus frutescens, Curcuma longa, Tinospora cordifolia, and Gymnema sylbestre are called '*valli-pañchamūla*'. The roots of Carissa carandas, Tribulus terrestris, Barleria cristata, Asparagus racemosus and Hygrophila spinosa are called '*kaṇṭaka pañcha-mūla*'. These two '*pañchamūlas*' relieve inflammation and gonorrhea.

XXXVII. *Diuretics* : The roots of Poa cynosuroides, Saccharum spontaneum, Phragmites communis, Imperata cylindrica and Saccharum officinarum are called *'tṛṇa pañcha-mūla'* and if given with milk, they are diuretic and cure urinary troubles." *Suśruta* I. 38. 2-36[187].

---

187. समासेन सप्तविंशद्द्रव्यगणा भवन्ति। तद्यथा—विदारिगन्धा विदारी सहदेवा विश्वदेवा श्वदंष्ट्रा पृथक्पर्णी शतावरी सारिवा कृष्णसारिवा जीवकर्षभकौ महासहा क्षुद्रसहा बृहत्यौ पुनर्नवैरण्डौ हंसपादी वृश्चिकाल्यृषभी चेति।

विदारिगन्धादिरयं गणः पित्तानिलापहः।
शोषगुल्माङ्गमर्दोर्द्ध-श्वासकासविनाशनः॥ २

आरग्वधमदनगोपधीघण्टाकण्टकीकुटजपाठापाटलामूर्व्वेन्द्रयव-सप्तपर्ण-निम्ब-कुरुण्टकदासीकुरुण्टक-गुडूचीचित्रकशार्ङ्गेष्टाकरञ्जद्वयपटोलकिराततिक्तकानि सुषवी चेति॥

आरग्वधादिरित्येष गणः श्लेष्मविषापहः।
मेहकुष्ठज्वरवमी-कण्डूघ्नो व्रणशोधनः॥ ३

वरुणार्त्तगलशिग्रुमधुशिग्रुतर्कारीमेषशृङ्गीपूतिकनक्तमालमोरटाग्निमन्थसैरीयकद्वय-बिम्बीवसुकवसिर-चित्रकशतावरी-बिल्वाजशृङ्गीदर्भा बृहतीद्वयञ्चेति।

वरुणादिर्गणो ह्येष कफमेदोनिवारणः।
विनिहन्ति शिरःशूलं गुल्माभ्यन्तरविद्रधीन्॥ ४

वीरतरुसहचरद्वयदर्भ-वृक्षादनीगुन्द्रानलकुशकाशाश्मभेदकाग्निमन्थमोरटावसुक-वसिरभल्लूककुरुण्टकेन्द्रीवरकपोतवङ्काः श्वदंष्ट्रा चेति।

वीरतर्वादिरित्येष गणो वातविकारनुत्।
अश्मरीशर्करामूत्रकृच्छ्राघातरुजापहः ५

सालसाराजकर्णखदिरकदरकालस्कन्धक्रमुकभूर्ज्जमेषशृङ्गीतिनिशचन्दनकुचन्दनशिंशपाशिरीषासनधवार्ज्जुनतालशाकनक्तमालपूतिकाश्वकर्णागुरूणि कालीयकञ्चेति।

Emetics : "Randia dumetorum, Wrightia antidysenterica, Andropogon serrata, Citrullus

---

सालसारादिरित्येष गणः कुष्ठविनाशनः ।
मेहपाण्डुामयहरः कफमेदोविशोषणः ॥ ६

रोध्रसावररोध्र, पलाशकुटन्नटाशोफफञ्जोकठ्फलैलवालुकसल्लकीजिङ्गिनीकदम्ब-सालाः कदली चेति ।

एष रोध्रादिरित्युक्तो मेदःकफहरो गणः ।
योनिदोषहरः स्तम्भी व्रण्यो विषविनाशनः ॥ ७

अर्कालर्क-करञ्जद्वय-नागदन्तीमयूरक - भार्गीरास्नेन्द्रपुष्पीक्षुद्रश्वेतामहाश्वेतावृश्चि-काल्यलवणास्तापसवृक्षश्चेति ।

अर्कादिको गणो ह्येष कफमेदोविषापहः ।
क्रिमिकुष्ठप्रशमनो विशेषाद् व्रणशोधनः ॥ ८

सुरसाश्वेतसुरसाफणिज्झकार्जकभूस्तृणसुगन्धकसुमुखकालमालकासमर्दकक्षवकखर-पुष्पाविड़ङ्गकट्फलसुरसीनिर्गुण्डीकुलाहलोन्दुरुकर्णिकाफञ्जीप्राचीवलकाकमाच्यो विष-मुष्टिकश्चेति ।

सुरसादिर्गणो ह्येष कफहृत् क्रिमिसूदनः ।
प्रतिश्यायारुचिश्वासकासघ्नो व्रणशोधनः ॥ ९

मुष्कक-पलाश-धव-चित्रक-मदनवृक्षक-शिंशपावज्रवृक्षास्त्रिफला चेति ।

मुष्ककादिर्गणो ह्येष मेदोघ्नः शुक्रदोषहृत् ।
मेहार्शःपाण्डुरोगघ्नः शर्कराश्मरीनाशनः ॥ १०

पिप्पलीपिप्पलीमूलचव्यचित्रकशृङ्गवेरमरिचहस्तिपिप्पलीहरेणुकैलाजमोदेन्द्रयव-पाठाजीरकसर्षपमहानिम्ब-फल-हिङ्गुभार्गीमधुरसातिविषावचाविड़ङ्गानि कटुरोहिणी-चेति ।

पिप्पल्यादिः कफहरः प्रतिश्यायानिलारुचीः ।
निहन्याद्दीपनो गुल्म-शूलघ्नश्चामपाचनः ॥ ११

colocynthis, Luffa pentandra, Luffa amara, Sinapis alba, Embelia ribes, Piper longum,

---

एलातगरकुष्ठमांसीध्यामकत्वक्पत्रनागपुष्प-प्रियङ्गु हरेणुकाव्याघ्रनख-शुक्तिचण्डास्थौणेयकश्रीवेष्टकचोचचोरकवालक-गुग्गुलु-सर्ज्जरसतुरुष्ककुन्दुरुकाऽगुरुस्पृक्कोशीरभद्रदारु-कुङ्कुमाणि पुन्नागकेशरञ्चेति।

एलादिको वातकफौ निहन्याद्विषमेव च।
वर्णप्रसादनः कण्डू-पिड़काकोठनाशनः॥ १२

वचामुस्तातिविषाभयाभद्रदारूणि नागकेशरञ्चेति। हरिद्रादारुहरिद्राकलशीकूटज-बीजानि मधुकञ्चेति।

एतौ वचाहरिद्रादी गणौ स्तन्यविशोधनौ।
आमातीसारशमनौ विशेषाद्दोषपाचनौ॥ १३

श्यामामहाश्यामात्रिवृद्दन्तीशङ्खिनी-तिल्वककम्पिल्लक-रम्यकक्रमुकपुत्रश्रेणी-गवाक्षी-राजवृक्ष-करञ्जद्वय-गुडूची-सप्तलाच्छगलान्त्रीसुधाः सुवर्णक्षीरी चेति।

उक्तः श्यामादिरित्येष गणो गुल्मविषापहः।
आनाहोदरविड्भेदी तथोदावर्त्तनाशनः॥ १४

वृहतीकण्टकारिकाकुटजफलपाठा मधुकञ्चेति।

पाचनीयो वृहत्यादिर्गणः पित्तानिलापहः।
कफारोचकहृद्रोगमूत्रकृच्छ्रविनाशनः॥ १५

पटोलचन्दनकुचन्दनमूर्व्वागुडूचीपाठाः कटुरोहिणी चेति।

पटोलादिर्गणः पित्त-कफारोचकनाशनः।
ज्वरोपशमनो व्रण्यश्छर्द्दिकण्डुविषापहः॥ १६

काकोलीक्षीरकाकोलीजीवकर्षभकमुद्गपर्णी-माषपर्णीमेदामहामेदा-छिन्नरुहा-कर्कटशृङ्गी-तुगाक्षीरी-पद्मक-प्रपौण्डरीकर्द्धि-वृद्धि-मृद्वीकाजीवन्त्यो मधुकञ्चेति।

काकोल्यादिरयं पित्त-शोणितानिलनाशनः।
जीवनो वृंहणो वृष्यः स्तन्यश्लेष्मकरस्तथा॥ १७

Pongamia glabra, Cassia tora, Bauhinia variegata, Cordia myxa, Melia azadrachta, Withania

---

ऊषकसैन्धवशिलाजतुकासीसद्वयहिङ्गूनि तुत्थकञ्चेति ।

ऊषकादिः कफं हन्ति गणो मेदोविशोषणः ।

अश्मरीशर्करामूत्र-कृच्छ्रगुल्मप्रणाशनः ॥ १८

सारिवामधुकचन्दनकुचन्दनपद्मककाश्मीरफल-मधुकपुष्पाण्युशीरञ्चेति ।

सारिवादिः पिपासाघ्नो रक्तपित्तहरो गणः ।

पित्तज्वरप्रशमनो विशेषाद्दाहनाशनः ॥ १९

अञ्जनरसाञ्जननागपुष्प-प्रियङ्गुनीलोत्पलनलदनलिनकेशराणि मधुकञ्चेति ।

अञ्जनादिर्गणो ह्येष रक्तपित्तनिवर्हणः ।

विषोपशमनो दाहं निहन्त्याभ्यन्तरं तथा ॥ २०

परूषक-द्राक्षा-कट्फल-दाड़िम-राजादनकतकफल-शाकफलानि त्रिफला चेति ।

परूषकादिरित्येष गणोऽनिलविनाशनः ।

मूत्रदोषहरो हृद्यः पिपासाघ्नो रुचिप्रदः ॥ २१

प्रियङ्गुसमङ्गाधातकीनागपुष्पचन्दनकुचन्दनमोचरसरसाञ्जन-कुम्भीकस्रोतोऽञ्जनपद्म-केशरयोजनवल्ल्यो दीर्घमूला चेति ।

अम्बष्ठाधातकीकुसुमसमङ्गाकट्वङ्गमधुकबिल्वपेशिकारोध्रसावररोध्रपलाशनन्दीवृक्षपद्म-केशरानि चेति ।

गणौ प्रियङ्ग्वम्बष्ठादी पक्वातीसारनाशनौ ।

सन्धानीयौ हितौ पित्ते व्रणानाञ्चापि रोपणौ ॥ २२

न्यग्रोधोडुम्बराश्वत्थप्लक्षमधुक-कपीतनककुभाम्रकोशाम्रचोरकपत्रजम्बुद्वयपियालमधुक-रोहिणीवञ्जुलकदम्बबदरीतिन्दुकीसल्लकीरोध्रसावररोध्रभल्लातकपलाशा नन्दीवृक्षश्चेति ।

न्यग्रोधादिर्गणो व्रण्यः संग्राही भग्नसाधकः

रक्तपित्तहरो दाह-मेदोघ्नो योनिदोषहृत् ॥ २३

somnifera, Rumex vesicarius, Pentapetes phœnicea, Clitorea ternatea, Crotolaria verru-

---

गुड़ूचीनिम्बकुस्तुम्बुरुचन्दनानि पद्मकञ्चेति।

एष सर्व्वज्वरान् हन्ति गुड़ूच्यादिस्तु दीपनः।
हृल्लासारोचकच्छर्द्दि-पिपासादाहनाशनः॥ २४

उत्पलरक्तोत्पलकुमुदसौगन्धिककुवलयपुण्डरीकाणि मधुकञ्चेति।

उत्पलादिरयं दाह-पित्तरक्तविनाशनः।
पिपासाविषहृद्रोग-छर्द्दिमूर्च्छाहरो गणः॥ २५

मुस्ताहरिद्रादारुहरिद्राहरीतक्यामलकविभीतक-कुष्ठहैमवती-वचापाठाकटरोहिणी शार्ङ्गष्टातिविषाद्राविड़ीभल्लातकानि चित्रकञ्चेति।

एष मुस्तादिको नाम्ना गणः श्लेष्मनिसूदनः।
योनिदोषहरः स्तन्य-शोधनः पाचनस्तथा॥ २६

हरीतक्यामलकविभीतकानीति त्रिफला।

त्रिफला तु त्रिदोषघ्नी मेहकुष्ठविनाशिनी।
चक्षुष्या दीपनी चैव विषमज्वरनाशिनी॥ २७

पिप्पलीमरिचशृङ्गवेराणीति त्रिकटुकम्।

त्र्यूषणं कफमेदोघ्नं मेहकुष्ठत्वगामयान्।
निहन्याद्दीपनं गुल्म-पीनसाग्न्यल्पतामपि॥ २८

आमलकी-हरितकी-पिप्पल्यश्चित्रकश्चेति।

आमलक्यादिरित्येष गणः सर्व्वज्वरापहः।
चक्षुष्यो दीपनो वृष्यः कफारोचकनाशनः॥ २९

त्रपुसीसताम्ररजतकृष्णलोहसुवर्णानि लोहमलञ्चेति।

गणस्त्रप्वादिरित्येष गरक्रिमिहरः परः।
पिपासाविषहृद्रोग-पाण्डुमेहहरस्तथा॥ ३०

लाक्षारेवतकुटजाश्वमारकट्फलहरिद्राद्वयनिम्बसप्तच्छदमालत्यस्त्रायमाणा चेति।

cosa, Coccinea indica, Acorus calamus, Pyrotheca lagenaria and Plumbago zeylanica are emetics. And of them, fruits are to be used of the plants mentioned above up to Cassia tora, and from Crodia myxa roots are to be employed.

कषायस्तिक्तमधुरः कफपित्तार्त्तिनाशनः ।

कुष्ठक्रिमिहरश्चैव दुष्टव्रणविशोधनः ॥ ३१

पञ्च पञ्चमूलान्यत ऊर्द्ध्वं वक्ष्यामः । तत्र त्रिकण्टकबृहतीद्वयपृथक्पर्ण्यौ विदारिगन्धा चेति कनीयः ।

कषायतिक्तमधुरं कनीयः पञ्चमूलकम् ।

वातघ्नं पित्तशमनं बृंहणं बलवर्द्धनम् ॥ ३२

विल्वाग्निमन्थटुण्टुकपाटलाकाश्मर्य्यश्चेति महत् ।

सतिक्तं कफवातघ्नं पाके लघ्वग्निदीपनम् ।

मधुरानुरसञ्चैव पञ्चमूलं महत् स्मृतम् ॥ ३३

अनयोर्दशमूलमुच्यते ।

गणः श्वासहरो ह्येष कफपित्तानिलापहः ।

आमस्य पाचनश्चैव सर्व्वज्वरविनाशनः ॥ ३४

विदारीसारिवारजनीगुड़ूच्योऽजशृङ्गी चेति वल्लीसंज्ञः ।

करमर्द्द त्रिकण्टकशैरीयकशतावरीगृध्रनख्य इति कण्टकसंज्ञः ॥

रक्तपित्तहरौ ह्येतौ शोफत्रयविनाशनौ ।

सर्व्वमेहहरौ चैव शुक्रदोषविनाशनौ ॥ ३५

कुशकाशनलदर्भकाण्डेक्षुका इति तृणसंज्ञकः ।

मूत्रदोषविकारञ्च रक्तपित्तं तथैव च ।

अन्त्यः प्रयुक्तः क्षीरेण शीघ्रमेव विनाशयेत् ॥ ३६

सुश्रुतसंहिता, सूत्रस्थानम, ३८ ।

Purgatives : Ipomoea turpethum, Ipomoæ nil, Baliospermum montanum, Salvinia cucullata, Jasminum sambac, Andropogon acicularis, Gymnema sylvesre, Lagenaria vulgaris, Argyreia speciosa, Euphorbia neriifolia, Cleome felina, Plumbago zeylanica, Achyranthes aspera, Poa cynosuroides, Saccharum spontaneum, Symplocos racemosa, Mallotus philippenensis, Trichosanthes dioica, Stereospermum suaveolens, Areca catechu, Terminalia chebula, Phyllanthus emblica, Terminalia belerica, Indigofera tinctoria, Cassia fistula, Ricinus communis, Guilandina bonducella, Euphorbia neriifolia, Alstonia scholaris, Calatropis gigantea and Cardiospermum halicacabum are purgatives. And of them roots should be used of the plants up to Saccharum spontaneum, the bark from symplocos racemosa to stereospermum suaveolens, the pigmented granules of the fruit of mallotus philippenensis, the fruits from Areca catechu to Ricinus communis, the leaves of Guilandina bonducella and Calotropis gigantica, and the gum-resins (milky exudations) of the rest.

Emetics and purgatives : Luffa amara, Stereospermum suaveolens, Andropogon acicularis, Luffa pentandra, and Memordica Charantica are emetics and purgatives combined.

Errhines: Piper longum, Embelia ribes, Achyranthes aspera, Moringa pterygosperma, Sinapis alba, Albizzia lebbek, Piper nigrum, Nerium odorum, Coccinea indica, Clitorea ternatea, Achyranthes fruticosa, Acorus calamus, Cardiospermum halicacabum, Pongamia glabra, Calotropis gigantea, Calotropis procera, Allium sativum, Aconitum heterophyllum, Zingiber officinale, Pinus webbiana, Garcinia xanthochymus, Ocimum sanctum, Ocimum album, Balanites roxburghii, Gymnema sylvestre, Citrus medica, Salvadora oleoides, Salvadora persica, Jasminum grandiflorum, Shorea robusta, Borassus flabelliformis, Bassia latifolia, lac, assafœtida, sodium chloride, wine, cow's urine and extract of cow's dung (ammonium) are errhines. Of these fruits should be taken from Piper longum to Piper nigrum, roots from Nerium odorum, bulbs from Allium sativum to Zingiber officinale, leaves from Pinus webbiana to Ocimum album, the bark from Balanites roxburghiana to Gymnema sylvestre, the flowers of the next three plants and the extracts of the following next three; lac and assfoetida are resinous exudates, sodium chloride an earthly matter (mineral substance), and the cow's urine and the dung are excretory products." *Suśruta* I. 39. 2-5[188].

Saccharine drugs : The Asclepias (the *kākoli* group, *Suśruta* I. 38. 17 led by Gymnema balsimicum), milk, butter, fat, bone-marrow, Oryza sativa, Oryza praecox, Hordeum hexa-

---

188. मदनकुटजजीमूतकेक्ष्वाकुधामार्गवकृतवेधनसर्षपविडङ्गपिप्पलीकरञ्जप्रपुन्नाड़कोविदारकर्व्वुदारारिष्टाश्वगन्धाविदुलबन्धुजीवकश्वेताशणपुष्पी-विम्बी-वचामृगेर्व्वारु-चित्राश्चेत्यूर्द्ध भागहराणि। तत्र कोविदारपूर्व्वाणां फलानि। कोविदारादीनां मूलानि ॥ २

त्रिवृता-श्यामा-दन्ती-द्रवन्ती-सप्तला-शङ्खिनी-विषाणिका-गवाक्षी-च्छगलान्त्रीस्नुक्-सुवर्णक्षीरीचित्रककिणिहीकुशकाशतिल्वककम्पिल्लक-रम्यक-पाटला-पूग -हरितक्यामलक-विभीतकनीलिनी-चतुरङ्गुलैरण्ड-पूतीकमहावृक्षसप्तच्छदार्कज्योतिष्मती चेत्यधोभाग-हराणि। तत्र तिल्वकपूर्व्वाणां मूलानि। तिल्वकादीनां पाटलान्तानां त्वचः। कम्पिल्लकफलरजः। पूगादीनामेरण्डान्तानां फलानि। पूतीका-रग्वधयोः पत्राणि। शेषाणां क्षीराणीति ॥ ३

कोशातकी सप्तला शङ्खिनी देवदाली कारवेल्लिका चेत्युभयतोभागहराणि। एषां स्वरसा इति ॥ ४

पिप्पली-विड़ङ्गापामार्गशिग्रुसिद्धार्थकशिरीषमरिचकरवीरविम्बीगिरिकर्णिकाकिणिही-वचा-ज्योतिष्मती- करञ्जार्कालर्कलशुनातिविषाशृङ्गवेर-तालीश-तमालसुरसार्ज्जकेङ्गुदीमेष-शृङ्गीमातुलुङ्गीमुरुङ्गी-पीलुजाती-शाल-ताल-मधूक - लाक्षाहिङ्गुलवणमद्यगोशकृद्रसमूत्र-णीति शिरोविरेचनानि। तत्र करवीरपूर्व्वाणां फलानि। करवीरादी-नामर्कान्तानां मूलानि। तालीशपूर्व्वाणां कन्दाः। तालीशादीनामर्ज्जकान्तानां पत्राणि। इङ्गुदीमेषशृङ्गीत्वचौ। मातुलुङ्गीमुरुङ्गीपीलुजातीनां पुष्पाणि। शालतालमधूकानां साराः। हिङ्गुलाक्षे निर्य्यासौ। लवणानि पार्थिवविशेषाः। मद्यान्यासवसंयोगाः। गोमूत्रशकृद्रसौ मलाविति ॥ ५ सुश्रुतसंहिता, सूत्रस्थानम्, ३९।

stichon, Triticum æstivum, phaseolus radiatus, fructus Trapa bispinosa, Scrypus kysoor, Cucumis sativus, Cucumis melo, Cucumis anguinus, Lagenaria vulgaris, Cucumis utilismus, Strychnos potatorum, Citrus aurantium, Buchanania latifolia, Nelumbium speciosum, Gmelina arborea, Bassia latifolia, Vitis vinifera, Phœnix sylvetris, Mimusops indica, Borassus flabelliformi, Cocos nucifera, Saccharum officinarum, Sida cordifolia, Mucuna pruriens, Batatas paniculata, Oxystelma esculentum, Tribulus terrestris, Sanseviera zeylanica, Fœnicum vulgare and Cucurbita pepo contain saccharine substances.

Acids : Punica granata, Phyllanthus embelica, Citrus medica, Spondias mangifera, Feronia elephantum, Carissa carondas, Peucedanum sowa, Zizyphus jujuba, Tamarindus indicus, Mangifera salvatica, Diospyros embryosterus, fructus Calamus rotang, Artocarpus lakucha, Rumex vesicarius, Citrus bergamia, curdled milk (lactic acid content), whey, sour wine, sour gruel, fermented rice and barley water and other acetous fermentation products belong to the acid group.

Salines : Rock-salt, carbonate of lime (from incinerated shells and the salt is recovered by lixiviation), soda, potash, '*raumaka*' (salt made from the water of the Roma lake, now known as Sambar), sea-salt, '*pakrima*' (salt obtained from the ashes of the grain spikes of barley), caustic soda, magnesia, alkaline earth (containing sodium carbonate) etc. belong to the saline class.

Pungents : Piperaceæ (led by Piper longum of the '*pippali*' group I. 38. 10), the Ocimum group (I. 38. 8.), vitex negundo, Moringa pterygosperma, Allium sativum, Cinnamomum camphora, Datura fastuosa, Cedrus deodara, Piper auranticum, Vernonia anthelminthica, Canscora decussata, Balsamodendron mukula, Cyperus rotundus, Gloriosa superba, Calosanthes indica, Sesbania grandiflora, Salvadora persica, etc. and the gum-resins of the Shorea robusta group (I. 38. 5) are pungent.

Bitters : The Cassia fistula (I. 38. 3) and Tinospora cordifolia (I. 38. 24) groups, and Hydroctyle asiatica, tops of Calamus rotang, Curcuma longa, Berberis asiatica, Holarrhena antidysenterica, Capparis trifolia, Flacourtia cataphracta, Alstonia scholaris, Solanum indicum, Solanum xanthocarpum, Canscora decussata, Salvinia cucullata, Ipomœa turpethum, Luffa amara, Momordica myxta, solanum melongena, Capparis aphylla, Nerium odorum, Jasminum grandiflorum, Andropogon acicularis, Achyranthes aspera, Ficus heterophyllum, Saraca indica, Herpestis monieria, Boerhaavia diffusa, Tragia involucrata, and Cardiospermum halicacabum are bitter.

Astringents : The groups led by Ficus bengalensis (I. 38. 23), Aglaia roxburghiana (I. 38. 21), Staphania hernandifolia (1. 38. 22), Symplocos racemosa, Terminalia chebula, Terminalia belerica, Phyllanthus embelica, Boswellia serrata, Eugenia jambu, Mangifera indica, Mimusops elengi, Diospyros embropteris, Strychnos potatorum, Stereospermum suaveolens, Barleria cristata, Bauhinia variegata, Caelogyne ovalis, Symplocos racemosa, Beta maritima, Marsilia quadrifolia etc., Oryza montana etc., Phaseolus mungo etc., these in brief belong to the astringent class. "*Suśruta* I. 42. 15-20[189].

Alkalies : Alkalies are obtained from the ashes

---

189. तद्यथा—काकोल्यादिः चीर-घृत-वसा-मज्ज-शालि-षष्टिक-यव-गोधूम-माषशृङ्गाटककसेरुकत्रपुसैर्व्वारुकालावुकालङ्कतकाङ्कलोड्यपियालपुष्करवीजकाश्मर्य्यमधूकद्राचाखर्ज्जुरराजादनतालनारिकेलेचुविकारवलातिवलात्मगुप्ताविदारी-पयस्यागोचुरकचीरमोरट मधूलिकाकुष्माण्डप्रभृतीनि समासेन मधुरो वर्गः ॥ १५

दाड़िमामालकमातुलुङ्गाम्रातककपित्थकरमर्द्दवदरकोलप्राचीनामलक-तिन्तिड़ीक-कोशाम्रभव्यपारावतवेत्रफललकुचाम्लवेतसदन्तशठ-दधि तक्र-सुराशुक्तसौवीरतुषोदकधान्याम्लप्रभृतीनि समासेनाम्लो वर्गः ॥ १६

of the following plants. "Holarrhena antidysenterica, Butea frondosa, Shorea robusta, Erythrina fulgens, Terminalia belerica, Cassia fistula, Symplocos racemosa, Asclepia gigantea, Euphorbia antiquorum, Achyranthes aspera, Bignonia suaveolens, Methonica superba, Justicia ganderussa, Musa paradisiaca, Plumbago zeylanica, Guilandina bonducella, Jasminum augustifolium, Nerium odorum, Alstonia scholaris, Premna spinosa, Abrus precatorius and Trichosanthes dioeco." *Suśruta* I. 11. 7[190].

सैन्धवसौवर्च्चल-विड़पाक्यरोमकसामुद्रकपक्किमयवक्षारोषप्रसूतसुवर्च्चिकाप्रभृतीनि समासेन लवणो वर्ग: ॥ १७

पिप्पल्यादि: सुरसादि: शिग्रुमधुशिग्रुमूलकलशुनसुमूखशीतशिवकुष्ठदेवदारु-हरेणुकावल्गुजफलचण्डागुग्गुलु-मुस्तलाङ्गलकीशुकनासापीलुप्रभृतीनि सालसारादिश्च प्रायश: कटुको वर्ग: ॥ १८

आरग्वधादिगुडूच्यादिर्मण्डूकपर्णीवेत्रकरीर-हरिद्राद्वयेन्द्रयववरुणस्वादुकण्टकसप्तपर्ण-बृहतीद्वय-शङ्खिनी-द्रवन्तीत्रिवृत्-कृतवेधनकर्कोटककारवेल्लकवार्त्ताक-करीर-करवीर-सुमन:शङ्खपुष्पापामार्गत्रायमाणाशोकरोहिणीवैजयन्ती सुवर्च्चलापुनर्नवावृश्चिकालीज्योतिष्मतीप्रभृतीनि समासेन तिक्तो वर्ग: ॥ १९

न्यग्रोधादिरम्बष्ठादि: प्रियङ्ग्वादी रोध्रादिस्त्रिफला शल्लकीजम्ब्वाम्रवकुलतिन्दुकफलानि कतकशाकफलपाषाणभेदकवनस्पतिफलानि सालसारादिश्च, प्रायश:, कुरुवककोविदारकजीवन्तीचिल्लीपालङ्क्यासुनिषण्णकप्रभृतीनि नीवारकादयो मुद्गादयो वैदलाश्च समासेन कषायो वर्ग: ॥ २०

सुश्रुतसंहिता, सूत्रस्थानम्, ४२।

190. अथानेनैव विधानेन कुटजपलाशाश्वकर्णपारिभद्रकविभीतकारग्वधतिल्वकार्कस्नुह्यपामार्ग-पाटला-नक्तमाल-वृषकदलीचित्रकपूतीकेन्द्रवृक्षास्फोताश्वमारकसप्तच्छदाग्निमन्थगुञ्जाश्चतस्त्रश्चकोशातकी: समूलफलपत्रशाखा दहेत् ॥ ७

सुश्रुतसंहिता, सूत्रस्थानम्, ११।

Antiparasital Oils: "The oils of Azadirachta indica, Linum usitatissimum, Carthamus tinctorius, Raphanus sativus, Andropogon serrata, Holarrhena antidysenterica, Luffa amara, Calotropis gigantea. Mallotus philipenensis, Butea frondosa, Elettaria cardamomum, Salvadora persica, Pongamia glabra, Balanites roxburghii, Moringa pterygospermum, Sinapis alba, Cleome viscosa, Embelia ribes and Cardiospermum halicacabum are acrid, irritant, pungent and they are beneficial in '*vāyu, kapha*', parasital (or intestinal worms), or syphilitic skin lesions and headache." *Suśruta* I. 45. 101[191].

Diuretic and laxative oils: "The oils of Ophelia chirayta, Eugenia dalbergioides, Terminalia belerica, Cocos nucifera, Zizyphus jujuba, Salvadora persica, Cælagyne ovalis, Buchanania latifolia, Bauhinia variegata, Gynandropsis pentaphylla, Cucumis sativus, Cucumis melo, Cucurbita pepo, and Benicassa cerifera are sweetish, sedative, non-irritant, diffusive, laxative, diuretic and dyspeptic.

---

191. निम्बासती-कुसुम्भ-मूलक-जीमूतक-वृचकक्षतवेधनार्ककम्पिल्लकहस्तिकर्ण-पृथ्वीकापीलु-करञ्जेङ्गुदीशिग्रुसर्षपसुवर्चलाविडङ्गज्योतिष्मतीफलतैलानि तीक्ष्णानि लघन्युष्णवीर्य्याणि कटूनि कटुविपाकानि सराण्यनिलकफक्रिमिकुष्ठप्रमेहशिरोरोगहराणि चेति ॥ १०१

सुश्रुतसंहिता, सूत्रस्थानम्, ४५।

The oils of Bassia latifolia, Gmelina arborea and Butea frondosa are sweetish astringent and they remove the excess of '*kapha*' and '*pitta*'.

Bactericidal emetics and purgatives : The oils of Hydrocarpus kurzii (*tuvara* is popularly known as '*chaulmoogra*'), and Semicarpus anacardium are of astringent sweetish bitter taste, are calorific, emetic, purgative and bactericidal, and are specific in leprosy, adiposis and syphilis (syphilitic cutaneous manifestations).

Oxidizing oils : The oils of turpentine obtained from oleoresins (by distillation) of Pinus longifolia, Cedrus deodara, Tithymallus antiquorium (?), Dalbergia sissoo and Aquilaria agallocha are of astringent bitterish pungent taste and are beneficial in indolent ulcers, intestinal worms, catarrhal affection (of the respiratory tract) and scrofula.

Antiseptic Oils : The fruit-oils of Lagenaria vulgaris, Mangifera sylvetica, Baliospermum montanum, Salvinia cucullata, Vernonia anthelminthica, Stereospermum suaveolens, Vitex negundo, Mallatus philippenensis and Andropogon aciculatus are of bitterish-pungent astringent taste, are purgative and are beneficial in intestinal worms, skin lesions and indolent ulcers." *Suśruta* I. 45. 106-110[192].

The therapeutic value of these drugs is also significant. Many of them are of unquestioned effectiveness in the symptomatic treatment of the diseases for which they have been described. It is not possible here to go into details as to the chemical principles contained in them, for it will not only encumber the book with an extraneous subject, but many of them have not yet been analized in a modern laboratory. However, in the popular pragmatic test, they have shown their fitness of survival in competition with the foreign drugs which unmistakably demonstrates

---

192. किराततिक्तकाऽतिमुक्तक-विभीतक-नारिकेर-कोलाक्षोड़जीवन्तो-पियाल-कर्व्वुदार-सूर्य्यवल्ली-त्रपुसैर्व्वारुक-कर्कारु-कुष्माण्डप्रभृतीनां तैलानि मधुराणि मधुरवीर्य्य-विपाकानि वातपित्तप्रशमनानि शीतवीर्य्याण्यभिष्यन्दीनि सृष्टविण्मूत्राण्यग्निसादनानि चेति ॥ १०६

मधूककाश्मर्य्यपलाशतैलानि मधुरकषायाणि कफपित्तप्रशमनानि ॥ १०७

तुवरकभल्लातकतैले उष्णे मधुरकषाये तिक्तानुरसे वातकफकुष्ठमेदोमेहक्रिमिहरे उभयतोभागदोषहरे च ॥ १०८

सरलदेवदारु-गण्डीर-शिंशपागुरुसारस्नेहास्तिक्त-कटु-कषाया दुष्टव्रणशोधनाः क्रिमि-कफकुष्ठानिलहराश्च ॥ १०९

तुम्बीकोशाम्रदन्तोद्रवन्तोश्यामासप्तलानीलिकाकम्पिल्लकशङ्खिनीस्नेहास्तिक्तकटुकषाया अधोभागदोषहराः क्रिमिकफकुष्ठानिलहरा दुष्टव्रणविशोधनाश्च ॥ ११०

सुश्रुतसंहिता, सूत्रस्थानम्, ४५।

their therapeutic worth.* Opotheraphy was known in its crude form (*Charaka* I. 1. 35). Of course it is too much to expect that it was known that the activating principles of the glands—the hormones, were not destroyed by gastric digestion or boiling at ordinary temperature, or they knew to extract chemically pure thyroidin, adrenalin, pancreatin or spermin, but they prescribed, never-the-less the testicles of goat and cock as potent aphrodisiac (*Charaka* VII. 2. 13.[193] ; VII. 2. 28.[194]). It is very

* Those who are further interested in the subject, will find in '*A Comparative Hindu Materia Medica*' which is under preparation, and which contains their synonyms, expressions in the vernacular provincial dialects, Arabic, Persian, Latin, Greek, English, French and German, their botanical order and classification, chemical analysis when known and their popular therapeutic uses, as well of the allied genera in other countries.

193. ईषत् सलवणं युक्तं धान्यजीरकनागरैः ।
एष वृष्यश्च बल्यश्च बृंहणश्च रसोत्तमः ॥
चरकसंहिता, चिकित्सास्थानम्, २ ।

194. तप्ते सर्पिषि नक्राण्डं ताम्रचूड़ाण्डमिश्रितम् ।
युक्तं षष्टिकचूर्णेन सर्पिषाभिनवेन च ॥
पक्वा पूपलिकाः खादेद्वारुणीमण्डपो नरः ।
य इच्छेदश्ववद्गन्तुं प्रसेक्तुं गजवच्च यः ॥
चरकसंहिता, चिकित्सास्थानम्, २ ।

likely that the biliary calculus (*rochanā*) was given in intestinal putrefaction, in case of insufficiency of biliary salts, and the cow's urine was used in cooking the alkalies in order to add the ammonium to the alkalies to make them more caustic (*Suśruta* I. 11. 6), and the dessiccated cow's dung was either used as a fuel for cautery or as heat-absorbent in which some liquid preparations were kept for ripening.

VII. SURGERY.

"There are eight kinds of surgical operations, namely, excision (*chhedya*), incision (*bhedya*) scarification (*lekhya*), puncturing (*vedya*), exploration (*eṣya*), extraction (*āhārya*), drainage (*visrāvya*) and suturation (*sīvya*). For any of these operations, the surgeon must have the following materials ready at hand and at his disposal, namely the blunt surgical instruments (*yantra*), sharp instruments (*śastra*), caustics (*kṣāra*), cautery (*agni*), probes (*śalākā*), speculum (*śṛṅga*), bottle-gourd (*alāvū*), bougie (*jāmvavauṣṭha*), cotton (*pichu*), pad or lint (*plota*), silkworm gut (*sūtra*), sponge (*patra*=leaf ?), bandage (*paṭṭa*), honey, clarified butter, fat, milk, oils, irrigator (*tarpaṇa*), disinfectants (*kaṣāya*), liniments (*ālepana*), paste or ointment (*kalka*) and other auxiliary requisites." *Suśruta* I. 5. 3 [195].

---

195. तत्र शस्त्रकर्म्माष्टविधम्। तद्यथा—छेद्यं भेद्यं लेख्यं वेध्यमेष्यमाहार्य्यं विस्राव्यं सीव्यमिति। अतोऽन्यतमं कर्म्म चिकीर्षता वैद्येन पूर्व्वमेवोपकल्पयितव्यानि भवन्ति—तद्यथा यन्त्रशस्त्रक्षाराग्निशलाकाशृङ्गजलौकालाबुजाम्बवौष्ठपिचुप्लोतसूत्रपत्रपट्ट-मधुघृतवसापयस्तैलतर्पणकषायालेपन-कल्कव्यजनशीतोष्णोदककटाहादीनि परिकर्म्मिणश्च स्निग्धाः स्थिरा बलवन्तः॥ ३

सुश्रुतसंहिता, सूत्रस्थानम्, ५।

"There are one hundred and one kinds of blunt instruments (*yantra*), of which the hand is the most important, for the hand controls the application of all the (surgical) instruments and without it (an adept hand), they can not be manipulated. Whatever (foreign body) causes pain to the body and the mind, is called '*śalya*' and the instruments that are necessary to extract the '*śalyas*' are called '*yantras*'. *Yantras* are of six kinds, namely (1) Cruciform forceps (*svastika yantra*), (2) pincer-like forceps (*sandaṃśa yantra*), (3) pick-lock forceps (*tāla yantra*), (4) cannula (*nāḍī yantra*), (5) probes (*śalākā yantra*) and (6) accessory appliances (*upayantra*). Of them the cruciform forceps are of forty kinds, pincer-like forceps of twenty kinds, pick-lock forceps two kinds, cannulata twenty kinds, probes twenty-eights kinds and accessory appliances are of twenty-five kinds. They are usually made of (steel) iron, but, (if it be not available, they can be also made) of similar (hard) metal. Their blades are shaped like those of the carnivorous animals, deer, or birds. Therefore likewise they should be manufactured, or according to the rules in the surgical text-books, or according to the instruction of an expert of surgical instruments. They should be of normal size, and according to the needs, either with sharp edges or with polished curbed ends, of firm structure, pleasant appearance and with a good handle.

Swastika Forceps :—The swastika forceps should be eighteen fingers' breadth long (about 12 inches) and their blades shaped like the jaws of a lion (*siṃha* : 1. Ferguson's lion-jaw bone-holding forceps—*osteophore*—with strong blades and teeth to crush and divide bone) ; tiger (*vyāghra* : 2. A bone-gnawing forceps with double-jointed, short, concave blades, having sharpened edges) ; wolf (*vṛka* : 3. Ferguson's bone-holding forceps, having long, strong handles, and short, straight or curved jaws serrated on their internal faces) ; hyena (*tarakṣu* : 4. Farabeuf's forceps with strong grasping teeth all along the inner surface of each blade) ; bear (*bhalluka* : 5. Bulldog forceps with sliding catch, concave, expanded and fenestrated extremities and at the tips, fine teeth) ; panther (*dvïpï* : 6. Gross's bullet forceps with one blade hooked and the other fenestrated and toothed) ; cat (*mārjāra* : 7. Mouse-tooth forceps, with one or two fine points at the tip of each blade, fitting into hollows between the points on the opposite side) ; jackal (*śṛgāla* : 8. Bone forceps, used for seizing and tearing away fragments of bone) ; deer (*hariṇa* ;

9. Bedford's obstetric forceps, short-handled, movable-jointed and having long, curved, fenestrated blades); stag (*ervvāruka*; 10. Bullet-forceps, single-jointed, having long delicate blades, the tips being expanded and concave on their internal side to correspond to the spherical shape of the bullet, or the tips are hooked, so that they may be forced into the bullet); crow (*kāka*), heron (*kaska*), osprey (*kurara*), golden jay (*chasa*), vulture (*bhāsa*), hawk (*śaśaghātī*), owl (*lūka*), kite (*chilli*), black vulture (*śyena*), falcon (*gṛdhra*), crane (*krauñcha*), '*vṛṅgarāja*, *añjalikarṇa*, *avabhañjana*, *nandimukha*' etc. (Dental forceps, double-jointed, having long handles of various curves, and short jaws set at various angles and shapes to hold and extract different teeth in the upper and the lower jaw, resembling the beak of birds). The blades (of the *swastika* forceps) should be joined by a lentil-like (Ervum lens) joint, and the handles should be curved like the elephant-driver's hook. The '*swastika* forceps' are used in extracting foreign bodies impacted in bones (foreign bodies were usually sharp-pointed iron-arrows, used in ancient Indian warfare, and though the comparative forceps, mentioned above, may be similar, they can not be the same, as it needed different kinds

of forceps to extract sharp-pointed, possibly thin-plated steel-arrows, impacted in bones ; the comparison has only been made to give an idea of the similarity of the construction of the forceps, used in ancient and modern surgery).

Pincer-like Forceps : The pincer-like forceps (*sandaṃśa yantra*) are of two kinds, jointed and with sliding catch-spring. They should be 16 fingers' breadth long (about 10 inches) and they are used in extracting foreign bodies in the skin, tissues, vessels and nerves (*śirā*) and tendons.

Pick-lock Forceps : Pick-lock forceps should be made 12 fingers' breadth long (about 8 inches), like the jaw of fish (dolphin), serrated either on one blade or both the blades and they are used in extracting foreign bodies from the aural and nasal passages (Alligator forceps, having delicate, straight or curved wide-opening jaws, for use in narrow canals).

Tubular instruments : Tubular instruments (*nāḍī yantra*) are many and they serve various purposes. Some of them have opening at one end, and others at both ends (or some are single-barrelled, and others are double-barrelled). They are used for the extraction of foreign bodies from vessels (Tubular forceps, with long and slender blades, intended for use through a cannula or other tubular instrument), for the exploration of (internal) lesions (*Bougie*, a cylindrical instrument, resembling a Sound, usually more or less flexible and yielding, and which is employed in the diagnosis and treatment of stricture of tubular passages, such as the urethra or the rectum ; *Probe*, a slender rod of silver or other flexible metal, with blunt bulbous tip, and which is used for exploring sinuses, fistulas or other cavities ; Sound, an elongated, cylindrical, usually curved instrument of metal and which is used for exploring the bladder or other cavities of the body, or for dilating strictures of the urethra or other canal ; with the general use of electricity, many devices have been perfected, by introducing a tiny incandescent bulb at the end of the tube and a reflector at the top, which projects the exact condition of the internal organs as larynx, pharynx or urethra, through laryngoscope, pharyngoscope and urethroscope), for suction of fluids (as *Catheter*, for draining away urine from the bladder, in case of its retention from any cause ; or *Trocar* for withdrawing fluid from any cavity, as in hydrocele), and for facilities for other operations (as Director in lithotomy). The breadth and the length of the tubular instrument should harmonize with the narrow canal (in which it is to be used). The tubular instruments that are used in fistula-in-ano, gummata, tumors, abscesses, for injection, irrigation, in hydrocele, ascites, for fumigation, in stricuture of urethra, and stricture of the rectum, and other instruments such as '*alāvu yantra*' (-bottle-gourd ?) and speculum will be mentioned later.

Probes : The probes (*ṣalākā yantra*) have various uses ; their dimension and their length are dependent on their requirements. They have their ends shaped like an earthworm, the feathered part of an arrow, the hood of a snake, or a fish-hook, and there are two varieties of each kind. They are used for exploration (*eṣaṇa*, such as Bougie, probe or sound), retraction (*vyūhana*, as by a Retractor), grafting (*chālana*) and extraction (*āharaṇa*, by a tubular forceps). For extraction of foreign bodies from vessels, two *śalākā* forceps (Haemostatic forceps) are used, whose ends are slightly flattened like those of a lentil (Ervum lens). Six are used for the drainage of pus having ends covered with cotton. For the application of caustics, three kinds are used whose ends are shaped like a spoon with a conical cavity. For cautery six kinds are used of which the orifice is shaped like the fruit of Eugenia jambolama, and the other like that of the elephant-driver's goad. For the removal of the nasal polypi, one kind is used whose orifice is shaped like half the stone of Ziziphus jujuba, of conical formation with sharp edges (Meyer's ring knife or Luc's forceps). One kind is used for the application of ointment (in the narrow aural or nasal passages) whose both extremities are shaped like a pea or a flowering-bud (as in Tilley's Burr). For the urethral passage one kind is used whose circumference is like the flower-stalk of Jasminum grandiflorum.

Accessory Appliances :—The accessory appliances are thread, twine, bandage, skin-gloves, (*charmmānta*), birch-skin (*valkala* = bark), (tendril of) creeper (for gently dislocating foreign bodies from delicate sensitive organs or abscess cavities), lint, a large rounded stone, hammer (for loosening foreign bodies impacted in bone), the palm of the hand, the sole of the foot, finger, tongue, tooth, nail, mouth (for suction of the fluid as in ascites), hair, horse-hair (for suturation), a branch (of a tree, for extracting foreign bodies, from superficial wounds), expectoration, fluxing (causing discharge in the eyes or throat to remove foreign bodies), cheerfulness, loadstones (used for finding out whether there are iron fragments in the wounds, as loadstones possess polarity and are attracted by iron), caustics, cautery and medicines (including disinfectants).

These instruments can be applied all over the body, any of the limbs, joints, viscera and vessels (including nerves).

Extraction (of foreign bodies with pulling : *nirghātana*), injection (of disinfectants in the bladder or enema in the rectum, *pūraṇa*) : bandaging (*vandhana*); retraction (of the lips of the wound by a '*Retractor*' for inspection, extraction of the foreign body and disinfection,(*vyūhana*) : replacement (of the lips of the wound in their proper place : *varttana*), grafting (principally cutaneous, to cover the wounded scar : *Chālana*), wrenching (of a foreign body, with a forceps to facilitate its extraction : *vivarttana*), dilatation (of any canal or cavity by a '*speculum*' for exploration : *vivaraṇa*), pressing (of the wounded parts to loosen the foreign body, or for the drainage of the pus, if suppuration has taken place : *pīḍana*),disinfection (of the wound, canal or cavity : *viśodhana*), extraction (with force : *vikarṣaṇa*), pulling out (*āharaṇa*), pulling gently to and fro (to loosen the foreign body : *āñchhana*), elevation (of the foreign body, in order to loosen it : *unnamana*), depression (of the fereign body : *vinamana*), pressure (by manipulation of neighboring tissues : *bhañjana*), suction (by a tube of the fluids, as in hydrocele or ascites : *āchūṣaṇa*) exploration (of canal or sinus : *eṣaṇa*), splitting up (a foregn body, to facilitate its removal : *dāraṇa*), straightening (of the foreign body, in order to loosen it : *rjukaraṇa*), irrigation (of the wound with an '*Irrigator*' : *prakṣālana*), blowing disinfectant powders, vulneraries or errhines to deep-seated wound, narrow canal or nasal passage : *pradhamana*), and rubbing (with hair-brush any wound cavity : *pramārjjana*)—these twenty-four are the uses of the '*yantra*' (blunt instruments).

As the foreign bodies can be of infinite varieties, so a wise surgeon must intelligently choose his instrument for each individual case.

Defects in Instruments : Too cumbersome or light, long or short appliances, the blades lacking the power of grasping, or grasping it badly, bent, shaky, too-high-jointed or loose-jointed, loose-bladed or loose-tipped appliances are the twelve defects in '*yantra*' (blunt instruments).

The instrument that is free from these defects, and which is eighteen fingers' breadth long, is the only proper one, which the surgeon must select in surgical operations. The surgeon shall extract, according to the surgical code, the visible missile (*śalya*) by the '*Lion-jaw forceps*' and the invisible missiles by '*kaṅka-mukha*' (*heron-beaked forceps* = dental forceps).

Among the '*yantras*', '*heron-beaked forceps*' is the best, as it can be easily introduced everywhere, and easily withdrawn with the extracted missile''. *Suśruta* I. 7. 2-18 [196].

---

196. यन्त्रशतमेकोत्तरमत्र हस्तमेव प्रधानतमं यन्त्राणामवगच्छ। यस्माद्धस्तादृते यन्त्राणामप्रवृत्तिरेव तदधीनत्वाद् यन्त्रकर्म्मणाम् ॥ २

तत्र मनःशरीराबाधकराणि शल्यानि, तेषामाहरणोपायो यन्त्राणि। तानि षट्-प्रकाराणि। तद्यथा, स्वस्तिकयन्त्राणि। सन्दंश-यन्त्राणि। तालयन्त्राणि। नाड़ी-यन्त्राणि। शलाकायन्त्राणि। उपयन्त्राणि चेति ॥ ३

तत्र चतुर्व्विंशतिः स्वस्तिकयन्त्राणि। द्वे सन्दंशयन्त्रे। द्वे एव तालयन्त्रे। विंशतिर्नाड्यः। अष्टाविंशतिः शलाकाः। पञ्चविंशतिरुपयन्त्राणि। तानि प्रायशो लौहानि भवन्ति तत्प्रतिरूपकाणि वा तदलाभे। तत्र नानाप्रकाराणां व्यालानां मृग-पक्षिणां मुखैर्मुखानि यन्त्राणां प्रायशः सदृशानि तस्मात् तत्सारूप्यादागमादुपदेशादन्य-यन्त्रदर्शनाद् युक्तितश्च कारयेत् ॥ ४

समाहितानि यन्त्राणि खरश्लक्ष्णमुखानि च।

सुदृढ़ानि सुरूपाणि सुग्रहाणि च कारयेत् ॥ ५

तत्र स्वस्तिकयन्त्राण्यष्टादशाङ्गुलप्रमाणानि सिंहव्याघ्रवृकतरक्षुऋक्षद्वीपिमार्जार-शृगालमृगैर्व्वारुककाककङ्ककुररचासभासशशघात्युलूकचिल्लिश्येन-गृध्रक्रौञ्च-भृङ्गराजाञ्जलि-कर्णावभञ्जन-नन्दिमुखमुखानि मसूराकृतिभिः कीलैरवबद्धानि मूलेऽङ्कुशवदावृत्तवारङ्गा-ण्यस्थिविनष्टशल्योद्धरणार्थमुपदिश्यन्ते ॥ ६

Sharp Instruments: Sharp instruments (*śastra*) are of twenty kinds. They are as follows: (1) *Circular knife* (*maṇḍalāgra*);

सनिग्रहोऽनिग्रहश्च सन्दंशौ षोड़शाङ्गुलौ भवतस्त्वङ्मांसशिरास्नायुगतशल्योद्धरणार्थमुपदिश्येते ॥ ७

तालयन्त्रे द्वादशाङ्गुले मत्स्यतालुवदेकतालद्वितालके कर्णनासानाड़ीशल्यानामाहरणार्थम् ॥ ८

नाड़ीयन्त्राणि अनेकप्रकाराण्यनेकप्रयोजनान्येकतोमुखान्युभयतोमुखानि च, तानि स्रोतोगतशल्योद्धरणार्थं रोगदर्शनार्थमाचूषणार्थं क्रियासौकर्य्यार्थञ्चेति। तानि स्रोतोद्वारपरिणाहानि यथायोगपरिणाहदीर्घाणि च। भगन्दरार्शोऽर्व्वुदव्रणवस्त्युत्तरवस्तिमूत्रवृद्धिदकोदरधूमनिरुद्धप्रकशसन्निरुद्धगुदयन्त्राण्यलावूशृङ्ग यन्त्राणि चोपरिष्टाद् वक्ष्यामः ॥ ९

शलाकायन्त्राण्यपि नानाप्रकाराणि नानाप्रयोजनानि यथायोगपरिणाहदीर्घाणि च। तेषां गण्डूपदशरपुङ्खसर्पफणवड़िशमुखे द्वे द्वे एषणव्यूहनचालनाहरणार्थमुपदिश्येते। मसूरदलमात्रमुखे द्वे किञ्चिदानताग्रे स्रोतोगतशल्योद्धरणार्थम्। षट् कार्पासकृतोष्णीषाणि प्रमार्ज्जनक्रियासु। त्रीणि दर्व्व्याकृतीनि खल्लमुखानि क्षारौषधप्रणिधानार्थम्। त्रीण्यन्यानि जाम्बववदनानि त्रीण्यङ्कुशवदनानि षड़ेवाग्निकर्म्मस्वभिप्रेतानि। नासार्व्वुदहरणार्थमेकं कोलास्थिदलमात्रमुखं खल्लतीक्ष्णोष्ठम्। अञ्जनार्थमेकं कलायपरिमण्डलमुभयतो मुकुलाग्रं। मूत्रमार्गविशोधनार्थमेकं मालतीपुष्पवृन्ताग्रप्रमाणपरिमण्डलमिति ॥ १०

उपयन्त्राण्यपि रज्जुवेणिकापट्टचर्म्मान्तवल्कल लतावस्त्राष्ठीलाश्ममुद्गर-पाणिपादतलाङ्गुलि-जिह्वादन्त-नखमुख-वालाश्व- कटकशाखाष्ठीवनप्रवाहणहर्षायस्कान्तमयानि क्षाराग्निभेषजानि चेति।

एतानि देहे सर्व्वस्मिन् देहस्यावयवे तथा।
सन्धौ कोष्ठे धमन्याञ्च यथायोगं प्रयोजयेत् ॥ १२

यन्त्रकर्म्माणि तु निर्घातनपूरणबन्धनव्यूहनवर्त्तनचालनविवर्त्तनविवरण-पीड़नमार्ग-

(2) *Saw* (*kara-patra*, resembling hand, that is, consisting of a thin blade with sharp teeth in the edge, as the hand has fingers) ; (3) *Lancet* (*vṛddhi-patra*, a short, wide, sharp-pointed and two-edged blade, resembling the leaf of '*vṛddhi*'—Batata edulis) ; (4) *Canalicular knife* (*nakha-śastra*, resembling nail-parer) ; (5) *Gum lancet* (*mudrikā*, a short lancet of the size and shape of the last phalanx of the index finger) ; (6) *Thumb lancet* (*utpala-patra*, resembling the petal of Nymphæa stellata) ; (7) *Amputating knife* (*arddha-dara*, a single-edged

---

विशोधनविकर्षणाहरणाच्छनोन्नमनविनमन-भञ्जनोन्मथनाचूषणैषणदारणर्ज्जुकरण-प्रक्षालन-प्रधमनप्रमार्ज्जनानि चतुर्व्विंशतिः ॥ १३

स्वबुद्ध्या चापि विभजेद् यन्त्रकर्म्माणि बुद्धिमान् ।
असंख्येयविकल्पत्त्वाच्छल्यानामिति निश्चयः ॥ १४

तत्रातिस्थूलमसारमतिदीर्घमतिह्रस्वमग्राहि विषमग्राहि वक्रं शिथिलमत्युन्नतं मृदुकीलं मृदुमुखं मृदुपाशमिति द्वादश यन्त्रदोषाः ॥ १५

एतैर्दोषैर्व्विनिर्म्मुक्तं यन्त्रमष्टादशाङ्गुलम् ।
प्रशस्तं भिषजा ज्ञेयं तद्धि कर्म्मसु योजयेत् ॥ १६

दृश्यं सिंहमुखाद्यैस्तु गूढ़ं कङ्कमुखादिभिः ।
निर्हरेत् तु शनैः शल्यं शस्त्रयुक्तिव्यपेक्षया ॥ १७

निवर्त्तते साध्वगाहते च शल्यं निगृह्योद्धरते च यस्मात ।
यन्त्रेष्वतः कङ्कमुखं प्रधानं स्थानेषु सर्व्वेष्वधिकारि चैव ॥१८

सुश्रुतसंहिता, सूत्रस्थानम्, ७।

cutting instrument); (8) *Needle* (*sūchī*, a slender, sharp-pointed instrument, used for puncturing the tissues, for guiding the thread in suturing or for passing a ligature round an artery); (9) *Bistoury* (*kuśa-patra*, a long, narrow-bladed knife, shaped like the '*kuṣa*' grass—Eragrotis cynosuroides); (10) *Hawk-bill scissor* (*āṭī-mukha*, an instrument with two blades, held together by a rivet, moving on the pivot and cutting against each other, resembling the bill of '*āṭī*' bird—Turdus Ginginianus); (11) *Scissor* (*sarārī-mukha*, resembling the long and slender beak of heron); (12) *Concave bistoury* (*antaramukha*, having curved blade inside); (13) *Trocar* (*trikūrchchaka*, an instrument for withdrawing fluid from a cavity or for use in paracentesis, consisting of a metal tube—'*cannula*', open at both ends, in which fits a rod with a sharp three-cornered tip, which is withdrawn after the instrument has been pushed into the cavity; trocar is derived from French '*trois*'—three, + '*carre*'—side, having the same meaning of '*tri-kūrchchaka*'); (14) Lenticular knife (*kuṭhārikā*, an axe-like knife, resembling cow's tooth): (15) *Aspirating needle* (*vrīhi-mukha*, a hollow needle, used for withdrawing fluid from a cavity, an aspirator tube being attached to one end, the other end, shaped like the rice grain, being thrust into the cavity) ; (16) *Iredectomy knife* (*ārā*, an arrow-headed knife, resembling an owl) ; (17) *Scalpel* (*vetasa-patra*) a pointed, long and slender knife with convex edge, resembling the rattan leaf) ; (18) *Hook* (*vaḍiṣa*, an instrument curved or bent near its tip, used for fixation of a part or traction) ; (19) *Scaler* (*danta śaṅku*, an instrument to remove tartar from the teeth) ; (20) *Fine-pointed probe* (*eṣaṇī*, used for dilating contracted lacrymal puncta or examining the lacrymal canals).

Uses : Of them, the Circular Knife and the Saw can be used for excision and scarification ; Lancet, Canalicular Knife, Gum Lancet, Thumb Lancet and the Amputating Knife for excision and incision ; Needle, Bistoury, Hawk-bill Scissor, Scissor, Concave Bistoury and the Trocar for drainage (of the fluid cavities) ; Lenticular Knife, Aspirating Needle, Iredectomy Knife and the Scalpel for puncturing ; the Needle can also be used for puncturing ; Hook and the Scaler for extraction(scraping of tartar from the teeth etc.) ; Fine-pointed Probe for finding out the passage and the direction of a sinus ; and Needles for suturation. In these eight kinds of action the use of '*śastra*' (sharp instruments) are described.

The way these instruments shall be handled, shall be described now. The lancet and other incising instruments should be held by the top and the middle of the handle. For scarification, the Lancet and the Circular Knife should be held with slightly bent hand. All the drainage instruments should be held by the top of the handle. For the drainage of the fluid cavities, children, the aged, the delicately constituted, the timid, women, kings and the princes, the Trocar should be employed. Of the Aspirating needle, the Aspirator should be held in the palm of the hand, and the needle between the thumb and the index finger. The handle of the Lenticular knife should be held in the left hand, and the index and middle fingers of the right hand should be pressed upon it during operation. Iredectomy Knife, Saw and the Fine-pointed Probe should be held by the root (middle of the handle.). The rest of the instruments should be held properly (as to give the most effective result).

The shapes of these instruments are indicated by their nomenclature. And the Canalicular Knife and the Fine-pointed Probe are eight fingers' breadth long (about 5 inches). Needles shall be described later. The extremity of the Hook and the Scaler is slightly curved, and it is sharp like the thorn or fine like the young leaf-blade of Hordeum hexastichum. The orifice of the Fine-pointed Probe is like that of an earthworm. The Gum Lancet is of the size of the top phalanx of the forefinger. The Scissor is ten fingers' breadth long (about 6 inches). And the rest of the instruments are about 6 fingers' breadth long (about 4 inches).

Good Instruments : The instruments which have good handles, are made of good iron (steel), are sharp, well-formed, and whose edges are fine and even, and without indentation, are the best.

Defective Instruments : The instruments that are bent, blunt, broken, jagged, too cumbersome, too light, too long or too short, are defective (these are the eight defects in sharp instruments). The sharp instruments that have the opposite qualities of these, are to be used, excepting that of the Saw, where the jagged sharpness is necessary for sawing bones, for which it is used.

Edges of the Instruments : The edge of the incising instruments should be like the thickness of the tip of Ervum lens, of the scarifying instruments, half the thickness of that of Ervum lens, of the puncturing and the draining instruments like that of hair, and of the excising instrument half the thickness of the tip of hair.

Sterilization of the Instruments: Sterilization (*pāyanā*) of the instruments can be accomplished in three ways: (1) by caustics; (2) by water (by boiling the instrument in water); (3) by oils (by immersing the instruments in antiseptic oils). The instruments that are used in the excision (extirpation) of missiles, foreign bodies and bone (saw) should be sterilized by caustics. The instruments for the excision and incision of the tissues should be sterilized in water. The instruments that are used for the excision of vessels and tendons, should be sterilized in (antiseptic and boiling) oils. For sharpening the instruments, pale, polished stone should be used, and to prevent the dullness of the edge (and rusting), they should be incased in a box, made out of the wood of silk-cotton tree (Bombax heptaphyllum).

The instruments that are very sharp and bright, and supplied with good handles and are of proper size, should only be used in operation." *Suśruta* I. 8. 2-10[197]

---

197. विंशतिः शस्त्राणि। तद्यथा। मण्डलाग्रकरपत्रवृद्धिपत्रनखशस्त्र-मुद्रिकोत्पलपत्रकार्द्धधार-सूची-कुशपत्राटीमुख-शरारिमुखान्तर्मुखत्रिकूर्चक-कुठारिकाव्रीहिमुखारावेतसपत्रक-बडिश-दन्तशङ्क्वेषण्य इति ॥ २

तत्र मण्डलाग्रकरपत्रे स्यातां छेदने लेखने च। वृद्धिपत्रनखशस्त्रमुद्रिकोत्पलपत्र-

Lesions that need Excision Operation: "Excision (or extirpation) should be performed

---

कार्द्धधाराणि छेदने भेदने च। सूचीकुशपत्राटीमुखशरारिमुखान्तर्म्मुखत्रिकूर्च्चकानि विस्रावणे। कुठारिकाव्रीहिमुखारावेतसपत्रकाणि व्यधने सूची च। वड़िशं दन्तशङ्कुश्चाहरणे। एषण्य एषणे आनुलोम्ये च। सूच्यः सेवने। इत्यष्टविधे कर्म्मण्युपयोगः शस्त्राणां व्याख्यातः॥ ७

तेषामथ यथायोगग्रहणसमासोपायः कर्म्मसु वक्ष्यते। तत्र वृद्धिपत्रं वृन्तफलसाधारणे भागे गृह्णीयाच्छेदनान्येवं सर्व्वाणि। वृद्धिपत्रं मण्डलाग्रञ्च किञ्चिदुत्तानपाणिना लेखने बहुशोऽवचार्य्यम्। वृन्ताग्रे विस्रावणानि। विशेषेण बालवृद्धसुकुमारभीरुनारीणां राज्ञां राजपुत्राणाञ्च विकूर्च्चकेन विस्रावयेत्। तलप्रच्छादितवृन्तमङ्गुष्ठप्रदेशिनीभ्यां व्रीहिमुखम्। कुठारिकां वामहस्तन्यस्तामितरहस्तमध्यमाङ्गुल्याङ्गुष्ठविष्टब्धयाभिहन्यात्। आराकरपत्रैषण्यो मूले। शेषाणि तु यथायोगं गृह्णीयात्॥ ४

तेषां नामभिरेवाकृतयः प्रायेण व्याख्याताः। तत्र नखशस्त्रैषण्यावष्टाङ्गुले, सूच्यो वक्ष्यन्ते। वड़िशं दन्तशङ्कुश्चानताग्रे तीक्ष्णकण्टकप्रथमयवपत्रमुखे। एषणी गण्डूपदाकारमुखी। प्रदेशिन्यग्रपर्व्वप्रदेशप्रमाणा मुद्रिका। दशाङ्गुला शरारिमुखी सा कर्त्तरीति कथ्यते। शेषाणि तु षड़ङ्गुलानि॥ ५

तानि सुग्रहाणि सुलोहानि सुधाराणि सुरूपाणि सुसमाहितमुखाग्राण्यकरालानि चेति शस्त्रसम्पत्॥ ६

तत्र वक्रं कुण्ठं खण्डं खरधारमतिस्थूलमत्यल्पमतिदीर्घमतिह्रस्वमित्यष्टौ शस्त्रदोषाः। अतो विपरीतगुणमाददीत अन्यत्र करपत्रात् तद्धि खरधारमस्थिच्छेदनार्थम्॥७

तत्र धारा भेदनानां मासूरी, लेखनानामर्द्धमासूरी, व्यधनानां विस्रावणानाञ्च कैशिकी, छेदनानामर्द्धकैशिकीति॥ ८

तेषां पायना त्रिविधा क्षारोदकतैलेषु। तत्र क्षारपायितं शरशल्यास्थिच्छेदनेषु। उदकपायितं मांसच्छेदनभेदनपाटनेषु। तैलपायितं सिराव्यधनस्नायुच्छेदनेषु। तेषां निशाणार्थं श्लक्ष्णशिला माषवर्णा, धारासंस्थापनार्थं शाल्मलीफलकमिति॥ ९

in fistula-in-ano, tubercles, suppurative tumors, non-suppurative tumors, gummata, wart, foreign bodies in bones and tissues, hairy moles, Sarcoma, tonsillitis, sloughing tendons-muscles and vessels, tumor of the palate, condylomata, myxoma of the gullet, chancre, fibroma and myoma.

Lesions that need Incision : Incision (lancing) should be made in all (suppurative) tumors, except those caused by the derangement of the three humors (non-suppurative tumors), erysipelas, oscheopyedema, bubo, diabetic boils, carbuncle, galactoposterma (or mastosyrinx), pustules of the penis, stye, pustules of the foot, fistula, suppurative tonsillitis, suppurative eruption of the penis, gumma of the cornea, pustular abscesses, abscess on the palate, gum-boils, the tumors or sinuses that develop after suppuration, cyst formed round the nucleus of a calculus, or any other kind of suppurative tumor.

Lesions that need Scarification : Scarification should be made in the four forms of throat inflammation, leucoderma, ranula, inflammation of the gum, tubercles, lachrymal fistula, epiglottitis,

---

यदा सुनिशितं शस्त्रं रोमच्छेदि सुसंस्थितम् ।
सुगृहीतं प्रमाणेन तदा कर्मसु योजयेत् ॥ १०

सुश्रुतसंहिता, सूत्रस्थानम्, ८ ।

gummata of the throat, psoriatic patches, and granulations.

Lesions that need Punctures: Punctures should be made in cirsoid aneurysm, hydrocele and ascites.

Lesions that need Probing : Probing should be made in fistulas, fistulas with foreign bodies, or those extending sideways.

Lesions that need Extraction : Extraction should be made in three kinds of gravel, tartar on the teeth, wax in the ears, calculi, foreign bodies (missiles), mal-presentation of the fetus and the impacted feces in the rectum.

Lesions that need Drainage :—Drainage should be performed in all kinds of (suppurating) tumors except those that develop by the derangement of the three humors (non-suppurative tumors), lepromata, painful abscess, carbuncle, otorrhea, elephantiasis, toxic blood (blood in the infected region), furuncle, erysipelas, cysts, three kinds of chancres (hard, mixed, and soft chancres), breast-abscess (or fistula), suppurative bubo, pyorrhea, abscess and gummata of the palate, dental caries (causing suppuration in the gum), gingivitis, epulis, ulocase, gumboil, chancre of the lips, and pustules.

Lesions that need Suturation ;—Suturation

should only be made in those places which have been opened and been completely drained off (the foreign matter), or the fresh wounds near the movable joints.

Wounds that are not fit for suturation: Sutures should not be applied to those wounds caused by caustics, cautery and toxins, or in those where there is discharge of gas, or in the interior of which there is sanies or foreign body. These should be at first disinfected ; dust, hair, nails, fragments of bone (any foreign body), when found in a wound, should be removed before sutures are applied, as otherwise they are likely to provoke suppuration and pain. Therefore they should at first be disinfected. The lips of the wound then should be raised and placed in proper apposition, and sutures applied slowly with the fine cotton thread, or the bark-fiber of Caesalpinia digynia, flax, catgut (*snāyu* = tendon), hair (horse hair), fibers of Sanseviera zeylanica, or Tinospora cordifolia, in any of these sutures, (1) Twisted suture (*vellitaka*), (2) Quilled suture (*gophṇikā*), (3) Continuous suture (*tunna-sevanī*), (4) Interrupted suture (*ṛju-granthi*) or any other kind best suited to the requirement, and after the suturation is over, the sewed parts should be gently pressed by the finger and levelled. In parts of the body covered with little flesh, or over joints, a full-curved suture needle, of two fingers' width long, should be used. For fleshy parts, a straight, three-edged, suture-needle, three fingers' breadth long, is proper. In the vital parts, scrotum and the abdomen, a half-curved suture-needle (curved like a bow) is good. These three varieties of needles should be sharp-pointed, their body rounded like the flower-stalk of Aganosma cargophyllatum, and should be capable of easy handling. Sutures should not be made either too far off or too close to the edges of the wound. In the former case, lips of the wound will become painful, and in the latter case, they may be torn off. Then the stitched part should be covered with cotton (as a surgical dressing) or linen (as a lint), and a powder compound of Aglaia roxburghii, antimony sulphide, Glycerrhiza glabra, and Symplocos racemosa, or the powder of Boswellia serrata or the ashes of burnt linen, should be sprinkled over it (as antisepsis). Then after proper bandaging, the patient shall be told the hygienic rules, he will have to observe." *Suśruta* I. 25. 2-12[198].

---

198. छेद्या भगन्दरा ग्रन्थिः श्लैष्मिकस्तिलकालकः ।
व्रणवर्त्मार्ब्बुदान्यर्शश्चर्म्मकीलोऽस्थिमांसगम् ॥

Caustics :—"For particular purposes, of all sharp or accessory instruments, caustics are the

---

शल्यं जतुमणिर्मांसत्सङ्घातो गलशुण्डिका ।
स्नायुमांससिराकोथो वल्मीकं शतपोनकः ।
अध्युषश्चोपदंशाश्च मांसकन्द्यधिमांसकः ॥ २
भेद्या विद्रधयोऽन्यत्र सर्व्वजाद् ग्रन्थयस्त्रयः ।
आदितो ये विसर्पाश्च वृद्धयः सविदारिकाः ॥
प्रमेहपिड़काशोफ-स्तनरोगाववमन्थकाः ।
कुम्भीकानुशयीनाड्यो वृन्दौ पुष्करिकालजी ॥
प्रायशः क्षुद्ररोगाश्च पुप्पुटौ तालुदन्तजौ ।
तुण्डिकेरी गिलायुश्च पूर्व्वं ये च प्रपाकिणः ।
वस्तिस्तथाश्मरीहेतोर्मेदोजा ये च केचन ॥ ७
लेख्यास्चतस्रो रोहिण्यः किलासम पजिह्विका ।
मेदोजो दन्तवैदर्भौ ग्रन्थिवर्त्माधिजिह्विका ॥
अर्शांसि मण्डलं मांस-कन्दी मांसोन्नतिस्तथा ॥ ४
वेध्याः शिरा वहुविधा मूत्रवृद्धिर्दकोदरम् ॥ ५
एष्या नाड्यः सशल्याश्च व्रणा उन्मार्गिणश्च ये ॥ ६
आहार्य्याः शर्करास्तिस्रो दन्तकर्णमलाश्मरी ।
शल्यानि मूढ़गर्भाश्च वर्चंश्च निचितं गुदे ॥ ७
स्राव्या विद्रधयः पञ्च भवेयुः सर्व्वजादृते ।
कुष्ठानि वायुः सरुजः शोफो यश्च कदेशजः ॥
पाल्यामयाः श्लीपदानि विषजुष्टञ्च शोणितम् ।
अर्व्वुदानि विसर्पाश्च ग्रन्थयश्चादितस्तु ये ॥
त्रयस्त्रयश्चोपदंशाः स्तनरोगा विदारिका ।
शौषिरो गलशालकं कण्टकाः क्रिमिदन्तकः ॥

best (when alkalies in concentrated form (caustics) are brought into contact with the animal

दन्तवेष्ट: सोपकुश: शीतादो दन्तपुप्पुट: ।
पित्तासृक्कफजाश्चौष्ठ्या: क्षुद्ररोगाश्च भूयश: ॥ ८
सीव्या मेद:समुत्थाश्च भिन्ना: सुलिखिता गदा: ।
सद्योव्रणाश्च ये चैव चलसन्धिव्यपाश्रिता: ॥ ९
न क्षाराग्निविषैर्जुष्टा न वा मारुतवाहिन: ।
नान्तर्लोहितशल्याश्च तेषु सम्यग्विशोधनम् ।
पांशुरोमनखादीनि चलमस्थि भवेच्च यत् ॥
अहृतानि यतोऽमूनि पाचयेयुर्भृशं व्रणम् ॥
रुजश्च विविधा: कुर्य्युस्तस्मादेतान् विशोधयेत् ॥ १०
ततो व्रणं समुन्नम्य स्थापयित्वा यथास्थितम् ।
सीव्येत् सूक्ष्मेण सूत्रेण वल्केनाश्मन्तकस्य वा ॥
शणजक्षौमसूत्राभ्यां स्नायुना वालेन वा पुन: ।
मूर्व्वागुड़ूचीतानैर्वा सीव्येद्वेल्लितकं शनै: ॥
सीव्येद्गोफणिकां वापि सीव्येद्वा तुन्नसेवनीम् ।
ऋजुग्रन्थिमथो वापि यथायोगमथापि वा ॥
देशेऽल्पमांसे सन्धौ च सूची वृत्ताङ्गुलद्वयम् ।
आयता त्र्यङ्गुला त्र्यस्रा मांसले चापि पूजिता ॥
धनुर्व्वक्रा हिता मर्म्म-फलकोषोदरोपरि ।
इत्येतास्त्रिविधा: सूचीस्तीक्ष्णाग्रा: सुसमाहिता: ॥
कारयेन्मालतीपुष्प-वृन्ताग्रपरिमण्डला: ।
नातिदूरे निकृष्टे वा सूचीं कर्म्मणि पातयेत् ।
दूराद्रुजो व्रणौष्ठस्य सन्निकृष्टेऽवलुञ्चनम् ॥ ११
अथ क्षौमपिचुच्छन्नं संस्यूतं प्रतिसारयेत् ।
प्रियङ्ग्वञ्जनयष्ट्याह्व-रोध्रचूर्णै: समन्तत

tissues, they enter into chemical combination with the oxygen present, and thus give rise to an active necrosis or destructive inflammation; alkalies are likewise solvents of albumin; these physical and chemical properties render the caustic alkalies active in producing counter-irritation, and their escharotic effects have been made use of in the destruction of morbid tissue, whether of neoplastic or inflammatory origin, and chronic synovitis). Due to the escharotic property of the (concentrated) alkalies, they are called caustics (*kṣāra*). They are acrid, irritant, pungent, (and their external use causes) destruction of the tissues (eschars), corrosion, disinfection, granulation, desiccation, hemostatis, scarification, (and their internal administration cures), intestinal worms, hyperacidity, eructation, cutaneous lesions, auto-intoxication; but their excessive use induces impotence.

Alkalies are of two kinds (concentrated which is strong, and non-concentrated which is mild), for external application (strong) and for internal administration (mild). Their external application

---

शल्लकीफलचूर्णैर्वा चौमध्यामेन वा पुनः।
ततो व्रणं यथायोगं वद्राचारिकमादिशेत् ॥ १२

सूश्रुतसंहिता, सूत्रस्थानम्, २५

is indicated in lepromes, keloid, ringworm, leucoderma, psoriasis guttata, fistula-in-ano, tumors, indolent ulcers, fistula, condyloma, mole, impetigo, lichen planus, warts, external sores, dermatophyte, poison-bites, and gummata ; besides these, the application of caustics in seven kinds of mouth diseases (tumor of the tongue, stomatitis ulcerosa, chancres of the lips and the tongue, etc.) and three kinds of throat-neoplasms, is appropriate. Internally alkalies may be administered in auto-intoxication, adenitis, tympanites, indigestion, dyspepsia, anorexia, constipation, gravel, calculus, abdominal tumors, intestinal worms, poisoning and gummata. However its (internal) use is counter-indicated in persons who have a tendency to hemorrhage, biliousness, in children, the aged or weak persons, or those who are suffering from giddiness, delirium, epilepsy and amaurosis." *Suśruta* I. 11. 2-5[198a].

---

198 (a). शस्त्रानुशस्त्रेभ्यः क्षारः प्रधानतमश्छेद्य-भेद्य-लेख्य-करणात् त्रिदोषघ्नत्वाद्विशेषक्रियावचारणाच्च ॥ २

तत्र क्षरणात् क्षणनाद्वा क्षारः। नानौषधिसमवायात् त्रिदोषघ्नः, शुक्लत्वात् सौम्यस्तस्य सौम्यस्यापि सतो दहनपचनदारणादिशक्तिरविरुद्धा, स खल्वाग्नेयौषधिगणभूयिष्ठत्वात् कटुक उष्णस्तीक्ष्णः पाचनो विलयनः शोधनो रोपणः शोषणः स्तम्भनो लेखनः क्रिम्यामकफकुष्ठविषमेदसामुपहन्ता पुंस्त्वस्य चातिसेवितः ॥ ३

स द्विविधः प्रतिसारणीयः पानीयश्च। तत्र प्रतिसारणीयः कुष्ठकिटिमदद्रुकिलास-

Cautery : "Cautery is more potent in its action than caustics. For once cauterized, lesions lose their sepsis, and even those which defy the medicinal, operative and caustic treatments, become hereby amenable." *Suśruta* I. 12. 2[199].

Leeches : "By leeches (*Hirudo*), bleeding (or removal of congestion) can be accomplished in the easiest way of kings, wealthy personages, women, children, the aged, timid, weak or delicately constitutioned individuals." *Suśruta* I. 13. 2.[200].

Enema : "As enema (*vasti*) serves multifarious purposes, according to the medical experts,

---

मण्डलभगन्दरार्बुददुष्टव्रणनाडीचर्म्मकीलतिल-कालक - न्यच्छव्यङ्ग - मशकबाह्यविद्रधि-क्रिमिविषार्शःसु उपदिश्यते सप्तसु च मुखरोगेषूपजिह्वोपकुशदन्तवैदर्भेषु तिसृषु च रोहिणीष्वेतेषु चैवानुशस्त्रप्रणिधानमुक्तम्। पानीयस्तु गरगुल्मोदराग्निसङ्गाजीर्णारोचकानाहशर्कराश्मर्य्याभ्यन्तरविद्रधिक्रिमिविषार्शःसूपयुज्यते ॥ ४

अहितस्तु रक्तपित्तज्वरितपित्तप्रकृतिबालवृद्धदुर्ब्बलभ्रममदमूर्च्छातिमिरपरीतेभ्योऽन्येभ्यश्चैवंविधेभ्यः। तद्धि तरच्छारवद्दग्ध्वा परिस्रावयेत्। तस्य विस्तारोऽन्यत्र ॥ ५

सुश्रुतसंहिता, सूत्रस्थानम्, ११।

199. क्षारादग्निर्गरीयान् क्रियासु व्याख्यातः। तद्दग्धानां रोगाणामपुनर्भावाद्भेषजशस्त्रक्षारैरसाध्यानां तत्साध्यत्वाच्च ॥ २

सुश्रुतसंहिता, सूत्रस्थानम् १२।

200. नृपाढ्यबालस्थविरभीरुदुर्ब्बलनारीसुकुमाराणामनुग्रहार्थं परमसुकुमारोऽयं शोणितावसेचनोपायोऽभिहितो जलौकसः ॥ २

सुश्रुतसंहिता, सूत्रस्थानम्, १३।

it is the best of all analeptic (*sneha*) remedies. If it be properly applied, it makes the weak strong (Stimulating enema), the lean stout (enema nutriens), the stout lean (enema purgans), strengthens eye-sight (by removing the decomposing materials from the intestine, the toxic products of which are absorbed in the system, and provoke reflexably various maladies) and prolongs youthfulness. It promotes the general health of the body, adds to its vigor, brightens complexion, is a restorative of health and conduces to the logevity of life ; and its use in fever (enema purgans), diarrhœa (enema adstringens), amaurosis, catarrh, cephalalgia, ophthalmia, hemiprosoplegia, mimic convulsion, apoplexy, general paresis, tympanites, hemiplegia, flatulence, gravel, hyperalgia, oschitis, syphilis, constipation, strangury, bubo, hemorrhage, hydrothionuria, fecal impaction, aspermia, menostasia, galactozemia, cardipalmus, lockjaw, torticollis, piles, calculus and abortion, is appropriate.

Fountain-syringe : For a boy one year old the tube (*netra*) shall be six fingers' breadth long, having the dimension of the little finger, and at the extremity of which, the nozzle (*karṇikā*) should be fixed, one and a half fingers' breadth long ; the orifice at the mouth of the tube should be like that of a heron's feather, and at the end, like Phaseolus mungo. For a boy of eight years of age, the tube shall be eight fingers breadth long having the dimension of the ring-finger, and at the extremity of it, the nozzle should be fixed two fingers' breadth long ; the orifice at the mouth of the tube shall be like the feather of the vulture, and at the end like Phaseolus radiatum. And for a person, sixteen years old, the tube shall be ten fingers' breadth long, having the dimension of the middle finger, and at the extremity of it, the nozzle should be three and a half fingers' breadth long ; the orifice at the mouth of the tube shall be like the peacock's feather, and at the end like that of a pea. The reservoir (*āsthāpana*) for the enema, for persons, one, eight or sixteen years of age shall be the size of their two handfuls, four handfuls, and eight handfuls of their individual hands respectively (the modern fountain-syringe is an apparatus, consisting of a rubber reservoir for holding fluid for the enema, to the bottom of which is attached a rubber tube, provided with a suitable nozzle, usually made of vulcanized rubber ; and it is used for rectal or vaginal injections, irrigating wounds, etc., the force of the flow being regulated by the height of the reservoir above the point of discharge).

The size of the tube and the reservoir is not only to be graduated according to the age (of the patient), but also in addition to it, his physical condition and vigor.

For a person, above twenty five years of age, the tube shall be twelve fingers' breadth long, having the dimension at the mouth like the thumb, and at the end like the little finger, and the nozzle shall be three fingers' breadth long ; the orifice of the tube at the mouth should be like the feather of a female vulture, and at the end like the stone of plum. The tube should be firmly fixed with the reservoir. And the reservoir should be capable of holding twelve handfuls of enema. After seventy, the tube shall remain just the same, but the quantity of the enema should be reduced to that of a person of sixteen years of age.

The tube should be made of gold, silver, copper, bronze, ivory. horn, glass or wood, polished, strong, shaped like the bovine tail with gradually reducing dimension, straight and with globular orifice. And the reservoir is made out of the bladder of the matured cow, buffalo, boar, goat or sheep, and it should be flexible, even strong and of the required size." *Suśruta* IV. 35. 2-7[201].

---

201. तत्र स्नेहादीनां कर्म्मणां वस्तिकर्म्म प्रधानतममाहुराचार्य्याः। कस्मात्? अनेककर्म्मकरत्वाद्वस्तेः। इहवस्तिर्नानाविधद्रव्यसंयोगाद्दोषाणां संशोधनसंशमनसंग्रहणानि करोति, क्षीणशुक्रं वाजीकरोति, कृशं बृंहयति, स्थूलं कर्षयति, चक्षुः प्रीणयति, वलीपलितमपहन्ति, वयः स्थापयति। शरीरोपचयं वर्णं बलमारोग्यमायुषः परिवृद्धिञ्च करोति वस्तिः सम्यगुपासितः; तथा ज्वरातीसार-तिमिरप्रतिश्याय-शिरोरोगाधिमन्थार्द्दिताक्षेपकपक्षाघातैकाङ्ग-सर्व्वाङ्गरोगाध्मानोदर-शर्कराशूल-वृद्ध्युपदंशानाहमूत्रकृच्छ्र-गुल्म-वातशोणित-वातमूत्रपुरीषोदावर्त्त-शुक्रार्त्तव-स्तन्य-नाशहृद्धनुमन्याग्रहार्शोऽश्मरीमूढगर्भप्रभृतिषु चात्यर्थमुपयुज्यते ॥ २

वस्तिर्वाते च पित्ते च कफे रक्ते च शस्यते ।
संसर्गे सन्निपाते च वस्तिरेव हितः सदा ॥ ३

तत्र सांवत्सरिकाष्टद्विरष्टवर्षाणां षडष्टदशाङ्गुलप्रमाणानि कनिष्ठिकानामिका-मध्यमाङ्गुलि-परिणाहान्यग्रेऽध्यर्द्धाङ्गुल-द्व्यङ्गुलार्द्ध-तृतीयाङ्गुलसन्निविष्टकर्णिकानि कङ्कश्येनबर्हिपत्रनाड़ीतुल्यप्रवेशानि मुद्गमाषकलायमात्रस्रोतांसि विदध्यान्नेत्राणि। तेषु त्वास्थापनद्रव्यप्रमाणमातुरहस्तसम्मितेन प्रसृतेन सम्मितौ प्रसृतौ द्वौ चत्वारोऽष्टौ विधेयाः ॥ ४

वर्षोत्तरेषु नेत्राणां वस्तिमानस्य चैव हि ।
वयोबलशरीराणि समीक्ष्य वर्द्धयेद्विधिम् ॥ ५

पञ्चविंशतेरूर्द्ध्वं द्वादशाङ्गुलं मूलेऽङ्गुष्ठोदरपरिणाहमग्रे कनिष्ठिकोदरपरिणाहमग्रे त्र्यङ्गुलसन्निविष्टकर्णिकं गृध्रपत्रनाड़ीतुल्यप्रवेशं कोलास्थिमात्रं छिद्रं, क्लिन्नकलायमात्रं छिद्रमित्येके। सर्व्वाणि मूले वस्तिनिबन्धनार्थं द्विकर्णिकानि। आस्थापनद्रव्यप्रमाणन्तु विहिता द्वादश प्रसृताः। सप्ततेरूर्द्ध्वं नेत्रप्रमाणमेतदेव, द्रव्यप्रमाणन्तु द्विरष्टवर्षवत् ॥ ६

तत्र नेत्राणि सुवर्णरजतताम्रायोरीतिदन्तशृङ्गमणितरुसारमयाणि श्लक्ष्णानि दृढानि

Fractures : "One suffering from fractures, should avoid salt (sodium chloride), pungents, alkalies, acids, sexual indulgence, exposure to the sun, exercise and desiccant food. He should take cooked fine rice, meat-broth, milk, milk-fat, pea soup, and stimulative foods and drinks. The bark of Glycyrrhiza glabra, Ficus glomerata, Ficus religiosa, Butea frondosa, Terminalea arjuna, Bambusae, Shorea robusta and Ficus indica for splint (*kuśa*). For liniment, Rubra manjista, Glycyrrhiza glabra, Pterocarpum santalinum, and buttered rice-paste which has been repeatedly washed in water (that is fat has been washed out from the surface of the rice paste) should be used. The wound should be bandaged every seventh day in the wintry season, every fifth day in the temperate season, every third day in the hot weather, or according to the urgency of the needs. But if the bandage (splint) is loose, reparation of the joints does not take place, and if too tight, it is apt to cause inflammation of the tissues, pain and suppuration ; therefore

---

गोपुच्छाकृतीन्यृज नि गुटिकामुखानि । वस्त्रयश्चाङ्गानां मृद्वो नातिबहला दृढ़ाः प्रमाणवन्तो गोमहिषवराहाजोरभ्राणाम्. ॥ ७

सुश्रुतसंहिता, चिकित्सितस्थानम्, २५।

it should be properly bandaged (The reparation of the bone in fractures depends on two factors : (1) The fragments of the fractured bone are to be placed in apposition to one another in the normal position, and kept in that condition from a week to eight weeks, according to the needs of the case, so that the bone can be repaired and consolidated. (2) The reparation principally takes place in the soft tissues surrounding the bone, and from the torn periosteum granulation tissue is formed, which when calcified forms callus and which by ossification is converted into bony structure ; therefore if the splint has been put on before the bones have been properly set, or if the bandage is loose, or due to movement, the fragments change their place, then of course reparation can not take place, and after three months time, they lose their recuperative power ; if on the other hand, the fragments of the bones are very rigidly fixed, face to face, without leaving any space between them, and the bandage is very tight, there will be then minimum of callus formation. Therefore for successful reparation, both these extremes are to be avoided, and this can be only faithfully determined by X-ray examination. In children normally, the reparation is rapid, especially in cancellous tissues)." *Suśruta* IV. 3. 2-8[202].

Fractures of the Phalanges or dislocation of the Metacarpo-Phalangeal joints: "Whether the phalanges are fractured or the joints are dislocated, they should be placed in the normal apposition and bandaged (Wyeth's finger-bandage or roller-bandage), and upon it (vulnerary) butter should be applied.

Metatarsal fractures: In the fractures of

---

202. लवणं कटुकं क्षारमम्लं मैथुनमातपम् ।
व्यायामञ्च न सेवेत भग्नो रुक्षान्नमेव च ॥ ७
शालिर्मांसरसः क्षीरं सर्पिर्यूषः सतीनजः ।
बृंहणञ्चान्नपानं स्याद्देयं भग्नाय जानता ॥ ४
मधुकोडुम्बराश्वत्थ-पलाशककुभत्वचः ।
वंशसर्ज्जवटानां वा कुशार्थमुपसंहरेत् ॥ ५
आलेपनार्थं मञ्जिष्ठां मधुकं रक्तचन्दनम् ।
शतधौतघृतोन्मिश्रं शालिपिष्टञ्च संहरेत् ॥ ६
सप्ताहादथ सप्ताहात् सौम्येष्वृतुषु वन्धनम् ।
साधारणेषु कर्त्तव्यं पञ्चमे पञ्चमेऽहनि ।
आग्नेयेषु त्र्यहात् कुर्य्याद्भग्नदोषवशेन वा ॥ ७
तत्रातिशिथिलं बद्धे सन्धिस्थैर्य्यं न जायते ।
गाढ़े नापि त्वगादीनां शोफो रुक् पाक एव च ।
तस्मात् साधारणं वन्धं भग्ने शंसन्ति तद्विदः ॥ ८

सुश्रुतसंहिता, चिकित्सित-स्थानम्, ३ ।

the metatarsus, (vulnerary) liniment should be applied, then bandaged, and upon it splint should be placed (to prevent motion and displacement of the bones).

Fractures of fibula and femur : In fractures of the fibula (tibia) and the femur, the parts should be massaged with a liniment and the fragmented bones brought to apposition ; then after fixing a splint, they should be bandaged. If the neck of the femur project, or the fragments of the bone tear out through the flesh, it should be given a circular bandage.

Fractures of the hip-bone : In the fracture of the os innominatum (usually in the neck), the raised part of the bone should be lowered, and the depressed part raised, and thus it should be bandaged. When the hip-joint has been put in its normal place, it should be irrigated (with a vulnerary or an antiseptic).

Fractures of the Ribs : If the ribs are fractured, they are to be rubbed with a salve, and then after placing a pin (*kavalikā*), the ribs are to be fixed by '*twisted suture*' (*nivandhanī*), and then bandaged ; later the patient is to be laid in an extension splint, simple (*droṇī*) or filled with (vulnerary) oil (*kaṭāha*).

Dislocation of the scapulo-humeral joint : In the dislocation of the scapulo-humeral joint, the humerus is raised, by using a hammer at the axilla, and when the bones are in their normal apposition, affixed by the '*spica bandage for the shoulder*' (*svastika-vandhana*).

Dislocation of the Elbow-joint : If the elbow joint is dislocated, it should be massaged, and then put in the normal position through extension and flexion movements ; when it is done, it should be salved. The same treatment is applicable in the dislocation of the knee-joint, ankle-joint and radio-carpal joints (wrist-joint).

Fractures of the metacarpus : In the fractures of the metacarpus after proper bandaging, it should be moistened with a (vulnerary) oil ; then to find out the strength of reparation, it should be gradually tested by holding upon the palm of the hand, a dried cow-dung ball (very light), clay-ball, and at last a stone.

Dislocation of the acromio-clavicular joint : In the dislocation of the acromio-clavicular joint, if the (outer end of the) clavicle be displaced upwards, or downwards (from the acromion), after fomentation, it should be raised in the former case by a hammer, and in the latter case, depressed, and bandaged with a strong support

(Dessault's bandage: in obstinate cases, if the displacement persist and cause discomfort, the bones should be held together by wiring).

Fracture of the Humerus: In the fracture of the humerus, the treatment is similar to that of the femur.

Sprain of the Cervical vertebral articulations: If the neck is bent or depressed, it should be brought to apposition by pressure upon the cervical vertebræ and (with the traction-aid of) maxillary bones; it should then be bandaged after splint, and the patient laid to bed on his back for a week.

Dislocation of the Temporo-Maxillary joint: In the dislocation of temporo-maxillary or temporo-mandibular joints, the bones should be put in proper apposition and held together by five-tailed (*pañchāṅgī*) bandage (used as four-tailed bandage now-a-days), and there should be nasal injection of errhine, made of a sedative drug-cooked in butter.

Pyorrhea alveolaris: If in young people, the teeth become loose, associated with bleeding gum, without any external injury, it should be treated by antiseptic cold wash and injections; and the patient shall drink milk (during the treatment) with the (tubular) stem of Nymphaea stellata.

In case of old men, the loose teeth should be extracted (by a forceps).

Injuries to the Nose: If the nasal bone caves in or is bent (by traumatism or syphilitic lesion), then it should be raised and straightened (by a speculum) and then for respiration, in two nasal cavities, two double-mouthed tubes should be inserted. When it is done, it is to be bandaged, and the bandage to be kept moistened by a (vulnerary) ointment.

Injuries to the Ear: If the (ossicles of the) ears are broken, they should be put in their apposition, then after an application of a (vulnerary) ointment, they should be bandaged and treated like ordinary wounds.

Injuries to the Cranium:—In the fracture of the frontal bone, if the brain matter has not come out (if the dura matter has not been penetrated or hurt), after liniment, the wound shall be bandaged, and the patient shall take clarified butter (?) for a week.

Inflammation: If due to an accidental fall or traumatism, any part of the body becomes inflamed without any (apparent) injury, it shall be treated by cold application and fomentation alternatively).

Fractures of the Femur and the leg bones:

In the fractures of the leg-bones (tibia and patella) or of the thigh (femur), the patient has to be lain in wooden extension bed, and for the maintenance of the steady traction (until the consolidation of the bone has taken place, and to prevent the tension of the muscles which prevents the reparation of the fracture), the leg or the thigh has to be fixed with five nails ; thus in the fracture of the leg bones, there should be two nails on each side of the leg, and against the sole, upon the wooden frame (to prevent movement, which interferes with consolidation of the fractured bones) ; in case of the fracture of the femur, two nails on each side of the thigh, and at the hip joint should be fixed. (This treatment in the fractures of the femur or the leg bones, is very similar to the modern practice by Hodgen's nail extension splint). This is also applicable in the fractures or dislocations of the pelvis, vertebrae and the clavicle If the dislocation is old, this treatment is to be preceded by embrocation to soften the ligaments.

Fractures of Patella : If the fractured patella (*kāṇḍa*) has consolidated in wrong apposition, it has to be broken up (artificially) and then to begin treatment, after putting it in the normal apposition.

Amputation of a dried bone : If the flesh has retracted from a protruded bone, leaving it dry, then the bone has to be amputated (by saw) carefully up to the fleshy part, and then it has to be treated like a fresh wound (by a recurrent bandage)." *Suśruta* IV. 3. 23-42[203].

---

203. भग्नां व. सन्धिमुक्तां वा स्थापयित्वाङ्गुलीं समम् ।
अणुनावेष्ट्य पट्टेन घृतसेकं प्रदापयेत् ॥ २२
अभ्यज्य सर्पिषा पादं तलभग्नं कुशोत्तरम् ।
वस्त्रपट्टेन वध्नीयान्नच व्यायाममाचरेत् ॥
अभ्यज्यायामयेज्जङ्घामूरुञ्च सुसमाहितः ।
दत्त्वा वृक्षत्वचः शीता वस्त्रपट्टेन वेष्टयेत् ॥ २३
मतिमांश्चक्रयोगेण आञ्छेदूर्व्वस्थि निर्गतम् ।
स्फुठितं पिच्चितञ्चापि वध्नीयात् पूर्व्ववद्भिषक् ॥ २४
आञ्छेदूर्द्ध्वमधो वापि कटीभग्नन्तु मानवम् ।
ततः स्थानस्थिते सन्धौ वस्तिभिः समुपाचरेत् ॥ २५
पर्शुकास्वथ भग्नासु घृताभ्यक्तस्य तिष्ठतः ।
दक्षिणास्वथ वा वामास्वनुमृज्य निबन्धनीः ॥
ततः कवलिका दत्त्वा वेष्टयेत् सुसमाहितः ।
तैलपूर्णे कटाहे वा द्रोण्यां वा शाययेन्नरम् ॥ २६
मुषलेनोत्क्षिपेत् कक्षामंससन्धौ विसंहते ।
स्थानस्थितञ्च वध्नीत स्वस्तिकेन विचक्षणः ॥ २७
कौर्परन्तु तथा सन्धिमङ्गुष्ठेनानुमार्ज्जयेत्।
कनुमृज्य ततः सन्धिं पीड़येत् कूर्पराश्रुतम् ।
प्रसार्य्याकुञ्चयेच्चैनं स्नेहसेकञ्च दापयेत् ॥ २८

Rhinoplasty : The portion of the nose to be covered over, is to be measured (exactly) with a

---

एवं जानुनि गुल्फे च मणिबन्धे च कारयेत् ॥ २९
उभे तले समे कृत्वा तलभग्नस्य देहिनः ।
बध्वा यादामतैलेन परिषेकश्च कारयेत् ॥
प्राग्गोमयमयं पिण्डं धारयेन्मृन्मयं ततः ।
हस्ते जालबले चापि कुर्य्यात् पाषाणधारणम् ॥ ३०
सन्नमुन्नमयेत् श्लिन्नमचकं मुषलेन तु ।
तथोन्नतं पीड़येच्च बध्नीयाद्गाढ़मेव च ॥ ३१
ऊरुवच्चापि कर्त्तव्यं बाहुभग्नचिकित्सितम् ॥ ३२
ग्रीवायान्तु विवृत्तायां प्रविष्टायामधोऽपि च ।
अवटावथ हन्वोश्च प्रगृह्योन्नमयेन्नरम् ।
तथा कुशान् समं दत्त्वा वस्त्रपट्टेन वेष्टयेत् ।
उत्तानं शाययेच्चैनं सप्तरात्रमतन्द्रितः ॥ ३३
हन्वस्थिनी समानीय हनुसन्धौ विसंहते ।
स्वेदयित्वा स्थिते सम्यक् पञ्चाङ्गीं वितरेद्भिषक् ॥
वातघ्नमधुरैः सर्पिः सिद्धं नस्ये च पूजितम् ॥ ३४
अभग्नांश्चलितान् दन्तान् सरक्तानवपीड़येत् ।
तरुणस्य मनुष्यस्य शीतैरालेपयेद्बहिः ॥
सिक्ताम्बुभिस्ततः शीतैः सन्धानीयैरुपाचरेत् ।
उत्पलस्य च नालेन क्षीरपानं विधीयते ॥
जीर्णस्य तु मनुष्यस्य वर्ज्जयेच्चलितान् द्विजान् ॥ ३५
नासां सग्नां विवृत्तां वा ऋज्वीं कृत्वा शलाकया ।
पृथङ्नासिकयोर्नाड्यौ द्विमुख्यौ संप्रवेशयेत् ।
ततः पट्टेन संवेष्ट्य घृतसेकं प्रदापयेत् ॥ ३६

leaf; and a flap of the required size is to be taken from the '*gaṇḍa*' (goitre or the cheek), to be grafted there, and to support it a metallic frame is to be inserted with two tubes in the nostrils to hold it in position, and then scraping the border (to which the grafting is to be joined),

---

भग्नं दार्व्यश्च बध्नीयात् समं कृत्वा घृतप्लुतम् ।
सद्यःक्षतविधानश्च ततः पश्चात् समाचरेत् ॥ ३७
मस्तुलुङ्गादिना भिन्ने कपाले मधुसर्पिषी ।
दत्त्वा ततो निबध्नीयात् सप्ताहञ्च पिबेद्घृतम् ॥ ३८
पतनादभिघाताद्वा शूनभङ्गं यदृच्छतम् ।
शीतान् प्रदेहान् सेकांश्च भिषक् तस्यावचारयेत् ॥ ३९
अथ जङ्घोरुभग्नानां कपाटशयनं हितम् ।
कीलका बन्धनार्थञ्च पञ्च कार्य्या विजानता ॥
यथा न चलनं तस्य भग्नस्य क्रियते तथा ।
सन्धेरुभयतो द्वौ द्वौ तले चैकश्च कीलकः ॥
श्रोण्या वा पृष्ठवंशे वा वक्षस्यक्षकयोस्तथा ।
भग्नसन्धिविमोक्षेषु विधिमेनं समाचरेत् ॥
सन्धींश्चिरविमुक्तांस्तु स्निग्धान् स्विन्नान् मृदूकृतान् ।
उक्तैर्विधानैर्बुद्ध्या च सम्यक् प्रकृतिमानयेत् ॥ ४०
काण्डभग्ने प्ररूढे तु विषमोल्बणसंहिते ।
आपोथ्य शमयेद्भग्नं ततो भग्नवदाचरेत ॥ ४१
कल्पयेन्निर्गतं शुष्कं व्रणान्तेऽस्थि समाहितः ।
सन्ध्यन्ते वा क्रियां कुर्य्यात् सव्रणे व्रणभग्नवत् ॥ ४२

सुश्रुतसंहिता, चिकित्सितस्थानम्, ३ ।

and making the surface fresh (to make the grafting successful), the flap is to be carefully sutured. When the grafting has been properly made, a powder made out of Ptercarpus santalinus, Glycyrrhiza glabra and sulphate of antimony should be sprinkled over the part, and then it should be covered with a lint, which is to be kept moistened with oleum Sesamum (until the complete grafting has taken place. The modern method of rhinoplasty is almost the same, except the two tubes inserted in the nostrils; to hold the metallic frame in position, the metallic frame is made to fit tight the scraped pocket in the nasal bone, and it is provided with a few nodules which are inserted into the nasal bony frame. As to the grafting, the English method consists in taking a flap from the cheek, as devised by Syme, who borrowed it from India; the Italian and the German methods consist of taking the flap from the arm; in osteoplastic rhinoplasty, there is a transplantation of a cartilaginous flap to replace the septum nasi. The very recent method in nasal prosthesis consists of subcutaneous injection of a mixture of solid and liquid paraffin, as introduced by Gersuny in 1910. But as it might partially melt in the body temperature, and thus emigrate and provoke embolism, it has been improved upon by Eckstein who uses pure paraffin, which melts only at 60 degree centigrade and solidifies after injection, which can be easily performed by Brockaert or Lermoyer's syringe. This has given very satisfactory results). *Suśruta* I. 16. 23[204].

---

204. नासाप्रमाणं पृथिवीरुहाणां पत्रं गृहीत्वा त्ववलम्बितस्य ॥
तेन प्रमाणेन हि गण्डपार्श्वादुत्कृत्य वद्धन्त्वथ नासिकाग्रम् ।
विलिख्य चाशु प्रतिसन्दधीत तत् साधुवन्धैर्भिषगप्रमत्तः ॥
सुसंहितं सम्यगथो यथावन्नाड़ीद्वयेनाभिसमीक्ष्य वद्धा ।
प्रोन्नम्य चैनामवचूर्णयेच्च पत्तङ्गयष्ठीमधुकाञ्जनैश्च ॥
संछाद्य सम्यक् पिचुना सितेन तैलेन सिञ्चेदसकृत् तिलानाम् ।
सुश्रुतसंहिता, सूत्रस्थानम, १६ ।

VIII—DIETETICS.

"It is apparent that food and drink act as fuel, in the process of metabolism. Vital process is sustained when metabolism is fed by this fuel. Proper dietary nourishes all the bodily elements, improves complexion and enlivens the senses. On the other hand improper dietary provokes disease." *Charaka* I. 27. 2[205].

"Vigor, health, longevity and life itself is based on oxidation. Food and drink increase and balance the oxidizing process." *Charaka* I. 27. 165[206].

"The physician that does not know the principles of '*Dietetics*', can not cure diseases." *Suśruta* I. 46. 3[207].

---

205. प्रत्यक्षफलदर्शनात् तदिन्धनात् ह्यन्तरग्नेः स्थितिः। तत् सत्त्वमूर्ज्जयति, तच्छरीरधात्वव्यूहबलवर्णेन्द्रियप्रसादकरम् यथोक्तमुपसेव्यमानं। विपरीतमहिताय सम्पद्यते।

चरक-संहिता, सूत्रस्थानम्, २७।

206. बलमारोग्यमायुश्च प्राणाश्चाग्नौ प्रतिष्ठिताः।
अन्नपानेन्धनैश्चाग्निर्दीप्यते शाम्यतेऽन्यथा॥

चरक-संहिता, सूत्रस्थानम्, २७।

207. नह्यजनवबुद्धस्वभावा भिषजः स्वस्थानुवृत्तिं रोगनिग्रहणञ्च कर्त्तुं समर्थाः॥३

सुश्रुत-संहिता, सूत्रस्थानम्, ४६

"Every organic body contains five substances as (1) Minerals and Nitrogenous compounds (*pṛthivī*), (2) Water (*ap*), (3) Hydro-carbons (*tejas*), (4) Carbo-hydrates (*vāyu*) and (5) Ethers (*ākāśa*) ; but it may be called '*pārthiva, āpya, taijasa, vāyavya* or *ākāśīya* according to the predominance of the substance contained in it.

Minerals and Nitrogenous Compounds (*protein*) : The substance that is gross (*sthūla*), dense (*sāra*), has a high specific gravity (*sāndra*), non-pungent (*manda*), inert (*sthira*), rough (*khara*= sharp-edged crystals by the different inclination of their axes), heavy (*guru*), hard (*kaṭhina*), odoriferous (*gandhavahula*=extractive substances of the meat-protein),slightly astringent (*iṣat kaṣāya*) and sweetish (*madhura*), is '*pārthiva*' (organic mineral bodies, and protein which contains about 16 p.c. of nitrogen). This produces firmness (of the bony structure by the minerals), physical vigor (by protein), hardness (of the bony structure by the minerals) muscular tissue-growth (by protein), and particularly it has a high specific gravity.

Aquatic substance : The substance that is cool (*śīta*), moistening (*stimita*), soft (*snigdha*), liquid (*manda*), heavy (*guru*), fluidic (*sara*), dense (*sāndra*), smooth (*mṛdu*),viscous (*pichchhila*), savory (*rasa-vahula*), slightly astringent, acid or saline (*kaṣāya-amlalavaṇa*) and sweetish (*madhura*), is *āpya*' (juice of vegetable or meat). It is fattening, refreshing, moistening, adhesive (by nature), and excretory (diuretic or sudorific in action).

Hydrocarbons : The substance that is calorific (*uṣṇa*), penetrative (*tīkṣṇa*), fine-textured (*sūkṣma*), desiccant (*rukṣa*), escharotic (*khara*), light (*laghu*, in molecular weight), transparent (*viśada*, particularly liquid oil, having forms and containing active principles (*rūpaguṇavahula*), slightly acid and saline (*īṣad amla-lavaṇa*) and pungent (*kaṭu-rasa*), is '*tejasa*' (hydrocarbon, that is fatty bodies which generate heat. It is very likely that the pungent spices were also regarded calorific, as the congestive phenomenon with its concomittant redness, heat and the burning sensation, provoked by its excessive uses, was mistaken for calorific energy). It causes combustion (oxidation), digestion, cleavage (of the food particles in the alimentary tube), heat, radiation (of heat), round face (corpulency) and bright complexion.

Carbohydrates : The substance that is fine, desiccant, rough (in tactile sensation, by different inclinations of the axes as in sugar crystals), crystalline, tactile, slightly bitter (?), and astringent, is *'vāyavya'* (energy-producers, that is carbohydrates). It causes corpulence, agility (muscular energy), relaxation, desiccation (by external application), and motion (as manifestation of muscular energy).

Ethers : The substance that is tenuous, rarefied, non-resistant (when a body passes through it), diffusive (a solid body has both size and shape ; a liquid body takes the shape of the vessel in which it is kept : therefore it lacks shape, but quantitatively it does not lack size : but a gaseous body has neither size nor shape, as it diffuses itself in the surrounding atmosphere, if it be not confined in a closed container), transparent, made of diffused particles, tasteless, and soniferous, is *'ākāśīya'* (ethers, volatile oils and gas). It causes pliancy, distension and lightness." *Suśruta* I. 41.2-7[208].

---

208. तत्र पृथिव्यप्तेजोवाय्वाकाशानां समुदायाद् द्रव्याभिनिर्वृत्तिरुत्कर्षस्त्वभिव्यञ्जको भवतीदं पार्थिवमिदमाप्यमिदं तैजसमिदं वायव्यमिदमाकाशीयमिति ॥ २

तत्र स्थूलसारसान्द्रमन्दस्थिरखरगुरुकठिनं गन्धबहुलमीषत्कषायं प्रायशो मधुरमिति पार्थिवम्। तत् स्थैर्य्यबलसंघातोपचयकरं विशेषतश्चाधोगतिस्वभावमिति ॥ ३

शीत-स्तिमित - स्निग्ध - मन्द - गुरुसरसान्द्रमृदुपिच्छिलरसबहुलमीषत्कषायाम्ललवणं मधुररसप्रायमाप्यम्। तत् स्नेहनप्रह्लादनक्लेदनबन्धनविष्यन्दनकरमिति ॥ ४

उष्ण-तीक्ष्ण-सूक्ष्मरूक्षखरलघुविशदं रूपगुणबहुलमीषदम्ललवणं कटुकरसप्रायं विशे-

I.—Carbohydrates.

Rice : "The autumnal rice (Oryza sativa) is sweetish, produces energy without (much) heat (a gram of carbohydrate or protein produces 4. 1 Calories, while a gram of fat liberates 9. 3 Calories), easily digestible, strengthening (dynamogenesis is due to glycogen, which can be most economically produced in the human system by the carbohydrate portion of the diet, and for glycogenesis, carbohydrate in one form or another is the staple indispensable food of almost all the human beings, except a few Eskimoes who mostly live on seal-meat and fat, and the primitive Indians of Tierra del Fuego who mainly subsist on shell fish and hunting), sedative, causes slight flatulence (in case of fermentation), fattening (excess of glycogen, produced by the habitual consumption of

---

यतश्चोर्ध्वगतिस्वभावमिति तैजसम् । तद्दहनपचनदारणतापनप्रकाशनप्रभावर्णकरमिति ॥ ५

सूक्ष्मरूक्षखरशिशिरलघुविशदं स्पर्शबहुलमीषत्तिक्तं विशेषतः कषायमिति वायवीयम् । तद्वैशद्यलाघवग्लपनविरूक्षणविचारणकरमिति ॥ ६

श्लक्ष्णसूक्ष्ममृदुव्यवायिविशदविविक्तमव्यक्तरसं शब्दबहुलमाकाशीयम् । तन्मार्दवशौषिर्यलाघवकरमिति ॥ ७

सुश्रुत-संहिता, सूत्रस्थानम्, ४१ ।

carbohydrate more than the bodily requirement, is at first deposited in the hepatic and the muscle cells; but if it be not used, it is converted into adipose tissues, as a stored energy in case of future needs), is constipative, and leaves very little residue (rice is poor in cellulose; husked rice contains about 12. 0 water, 7. 12 protein, 1. 0 fat, 76. 8 carbohydrates, 1. 0 cellulose and 1. 0 p. c. minerals)." *Suśruta* I. 46. 6 [209].

"*Barley*: Barley (Hordeum distichon) is astringent-sweetish, produces energy without much heat generation, acidifying (by fermentation), removes '*kapha* and *pitta*', acts as vulnerary like the sesame (oil) and in abscesses (by external application), a daily food, diminishes urinary secretion (oliguria), produces flatulence (in fermentation), laxative having a large residue (3. 8 cellulose), promotes longevity, enhances metabolism, improves memory, voice and complexion, viscous (when barley powder is dissolved or cooked in water), reduces corpulency, adiposis (by increased metabolism),

---

209. मधुरा वीर्यतः शीता लघुपाका बलावहाः ।
पित्तघ्नाल्पानिलकफा स्निग्धा बद्धाल्पवर्चसः ॥ ६

सुश्रुत-संहिता, सूत्रस्थानम्, ४६ ।

refrigerent (when drunk internally as a decoction), desiccant (by external application) and is a purifier of blood and of bilious secretion (barley contains about 12. 3 p. c. water, 10. 1 protein, 1. 9 fat, 3. 8 cellulose, 2. 4 mineral matter)." *Suśruta* I. 46. 40[210].

Wheat : Wheat (Triticum sativum) is sweetish, heavy to digest (when not properly cooked), energizing, promotes vigor, aphrodisiac, appetizing, fattening, produces energy without much heat generation, sedative, vulnerary in fractures, diuretic and laxative (wheat contains about 12. 0 p. c. water, 11. 0 protein, 1. 7 fat, 71. 2 carbohydrates, 2. 2 cellulose and 1. 9 mineral matter.)" *Suśruta* I. 46. 42[211].

---

210. यवः कषायो मधुरो हिमश्च
कटर्विपाकि कफपित्तहारी ।
व्रणेषु पथ्यस्तिलवच्च नित्यं
प्रबद्धमूत्रो बहुवातवर्चाः ॥
स्थैर्य्याग्निमेधास्वरवर्णकृच्च
स पिच्छिलः स्थूलविलेखनश्च
मेदोमरुत्तृड्हरणोऽतिरूक्षः
प्रसादनः शोणितपित्तयोश्च ॥ ४०
सुश्रुत-संहिता, सूत्रस्थानम, ४६ ।

211. गोधूम उक्तो मधुरो गुरुश्च
बल्यः स्थिरः शुक्ररुचिप्रदश्च ।

II.—*Legumes.*

Legumes: "Phaseolus mungo (*mudga*), Phaseolus lobatus (*vana-mudga*), Pisum sativum (*kalāya*), Phaseolus aconotifolius (*makuṣṭa*), Ervum lens (*masūra*), Cicer lens (*maṅgalya*), Cicer arietinum (*chaṇaka*), Pisum arvense (*satïna*), Convolvolus turpethum album (*tripuṭa*), Lathyrus sylvestris (*hareṇu*), Cajan cajan (*udakï*). etc. are the legumes.. They are astringent-sweetish, energizing without production of heat, acidifying (in fermentation), productive of flatulence, constipation and oliguria (Legumes hold an intermediate place between carbohydrates and proteids, having nearly 18 to 25 p. c. of vegetable protein-legumin, (soy bean of Soia soja has about 32. 9 p. c. of protein, 18. 1 of fat, 28. 7 of carbohydrates, 4. 9 of minerals), half to one and half per cent of fat, 50 to 60 p. c. of carbohydrates. But unfortunately much of this rich food contents can not be absorbed, as they are confined in the cellulose, and the human stomach lacks sufficient enzymic potency to

---

स्निग्धोऽतिशीतोऽनिलपित्तहन्ता
सन्धानकृत् श्लेषकरः सरश्च ॥ ४२

सुश्रुत-संहिता, सूत्रस्थानम ; ४६ ।

burst open the cellulose shell. However, if it be taken in the pure form, enough of it can be assimilated to make it a valuable addition to the dietary)." *Suśruta* I. 46. 25-26[212].

III.—*Proteids.*

Meat : Meat can be had from six classes of animals —(1) Aquatic (*jaleśaya*), (2) Marshy (*ānūpa*), (3) Domesticated (*grāmya*). (4) Carnivorous (*kravyāda*), (5) Perissodactyla (*ekaśapha*, distinguished from arisodactyla), and (6) Wild (*jāṅgala*). (Meat supplies the protein needs of the organism, which is about from half to one gram for each kilo body weight per diem, in the most assimilable, tonic and appetizing manner)." *Suśruta* I. 46. 53[213].

Domesticated Animals : "The meat of domesticated animals, relieve flatulence, is nourishing, produces '*kapha* and *pitta*', is sweetish in taste, non acidifying in reaction, enhances metabolism and is stimulating.

212. मुद्गवनमुद्ग कलायमकुष्ठ - मसूरमङ्गल्यचणकसतीनत्रिपुटहरेणवाढकीप्रभृतयो वैदलाः ॥ २५

कषायमधुराः शीताः कटुपाका मरुत्कराः ।
बद्धमूत्रपुरीषाश्च पित्तश्लेष्महरास्तथा ॥ २६

सुश्रुत-संहिता, सूत्रस्थानम्, ४६ ।

213. जलेशया आनूपा ग्राम्याः क्रव्यभुज एकशफा जाङ्गलाश्चेति षण्मांसवर्गाः ।

सुश्रुत-संहिता, सूत्रस्थानम्, ४६ ।

Goat : Goat-meat is oxidized without the generation of excessive heat, is heavy (if old, tough or fatty), fattening, moderates '*pitta* and *kapha*', cures constipation and catarrh (goat's meat is not liked by some for its peculiar odor due to '*hircine*', otherwise if the animal is young and the meat is not fatty, it is easily digestible).

Mutton : Mutton is nourishing, produces '*pitta* and *śleṣma*'. is hard to digest (especially if it be of tough fiber or fatty, as the mutton fat has a very high melting point).

Mutton : The mutton of the broad-tailed sheep (*medaḥ-puchchha*) is a muscle-builder, and in other characteristics, it resembles the (ordinary) mutton.

Beef : The beef cures tuberculosis, respiratory diseases, catarrh, and typhoid ; it is very beneficial to the hard-workers and for those who have good digestion ; it is purifying and relieves flatulence." *Suśruta* I. 46. 45-89 [214].

---

214. ग्राम्या वातहरा: सर्व्वे वृंहणा: कफपित्तला: ।
मधुरा रसपाकाभ्यां दीपना बलवर्द्धना: ॥ ८५
नातिशीतो गुरु: स्निग्धो मन्दपित्तकफ: स्मृत: ।
छगलस्त्वनभिष्यन्दी तेषां पीनसनाशन: ॥ ८६
वृंहणं मांसमौरभ्रं पित्तश्लेष्मावहं गुरु ॥ ८७
मेद:पुच्छोद्भवं वृष्यमौरभ्रसदृशं गुणै: ॥ ८८

Venison : The venison is astringent-sweetish, easily digestible, relieves flatulence and biliousness, oxidizes with rapid heat production, is a cardiac stimulant, and relieves vesical troubles." *Suśruta* I. 46. 53[215].

Boar's meat : "Boar's (Sus scrofa) meat is sudorific, nourishing, muscle-builder, refrigerant (reflex reaction of perspiration), appetizing, hard to digest (especially fatty and coarse meat) fattening, relieves fatigue, flatulence, and is strengthening." *Suśruta* I. 46. 102[216].

"The meat of boar and pig is fattening, stimulating, tissue-builder, tonic (removes lassitude), carminative, strengthening, appetizing, sudorific and heavy " 2. 27. 32 [216a].

Fowls : "Partridge (perdix chinensis) is

श्वासकासप्रतिश्याय-विषमज्वरनाशनम् ।
अत्यग्निहितं गव्यं पवित्रमनिलापहम् ॥ ८९

सुश्रुत-संहिता, सूत्रस्थानम्, ४६ ।

215. मृगाः कषाया मधुरा लघवो वातपित्तहरास्तीक्ष्णा हृद्या वस्तिशोधनाश्च ॥ ५३ सुश्रुतसंहिता, सूत्रस्थानम्, ४६ ।

216. स्वेदनं बृंहणं वृष्यं शीतलं तर्पणं गुरु ।
स्निग्धं श्रमानिलहरं वाराहं बलवर्द्धनम् ॥ १०२

सुश्रुतसंहिता, सूत्रस्थानम्, ४६ ।

216.(a) स्नेहनं बृंहणं वृष्यं श्रमघ्नमनिलापहम् ।
वराहपिशितं बल्यं रोचनं स्वेदनं गुरु ॥

चरक-संहिता, सूत्रस्थानम्, २७ ।

restorative, enhances metabolism, astringent-sweetish, is oxidized with pungency, and is a good diet (during convalescence) in acute complicated cases." *Suśruta* I. 46-59[217].

"Snow-partridge (Tetraogallus himalayaensis) is slightly heavy, is oxidized with excessive heat production, sweetish, is a muscle-builder, improves memory (by accelerated circulation) and enhances metabolism, tonicises the entire system, is laxative and improves the complexion. Particularly its white variety cures hiccup, respiratory lesion and flatulence." *Suśruta* I. 46. 60[218].

"Chicken is fattening, is oxidized with excessive production of heat, relieves flatulence, builds muscles, improves voice, is strengthening and stimulating; the domesticated chicken is heavier than its wild variety, and is beneficial in (fermentative) flatulence, consumption, (acid)

---

217. संग्राही दीपनश्चैव कषायमधुरो लघुः ।
लावः कटुविपाकश्च सन्निपाते च पूजितः ॥ ५९

सूश्रुतसंहिता, सूत्रस्थानम्, ४६ ।

218. ईषद्गुरूष्णमधुरो वृष्यो मेधाग्निवर्द्धनः ।
तित्तिरिः सर्व्वदोषघ्नो ग्राही वर्ण्णप्रसादनः ॥
हिक्काश्वासानिलहरो विशेषाद्गौरतित्तिरिः ।

सुश्रुतसंहिता, सूत्रस्थानम्, ४६ ।

vomitings, and (chronic malarial) intermittent fever." *Suśruta* I. 46.63[219].

"Pigeons etc. are astringent-sweetish, desiccant, frugivorous, provoke flatulenee, *pitta* and *śleṣma*, are oxidized without much heat, produce oliguria and leave a very scanty residue. Of them, *bhedāśī* causes all kinds of disturbances and intestinal decomposition. The wild pigeon is astringent sweetish-saline (in taste) and is heavy. The domesticated pigeon is beneficial in gastrorrhagia, is astringent, stimulating, non-acidifying in reaction, and is heavy. The wild sparrow is sweetish, fattening, increases '*kapha*' and is aphrodisiac. The garden sparrow is beneficial in gastrorrhagia, and is a strong aphrodisiac." *Suśruta* I. 46. 65-69[220].

---

219. स्निग्धोष्णोऽनिलहा वृष्यः स्वेदस्वरबलावहः ।
बृंहणः कुक्कुटो वन्यस्तद्वद्ग्राम्यो गुरुस्तु सः ।
वातरोगक्षयवमी-विषमज्वरनाशनः ॥ ६३
सुश्रुत-संहिता, सूत्रस्थानम्, ४६ ।

220. कषायमधुरा रूक्षाः फलाहारा मरुत्कराः ।
पित्तश्लेष्महराः शीता बद्धमूत्राल्पवर्च्चसः ६५
सर्व्वदोषकरस्तेषां भेदाशी मलदूषकः ॥ ६६
कषायस्वादुलवणो गुरुः काणकपोतकः ॥ ६७
रक्तपित्तप्रशमनः कषायो विशदोऽपि च ।
विपाके मधुरश्चापि गुरुः पारावतः स्मृतः ॥ ६८

"Goose, crane, heron, ruddy goose, osprey, teal, duck, pheasant, a variety of crane (Ardea nivea), small crane, duck (Pelicanus fusicallus), heron, drake, bar-headed goose (Anser indicus), Chinese goose (Cygnopsis cygnoides), Turdus ginginianus, Corvus aquaticus, 4 members of the Antidæ family, water cock, Cocculus melanoleucus and the wild goose are called *'plava'* (aquatic floating birds) and they are gregarious. They are beneficial in gastrorrhagia, are oxidized without the production af excessive heat, fattening, muscle-builder, relieve flatulence, laxative and diuretic, sweetish, and non-acidifying in reaction. But of them the goose is hard to digest, is oxidised with the production of an excessive heat, sweetish, fattening, improves voice and complexion, strengthening, stimulating, aphrodisiac and carminative." *Suśruta* I. 46. 105-107[221].

Mollusca : Conch (Strombus gigas), mussel,

कुलिङ्गो मधुरः स्निग्धः कफशुक्रविवर्द्धनः ।
रक्तपित्तहरो वेश्म-कुलिङ्गस्त्वतिशुक्रलः ॥ ९९

सुश्रुत-संहिता, सूत्रस्थानम्,

221. हंससारसक्रौञ्चचक्रवाक-कुरर-कादम्ब-कारण्डव-जीवञ्जीवक-वक-वलाका-पुण्डरीकप्लवशरारीमुख-नन्दीमुख-मद्गूत्क्रोश-काचाक्ष-मल्लिकाक्ष-शुक्लाक्ष - पुष्करायिका-कोनालकाम्बुकुक्कुटिका-मेघराव-श्वेतचरण-प्रभृतयः प्लवाः संघातचारिणः ॥ १०५

oyster, snail (Helix pomatia), and large-shelled snail or cockle are called '*kośastha*' (mollusca).

Amphibia : Turtle, crocodile, red crab (cancer pagurus), shore crab (carcinus moenus), and porpoise (Delphinus gangeticum) are called '*pādī*' (footed).

They are sweetish, non-acidifying in reaction, carminative, are oxidized without the production of much heat, fattening, sedative, laxative and increases *kapha*." ***Suśruta*** **I. 46.108-110**[222].

Fish : "Fishes are of two kinds—fresh-water and marine. "***Suśruta*** **I.46.112**[223].

"Fresh-water fishes are sweetish, heavy,

रक्तपित्तहराः शीताः स्निग्धा वृष्या मरुज्जितः ।
सृष्टमूत्रपुरीषाश्च मधुरा रसपाकयोः ॥ १०६
गुरूष्णमधुरः स्निग्धः स्वरवर्ण बलप्रदः ।
वृंहणः शुक्रलस्तेषां हंसो वातविकारनुत् ॥ १०७

सुश्रुतसंहिता, सूत्रस्थानम्, ४६ ।

222. शङ्खशङ्खनखशुक्तिशम्बूकभल्लूकप्रभृतयः कोशस्थाः ॥ १०८
कूर्म्मकुम्भीरकर्कटककृष्णकर्कटकशिशुमारप्रभृतयः पादिनः ॥ १०९
शङ्खकूर्म्मादयः स्वादु-रसपाका-मरुन्नुदः ।
शीताः स्निग्धा हिताः पित्ते वर्चस्याः श्लेष्मवर्द्धनाः ॥ ११०

सुश्रुत-संहिता, सूत्रस्थानम्, ४६ ।

223. मत्स्यास्तु द्विविधा नादेयाः सामुद्राश्च ।

सुश्रुत-संहिता, सूत्रस्थानम्, ४६ ।

carminative, hemorrhagic, are oxidized with production of excessive heat, aphrodisiac, fattening, and leave little residue. "*Suśruta* I.46. 113[224].

"Sea-fishes are heavy, fattening, sweetish, do not increase '*pitta*' excessively, are oxidized with an excessive production of heat, carminative, muscle-builder, and increase '*śleṣma*'." *Suśruta* I. 46.120[225].

Milk : "There are eight kinds of milk (available for general uses, viz. : cow's milk, goat's milk, camel's milk, sheep's milk, buffalo's milk, mare's milk, woman's milk and elephant's milk. As these animals eat various kinds of food-stuffs, and their milk is the essence of the product of their metabolism (during lactation), therefore the milk is vitalizing, heavy (?), sweet, viscid, refrigerant, fattening, emollient, laxative and demulcent ; so the milk is regarded as the vital fluid (product) of the animal.

224, नादेया मधुरा मत्स्या गुरवो मारुतापहाः ।
रक्तपित्तकराश्चोष्णा वृष्याः स्निग्धाल्पवर्चसः ॥ ११३

सुश्रुत-संहिता, सूत्रस्थानम, ४६ ।

225. सामुद्रा गुरवः स्निग्धा मधुरा नातिपित्तलाः ।
उष्णा वातहरा वृष्या वर्चस्याः श्लेष्मवर्द्धनाः ॥ १२०

सुश्रुत-संहिता, सूत्रस्थानम, ४६ ।

As milk is beneficial to the (young) animal (for growth and development), so all kinds of milk are good for the animal life. Only it is counter-indicated in the derangements of '*vāta, pitta, blood and mind*'. It is beneficial in chronic fever, bronchitis, dyspnea, consumption, tuberculosis, cancers, insanity, tymphanites, epilepsy, vertigo, intoxication, hyperæmia. polydipsia, cardiac troubles, vesical lesions, anemia, chronic dysentery, piles, colic, ascites, diarrhœa, leucorrhœa, diseases of the female genital apparatus (gonorrhea), abortion, gastrorrhagia, fatigue, and pleurisy. Milk is depurant, strengthening, muscle-builder, oxidizer, fattening, restorative, analeptic, delays senility, promotes longevity, vitalizing, stimulating, emetic, laxative, and having the same quality of the bone-marrow, it increases hematogenesis. It is a good diet for the children, the aged, wounded, emaciated, starved, or those exhausted by sexual excess.

Cow's milk : Cow's milk is non-salivant, fattening, heavy (?), oxidizer, beneficial in gastrorrhagia, refrigerant, sweetish, non-acidifying in reaction (?), vitalizing and very hypotensive.

Goat's milk : Goat's milk possesses the same

properties as cow's milk ; but it is specially beneficial in tuberculosis, is light, restorative and cures dyspnea, bronchitis and gastrorrhagia ; as the goats are of small size, feed upon pungent-bitter substances, drink little water and take constant exercise, their milk is good in all diseases.

Camel's milk : Camel's milk is desiccant (?), calorific, slightly saline, of pleasant taste, light, and is beneficial in inflammation, cancers, ascites, piles, intestinal worms, skin lesions and poisonings.

Ewe's milk : Ewe's milk is sweetish, fattening, heavy (fat : 6.18), and moderates '*kapha and pitta*' ; it is a good diet in rheumatism and hebetic cough.

Buffalo's milk : Buffalo's milk is salivant, sweetish, lowers metabolism (?), somnifacient and induces chills (as the buffalo abounds in marshy places, where the malaria is rampant, the symptoms-complex, especially the chills and the metabolic derangements of malaria have been mistakenly attributed to the buffalo's milk); the buffalo's milk contains more fat than the cow's milk, and is heavier.

Mare's milk : Mare's milk is strengthening, beneficial in the rheumatism of the extremities, of acidulated sweetish saline taste, desiccant and light.

Woman's milk : Woman's milk is sweetish, astringent, refrigerant, can be used for irrigation of the nose and the eye-lids, promotes health, is light and oxidizing.

Elephant's milk : Elephant's milk is sweetish, astringent, muscle-builder, heavy, fattening, increases vigor, is beneficial to the eyes and is strengthening.

The milk, milked in the morning, due to the cooling influence of the night, and lack of exercise of the animals, is heavy, constipative and refrigerant ; the evening milk, on the other hand, as the animals are warmed by the sun, exercise and respiration, relieves rheumatism and fatigue and is beneficial to the eyes.

Raw milk is salivant and heavy, but if it be boiled, it becomes lighter (milk if exposed, especially in a tropical country, becomes soon contaminated, and it is a good precaution to boil it before using it) ; but this does not apply to woman's milk, where it is beneficial when it is fresh. Milk becomes contaminated, if after milking, it be exposed to cool itself ; but if it be too much boiled, it becomes heavy, but retains its tissue-building property.

The milk that is foul-smelling, sourish, discolored, or of perverted taste, or if it be mixed with salt, or coagulated, should not be used. *Suśruta* I. 45. 44-57[226].

---

226. गव्यमाजं तथा चौष्ट्रमाविकं माहिषञ्च यत् ।
अश्वायाश्चैव नार्य्याश्च करेणूनाञ्च यत् पयः ॥
तत्त्वनेकौषधिरस-प्रसादं प्राणदं गुरु ।
मधुरं पिच्छिलं शीतं स्निग्धं श्लक्ष्णं सरं मृदु ॥
सर्व्वप्राणभृतां तस्मात् सात्म्यं क्षीरमिहोच्यते ॥ ४४

तत्र सर्व्वमेव क्षीरं प्राणिनामप्रतिषिद्धं जातिसात्म्यात्। वातपित्तशोणितमानसविकारेष्वविरुद्धम्। जीर्णज्वरकासश्वासशोषक्षयगुल्मोन्मादोदरमूर्च्छाभ्रममददाहपिपासाहृद्वस्तिपाण्डुरोगग्रहणीदोषार्शः - शूलोदावर्त्तातिसार -प्रवाहिकायोनिरोगगर्भास्रावरक्तपित्तश्रमक्लमहरं पाप्मापहं बल्यं वृष्यं वाजीकरणं रसायनं मेध्यं सन्धानमास्थापनं वयःस्थापनमायुष्यं जीवनं बृंहणं वमनं विरेचनञ्च तुल्यगुणत्वाच्चौजसो वर्द्धनमिति बालवृद्धक्षतक्षीणानां क्षुद्व्यवायव्यायामकर्शितानाञ्च पथ्यतमम् ॥ ४५

गोक्षीरमनभिष्यन्दि स्निग्धं गुरु रसायनम् ।
रक्तपित्तहरं शीतं मधुरं रसपाकयोः ॥
जीवनीयं तथा वात-पित्तघ्नं परमं स्मृतम् ॥ ४६
गव्यतुल्यगुणन्त्वाजं विशेषाच्छोषिणे हितम् ।
दीपनं लघु संग्राहि श्वासकासास्रपित्तनुत् ॥
अजानामल्पकायत्वात् कटुतिक्तनिषेवणात् ।
नात्यम्बुपानाद्व्यायामात् सर्व्वव्याधिहरं पयः ॥ ४७
रूक्षोष्णं लवणं किञ्चिदौष्ट्रं स्वादुरसं लघु ।
शोफगुल्मोदरार्शोघ्नं क्रिमिकुष्ठविषापहम् ॥ ४८
आविकं मधुरं स्निग्धं गुरु पित्तकफावहम् ।
पथ्यं केवलवातेषु कासे चानिलसम्भवे ॥ ४९

Sour-milk : "Sour milk of cow is fattening, sweet in reaction (lactic acid in reaction) oxidizer, carminative, depurant (anti-putrefactive), and appetizing," *Suśruta* I. 45. 61[227].

महाभिष्यन्दि मधुरं माहिषं वह्निनाशनम् ।
निद्राकरं शीतकरं गव्यात् स्निग्धतरं गुरु ॥ ५०
उष्ट्राश्च कशफं वल्यं शाखावातहरं पयः ।
मधुराम्लरसं रूक्षं लवणानुरसं लघु ॥ ५१
नार्य्यास्तु मधुरं स्तन्यं कषायानुरसं हिमम् ।
नस्याश्च्योतनयोः पथ्यं जीवनं लघु दीपनम ॥ ५२
हस्तिन्या मधुरं वृष्यं कषायानुरसं गुरु ।
स्निग्धं स्थैर्य्यकरं शीतं चक्षुष्यं बलवर्द्धनम् ॥ ५३
प्रायः प्राभातिकं क्षीरं गुरु विष्टम्भि शीतलम् ।
रात्रौ सोमगुणत्वाच्च व्यायामाभावतस्तथा ।
दिवाकराभितप्तानां व्यायामानिलसेवनात् ।
वातानुलोमि श्रान्तिघ्नं चक्षुष्यञ्चापराह्णिकम् ॥ ५४
पयोऽभिष्यन्दि गुर्व्वामं प्रायशः परिकीर्त्तितम् ।
तदेवोक्तं लघुतरमनभिष्यन्दि वै शृतम् ।
वर्ज्जयित्वा स्त्रियाः स्तन्यमाममेव हि तद्धितम् ॥ ५५
धारोष्णं गुणवत् क्षीरं विपरीतमतोऽन्यथा ।
तदेवातिशृतं सर्व्वं गुरु वृंहणमुच्यते ॥ ५६
अनिष्टगन्धमम्लञ्च विवर्णं विरसञ्च यत् ।
वर्ज्यं सलवणं क्षीरं यच्च विग्रथितं भवेत् ॥ ५७
सुश्रुत-संहिता, सूत्रस्थानम्, ४५ ।

227. स्निग्धं विपाके मधुरं दीपनं बलवर्द्धनम् ।
वातापहं पवित्रञ्च दधि गव्यं रुचिप्रदम् ॥ ६१
सुश्रुत-संहिता, सूत्रस्थानम्, ४५

Whey : "Whey is acidulated sweetish astringent, is oxidized rapidly, light, pungent, oxidizer, antitoxic, is beneficial in (intestinal) inflammation, diarrhœa, chronic dysentery, piles, splenitis, tumors, intermittent fever, polydipsia, vomiting, stomatitis, colic, adiposis, catarrh and flatulence ; it is non-acidifying in reaction (?), cardiac stimulant, beneficial in strangury, adipositis, and is not a tissue builder. *Suśruta* I. 45. 77[228].

III.—*Fats.*

Butter : "Fresh-churned butter is energizing, calorific (*dïpana*) and cardiac stimulant, and is benefical in chronic dysentery, piles, trismus and anorexia." *Charaka* I. 27. 100[229].

Oil ; Sesame oil is slightly astringent, of pleasant taste, minute (of minute fat globules), calorific, diffusive, increases *'pitta'* (*pitta* is regarded as the humor and the seat of com-

---

228. तक्रं मधुरमम्लं कषायानुरसमुष्णवीर्य्यं लघु रूक्षमग्निदीपनं गरशोफाती-सार-ग्रहणी-पाण्डुरोगार्शः-प्लीह-गुल्मारोचक-विषमज्वर-तृष्णाच्छर्दि प्रसेकशूलमेदःश्लेष्मानिलहरं मधुरविपाकं हृद्यं मूत्रकृच्छ्रस्नेहव्यापत्प्रशमनमवृष्यञ्च ॥ ७७

सुश्रुत-संहिता, सूत्रस्थानम्, ४५ ।

229. संग्राहि दीपनं हृद्यं नवनीतं नवोद्धृतम् ।
ग्रहण्यर्शोविकारघ्नमर्द्दितारुचिनाशनम् ॥

चरक-संहिता, सूत्रस्थानम्, २७ ।

bustion energy and heat-metabolism), is laxative and diuretic. It does not increase phlegma, but is the best carminative ; it is energizing, beneficial to the skin, increases fat (*medas*) and heat (*agnivarddhna*)." *Charaka* I. 27. 137[230].

IV.—*Vegetables.*

Vegetables : "The cucumber, (Cucumis sativus), field-cucumber (Cucumis utilissimus), gourd (Benincasa cerifera), water-melon etc. are indigestible, retards digestion (of other foods), refrigerant, savorous, phlegmatic, laxative, diuretic, contain potash and are sweetish.." *Suśruta* I. 46. 227[231].

"The lotus root, the lotus, esculent root of the lotus, fibers of the stalk of the lotus, root of Scripus kysoor, Trapa bisponosa and water weeds are indigestible, arrest digestion and are

---

230. कषायानुरसं स्वादु सूक्ष्ममुष्णं व्यवायि च ।
पित्तलं बद्धविन्मूत्रं न च श्लेष्माभिवर्द्धनम् ॥
वातघ्नेषूत्तमं वल्यं त्वच्यं मेधाग्निवर्द्धनम् ।
चरक-संहिता, सूत्रस्थानम्, २७

231. त्रपुसैर्व्वारुककर्कारुकशीर्षहन्तप्रभृतीनि ॥ २२६
गुरुविष्टम्भिशीतानि स्वादूनि कफकन्ति च ।
सृष्टमूत्रपुरीषाणि सक्षारमधुराणि च ॥ २२७
सुश्रुत-संहिता, सूत्रस्थानम्, ४६ ।

refrigerant ; the stalk, flower and fruit of white and blue water-lilies (Nymphæa esculenta and Nymphæa stellata) are savorous, astringent, refrigerant, and provoke *'phlegma'* and flatulence. *Charaka* I. 27. 54[232].

Fruits : "*Pomegranate* is astringnt, non-calorific, oxidizer, appetizing, refreshing and constipative. *Suśruta* I. 46. 144[233].

"*Prune* provokes excessive flatulence, is laxative and reduces *'kapha and pitta'*." *Suśruta* I. 46. 169[234].

"*Fig* retards digestion, is sweet, fattening, refreshing and indigestible." *Suśruta* I. 46. 134[235].

"*Cocoa-nut* is indigestible, fattening, moderates *'pitta'*, sweetish, refrigerant, energizing, refresh-

---

232. तरुठविसशालूकक्रौञ्चादनकशेरुकम् ॥
शृङ्गाटकमङ्कलोड्यञ्च गुरुविष्टम्भिशीतलम् ।
कुमुदोत्पलनालास्तु सपुष्पाः सफलाः स्मृताः ।
शीताः स्वादुकषायास्तु कफमारुतकोपनाः ॥
चरक-संहिता, सूत्रस्थानम्, २७ ।

233. कषायानुरसं तेषां दाड़िमं नातिपित्तलम ।
दीपनीयं रुचिकरं हृद्यं वर्च्चोविवन्धनम् ॥
सुश्रुत-संहिता, सूत्रस्थानम्, ४६ ।

234. अत्यर्थं वातलं ग्राहि जाम्बवं कफपित्तजित् ॥ १६९
सुश्रुतसंहिता, सूत्रस्थानम्, ४६ ।

235. विष्टम्भि मधुरं स्निग्धं फल्गुजं तर्पणं गुरु ॥ १७६
सुश्रुत-संहिता, सूत्रस्थानम्, ४६ ।

ing, stimulating and diuretic." *Suśruta* I. 46. 184[236].

Grape is laxative, improves voice, sweet, fattening, refrigerant, and relieves gastrorrhagia, febricula, dyspnea, polydipsia, hyperemia and emaciation." *Suśruta* I. 27. 146[237].

V.—*Stimulants.*

Salt is appetizing, digestive, laxative and carminative." *Charaka* I. 27. 146[238].

Spices : "Foeniculum Nigella indica, Ptychotis ajowan, Cumminum cyminum, Coriandrum sativum and the leaf of Piper longum are digestive, oxidizing, carminative, antitoxic (relieves '*kapha*') and is deodorant." *Charaka* I. 27. 148[239].

---

236. नारिकेलं गुरु स्निग्धं पित्तघ्नं स्वादु शीतलम् ।
वलमांसप्रदं हृद्यं वृंहणं वस्तिशोधनम् ॥ १८४
सुश्रुत-संहिता, सूत्रस्थानम्, ४६ ।

237. तेषां द्राक्षा सरा स्वर्य्या मधुरा स्निग्धशीतला ।
रक्तपित्तज्वरश्वास-तृष्णादाहक्षयापहा ॥ १८८
सुश्रुत-संहिता, सूत्रस्थानम्, ४६ ।

238 रोचनं लवणं सर्व्वं पाकि संस्यनिलापहम् ॥
चरक-संहिता, सूत्रस्थानम्, २७ ।

239. कारव्य: कुञ्चिकाजाजी कवरी धान्यतुम्बुरु ।
रोचनं दीपनं वातकफदौर्गन्ध्यनाशनम् ॥
चरक-संहिता, सूत्रस्थानम्, २७ ।

Liquors : "All acidulated wines cause biliousness, increase digestive power, are appetizing, emetic, desiccant, carminative, cardiac stimulant, vesical disinfectant (?), easily oxidized, irritant, are oxidized with liberation of excessive heat, pungent, excitant of the senses, exhilarant, laxative and diuretic." *Suśruta* I. 45. 155 [240].

"*New Wine* is salivant, heavy, provokes flatulence, has disagreeable flavor, non-savorous, non-refreshing and irritant.

Old Wine has fine aroma, stimulates digestion, is refreshing, appetizing, anthelmintic (or bactericidal), depurant (?), quickly oxidized, desiccant and carminative." *Suśruta* I. 45. 179-180[241].

---

240. सर्व्वं पित्तकरं मद्यमम्लं दीपनरोचनम् ।
भेदनं कफवातघ्नं हृद्यं वस्तिविशोधनम् ॥
पाके लघु विदाह्युष्णं तीक्ष्णमिन्द्रियबोधनम् ।
विकासि सृष्टविण्मूत्रं श्रृणु तस्य विशेषणम् ॥ १५५

सुस्रुत-संहिता, सूत्रस्थानम्, ४५

241. नवं मद्यमभिष्यन्दि गुरु वातादिकोपनम् ।
अनिष्टगन्धि विरसमहृद्यञ्च विदाहि च ॥ १७९
सुगन्धि दीपनं हृद्यं रोचिष्णु क्रिमिनाशनम् ।
स्फुटस्रोतस्करं जीर्णं लघु वातकफापहम् ॥ १८०

सुश्रुत-संहिता, सूत्रस्थानम्, ४५ ।

"The wine that is opaque, irritant, malodorous, insipid, with yeast fermentation, heavy, non-enlivening, new, sharp (with a high percentage of alcohol), oxidized with a great amount of heat, which has been kept in a foul vessel, which has been made with insufficient materials, which has been kept exposed in an open bowl over night, colorless, should not be taken, as well as the wine left over from another person." *Suśruta* I. 45. 185[242].

"Wine is prescribed in emaciation, strangury, chronic dysentery, or for the person who has lost blood ; it is a carminative and a galactagogue. It is beneficial in hiccup, dyspnea, catarrh, bronchitis, constipation, anorexia, vomiting, tympanites, fecal impaction, and flatulence. "*Suśruta* I. 27. 93[243].

---

242. सान्द्रं विदाहि दुर्गन्धं विरसं क्रिमिलं गुरु ।
अहृद्यं तरुणं तीक्ष्णमुष्णं दुर्भाजनस्थितम् ॥
अल्पौषधं पर्य्युषितमत्यच्छं पिच्छिलञ्च यत् ।
तद्वर्ज्यं सर्व्वदा मद्यं किञ्चिच्छेषन्तु यद्भवेत् ॥ १८५
सुश्रुत-संहिता, सूत्रस्थानम्, ४५ ।

243. कृशानां सक्तमूत्राणां ग्रहण्यर्शोविकारिणाम् ।
सुरा प्रशस्ता वातघ्नी स्तन्यरक्तक्षयेषु च ॥
हिक्काश्वासप्रतिश्यायकासवर्च्चोग्रहारुचौ ।
वम्यानाहविबन्धेषु वातघ्नी मदिरा हिता ॥
चरक-संहिता, सूत्रस्थानम्, २७।

VI.- Water.

"The water falling from the clouds is tasteless (without any distinct taste), vitalizing (acts as an ambrosia), beneficial to life, refreshing, sustaining, circulatory (entering into every tissue metabolism), and removes lassitude, fatigue, thirst, intoxication, vertigo, somnolence, sleep and hyperemia.

The water-vapor of the sky falling upon the earth takes the taste of the place where it falls, and the water of the river, rivulet, lake, pond, dam, well, pool, fountain, vegetable sap, subterranean stream, field inundation, and pond in a swampy region covered with algae and filled with water-weeds, is sweetish." *Suśruta* I. 45. 2-3[244].

"The water vapor of the sky falls upon the earth in different ways, viz. : as (1) rain ; (2) hail ; (3) dew ; and (4) snow. Of them, the rain-water is the best for its lightness. The rain

---

244. पानीयमान्तरीक्षमनिर्द्देश्यरसममृतं जीवनं तर्पणं धारणमाश्वासजननं श्रमघ्नं क्लमपिपासामदमूर्च्छातन्द्रानिद्रादाहप्रशमनमेकान्ततः पथ्यतमञ्च ॥ २

तदेवावनीपतितमन्यतमं रसमुपलभते स्थानविशेषान्नदी-नद-सरस्तड़ागवापी-कूप-चुण्ढी-प्रस्रवणोद्भिदिकिरकेदार-पल्वलादिषु स्थानेष्ववस्थितमिति ॥

सुश्रुत-संहिता, सूत्रस्थानम्, ४५ ।

also comes from (the vapor of) two sources—Gangetic (sweet) and oceanic (saline)." *Suśruta* I. 45. 5[245].

"Of them, rain from the Gangetic (vapor) is the best." *Suśruta* I. 45. 5[246].

Polluted Water: "The water swarming with bacteria, polluted by their toxins, or by (human) excreta, decomposed egg or dead body, covered with grasses and (fallen) leaves, contaminated or poisoned, or the inundation water of the first rainy season, if bathed in, or drunk by a person, makes him suffer soon from external lesion, (skin-diseases for bathing) and internal troubles (intestinal disorders for drinking).

The water that contains slime, mud, or is covered with algae, water-weeds and lotus-leaves etc. and in which (the rays of) the sun, (the beams of) the moon, and air (aeration can not take place) can not penetrate, and which is distinguished by any smell, color or taste, that water is to be regarded as contaminated.

The contaminated water is marked by six

---

245. तत्रान्तरीक्षं चतुर्व्विधम्। तद्यथा—धारं कारं तौषारं हैममिति। तत् पुनर्द्विविधं गाङ्गं सामुद्रञ्चेति। तेषां धारं प्रधानं लघुत्वात्। सुश्रुत-संहिता, सूत्रस्थानम्, ४५।

246. गाङ्गं पुनः प्रधानम्। सुश्रुत-संहिता, सूत्रस्थानम्, ४५।

faults—in touch, appearance, taste, smell, action and reaction Roughness (due to the presence of sand or grit) viscosity (bacterial decomposition especially of the vegetable matter), warmth (due to carbonic acid gas), tooth-sensibility (due to astringency or any other chemical agent or bacterial product) are the touch-faults of contaminated water. Mud, sand, slime and colorings (chlorophyl) are the appearance faults. Any pronounced taste is the taste-fault. Foul-smelling is the smell-fault. If, when drunk, the water causes thirst, heaviness (in the stomach), colic, and expectoration, it is due to its action-fault. If when drunk, the water takes a long time for its digestion (passage, absorption and excretion) and is retained in the alimentary canal, it is the reaction fault. These faults are not found in the water (that falls upon the earth from condensation of the water- vapors) of the sky.

Sterilization of Water : Water should be sterilized, if of contaminated source, by boiling, warming in the sun, or by throwing into it, red-hot iron-balls, sand and stones. For its deodorization, flowers of Rotleria tinctoria, Michelia champaca, Nymphæa cerula, and Bignonia suaveolens should be kept in water over-night.

The water saturated with the fragrance of the flower, should be drunk in a gold, silver, copper, bronze, crystal or earthen bowl. Polluted water, or untimely rain water should be always avoided. He who drinks water not sterilized by boiling etc., is apt to suffer from inflammation, anemia, diseases, indigestion, bronchitis, dyspnea, catarrh, colic, tumor, ascites and other malignant diseases." *Suśruta* I. 45, 6-11[247].

---

247. कीटमूत्रपुरीषाण्ड-शवकोथप्रदूषितम् ।
तृणपर्णोत्करयुतं कलुषं विषसंयुतम् ॥
योऽवगाहेत वर्षासु पिवेद्वापि नवं जलम् ।
स वाह्याभ्यन्तरान् रोगान् प्राप्नुयात् चिप्रमेव तु ॥ ६

तत्र यत् शैवालपङ्कहटतृणपद्मपत्रप्रभृतिभिरवच्छन्नं शशिसूर्य्यकिरणानिलैर्नाभिजुष्टं गन्धवर्णरसोपसृष्टञ्च तद्व्यापन्नमिति विद्यात् ॥ ७

तस्य स्पर्शरूपरसगन्धवीर्य्यविपाकदोषाः षट् सम्भवन्ति ॥ ८

तत्र खरता पैच्छिल्यमौष्ण्यं दन्तग्राहिता च स्पर्शदोषः। पङ्कसिकताशैवालवहुवर्णता रूपदोषः। व्यक्तरसता रसदोषः। अनिष्टगन्धता गन्धदोषः यदुपयुक्तं तृष्णागौरवशूलकफप्रसेकानापादयति स वीर्य्यदोषः। यदुपयुक्तं चिराद्विपच्यते विष्टम्भाति वा स विपाकदोष इति। त एते आन्तरिचे न सन्ति ॥ ९

व्यापन्नानामग्निक्वथनं सूर्य्यातपप्रतापनं तप्तायःपिण्डसिकतालोष्ट्राणां वा निर्व्वापणं प्रसादनञ्च कर्त्तव्यं, नागचम्पकोत्पलपाटलापुष्पप्रभृतिभिश्चाधिवासनमिति ॥ १०

सौवर्णे राजते ताम्रे कांस्ये मणिमयेऽपि वा ।
पुष्पावतंसं भौमे वा सुगन्धि सलिलं पिवेत् ॥

Pure water : "The water that is without smell, distinct taste, that quenches thirst, that is pure, cool, transparent, light and refreshing, is to be regarded as '*pure water*'." *Suśruta* I. 45. 13[248].

व्यापन्नं वर्ज्जयेन्नित्यं तोयं यद्वाप्यनार्त्तवम् ।
दोषसञ्जननं ह्येतन्नाददीताहितन्तु तत् ॥
व्यापन्नं सलिलं यस्तु पिबतीहाप्रसाधितम् ।
श्वयथुं पाण्डुरोगञ्च त्वग्दोषमविपाकताम् ॥
श्वासकासप्रतिश्याय-शूलगुल्मोदराणि च ।
अन्यान् वा विषमान् रोगान् प्राप्नुयात् चिप्रमेव च ॥ ११

सुश्रुत-संहिता, सूत्रस्थानम्, ४५ ।

248.] निर्गन्धमव्यक्तरसं तृष्णाघ्नं शुचि शीतलम् ।
अच्छं लघु च हृद्यञ्च तोयं गुणवदुच्यते ॥ १२

सुश्रुत-संहिता, सूत्रस्थानम्, ४५ ।

IX. HYGIENE.

Hospital : "By an expert architect, a large house should be built; it should be strong, but not drafty, except the current of air shall pass in one direction; it should be so built that one can easily move about within it; it should be built on an elevated place (having nothing higher than it in the locality), and within, it should be free from smoke, sun (exposure to the sun was regarded injurious; its disinfectant and sterilizing property was not understood), dust, noise, (sensual) touch, (exciting) ocular impressions, (spicy) taste, and (penetrating) smell (that is, whatever excites the nerves and disturbs the nervous quietude); and it should be provided with staircase, mortar, pestle, toilet, bath-room and kitchen.

There attendants (interns) for nursing the sick, should be appointed, who are of good character, are pure (free from any disease), obedient, clever, kind-hearted, fit for any kind of work (associated with nursing hospital duties), expert in cooking, in bath-attendance, massage, capable of lifting and putting the sick into bed, and who do not show unwillingness for any kind of work. There experts should be engaged who are well-versed in singing, music, (in recitation of) prayers, poems, hymns, stories, history and contemporary events ;(for the distraction of the mind and entertainment of the sick).

There should be also kept (in the enclosure) Tetraoperdix himalayensis, Galloperdix spadiceus, hare, stag (Cervus elaphus), black deer, black-tailed deer (Cervus cashmirianus), Dama platyceros, and sheep. As well as gentle, milking cows with calves, free from diseases should be kept, and for them feed, sleeping places (stable) and drinking water should be provided.

There should be also cistern, pail, tub, cask, keg, pitcher, jar, ewer, platter, dipper, cooking-pot, double-boiler, bandage, thread, cotton, animal thread (horse-hair for suturation), a comfortable bed with all accessories, jug, spittoon, and all that are necessary for leaning (easy chair), sitting, (for the application of) ointment, sweating, massage, emplastrum, fomentation, embrocation, emetics, sedatives, vulnerary enemata, oily enemata, errhines, urination and purgation." *Charaka* I. 15, 5-9[249].

Qualifications of a Surgeon: "For the practice of operative surgery, a physician has to get the *license* from the king, and for this he has to acquire a thorough knowledge of the medical science and surgery, must have keen observation and experience of operations (under a licensed preceptor or in a hospital); and before an operation, he has to pair his nails (to prevent sepsis, and to carry pathogenic

---

249. दृढ़ं निवातं प्रवातैकदेशं सुखप्रविचारमनुपत्यकं धूमातपरजसामनभिगमनीयमनिष्टानाञ्च शब्दस्पर्शरसरूपगन्धानां सोपानोदूखल मूषलवर्च्चः स्थानस्नानभूमिमहानसोपेतं वास्तुविद्याकुशलः प्रशस्तं गृहमेव तावत् पूर्व्वमुपकल्पयेत् ॥

ततः शीलशौचानुरागदाक्ष्यप्रादक्षिण्योपपन्नानुपचारकुशलान् सर्व्वकर्म्मसु पर्य्यवदातान् सूपौदनपाचक-स्नापक-संवाहकोत्थापक-सम्वेशकौषधपेषकांश्च परिचारकान् सर्व्वकर्म्मस्वप्रतिकूलान्। तथा गीतवादित्रोल्लापक - श्लोकगाथाख्यायिकेतिहासपुराणकुशलानभिप्रायज्ञाननुमतांश्च देशकालविदः पारिषद्यांश्च।

तथा लावकपिञ्जलशशहरिणैनकालपुच्छकमृगमातृकोरभ्रान्। गाञ्च दोग्ध्रीं शीलवतीमनातुरां जीववत्सां सुप्रतिविहिततृणशरणपानीयान् ॥

जलपात्राचमनोदकोष्ठमणिकपिठरघटकुम्भी कुम्भ कुण्डशरावदर्व्वीक परिपचन मन्थान चर्म्मसूत्रकार्पासोर्णादीनिच शयनासनादीनि चोपन्यस्त - भृङ्गारप्रतिग्रहाणि सुप्रयुक्तास्तरणोत्तरप्रच्छदोपधानानि स्वापाश्रयाणि सम्वेशनोपवेशनस्नेहस्वेदाभ्यङ्ग प्रदेहपरिषेकानुलेपनवमनविरेचनास्थापनानुवासनशिरोविरेचनमूत्रोच्चारसुखानि ॥

चरक-संहिता, सूत्रस्थानम्, १५।

germs and spread infection from patient to patient), to cut short his hair (shaving for the same purpose), become purified (free from any disease, and disinfected) and shall put on (washed, disinfected) white robes, (and shall go to the operation) with umbrella (on his head), stick in his hand, sandals (in his feet), robes not highly raised (gracefully attired), having pleasant speech, uprighteous conduct, friendly to all living beings, and succor of the good." *Suśruta* I. 10. 2[25] .

I.—*Dietetic Hygeine*.

"Desiccated (for losing flavor and savor), or decomposed meat (to prevent ptomaine poisoning), or meat from a deceased animal (to prevent the infection of the pathogenic germs of the disease from which the animal has died), or killed by poisoning, or by a venomous snake, or by an instrument which has been covered

---

250. अधिगततन्त्रेणोपासिततन्त्रार्थेन दृष्टकर्म्मणा कृतयोग्येन शास्त्रं निगदता राजानुज्ञातेन नीचनखरोम्णा शुचिना शुक्लवस्त्रपरिहितेन छत्रवता दण्डहस्तेन सोपानत्केनानुद्धतवेशेन सुमनसा कल्याणाभिव्याहारेणाकुहकेन बन्धुभूतेन भूतानां सुसहायवता वैद्येन विशिखानुप्रवेष्टव्या ॥ २

सुश्रुत-संहिता, सूत्रस्थानम्., १० ।

with poisons, too old (the meat of an old animal is not only tough and unsavorous, but it also contains an excessive amount of metabolic wastes, due to the deficiency of glandular secretions and incomplete oxidation), or too young (the meat of a young animal contains an excessive amount of purine bodies, and extractives are not yet formed, which exert a tonic effect on the organism)." *Suśruta* I. 46. 129 [251].

Evil Effects of Over-Nutrition : Any one who with sedentary habits, indulges in fatty, sweet, heavy, viscid foods, new rice, new wine, meat of animals of marshy region, or aquatic creatures, milk, and milk-products, sugar-preparations, and cakes excessively, is subject to diathesis of various lesions, and if he does not take precautionary measures against them, he suffers from diabetes, pruritus, eczema, impetigo, jaundice, fever ; skin diseases, hyperacidity, strangury, anorexia, somnolence, impotence, adiposis, lassitude, foul-emanation from the body, encrusting (calcification) of the vascular system,

---

251. शुष्कव्याधिविषसर्प हतदिग्धविद्धजीर्ण कृशबालानामसात्म्यचारिणां मांसान्यभक्ष्याणि ।

सुश्रुत-संहिता, सूत्रस्थानम्, ४६ ।

intellectual fatigue, enervation, ascites and other diseases." *Charaka* I. 23. 2 [252].

"A stimulant taken in proper dose increases the strength and weight of the body, but taken excessively, it reduces the body-weight (by inducing hyper-metabolism)." *Charaka* I. 22. 25 [253].

Seasonal dietetic variations : "He who understands and follows the hygienic and dietetic regulations for each season, by his seasonal vari-

---

252. सन्तर्पयति यः स्निग्धैर्मधुरैर्गुरुपिच्छिलैः ।
नवान्नैर्नवमद्यैश्च मांसैश्चानूपवारिजैः ॥
गोरसैर्गौड़िकैश्चान्यैः पिष्टकैश्चातिमात्रशः ।
चेष्टाद्वेषी दिवास्वप्नशय्यासनसुखे रतः ॥
रोगास्तस्योपजायन्ते सन्तर्पणनिमित्तजाः ।
प्रमेहपिड़काकोठकण्डू-पाण्ड्वामयज्वराः ॥
कुष्ठान्यामप्रदोषाश्च मूत्रकृच्छ्रमरोचकः ।
तन्द्रा क्लैव्यमतिस्थौल्यमालस्यं गुरुगात्रता ॥
इन्द्रियस्रोतसां लेपो बुद्धेर्मोहः प्रमीलकः ।
शोथाश्चैवं विधाश्चान्ये शीघ्रमप्रतिकुर्व्वतः ॥

चरक-संहिता, सूत्रस्थानम्, २३ ।

253. बलं पुष्ट्युपलम्भश्च कार्श्यदोषविवर्ज्जनम् ।
लक्षणं बृंहिते स्थौल्यमति चात्यर्थबृंहिते ॥

चरक-संहिता, सूत्रस्थानम्, २२ ।

ation of diet improves his complexion and increases his vigor." *Charaka* I 6. 2 [253]*a*.

Seasonal variation of food is conducive to health and vitality. In the summer one does not need so much fat as in the winter, as the caloric needs of the organism is much less, owing to the less radiation of heat from the body surface to the surrounding atmosphere. And as the cold air contains more oxygen, the increased oxygen intake naturally enhances metabolism, and therefore one has in the winter better appetite, and can digest a large quantity of meat and other nitrogenous food, which in the summer may easily cause gastro-intestinal troubles. Carbohydrate needs of the body are also increased, as to keep the body warm, one is apt to move and to take exercise, which naturally eonsumes more glycogen than in the summer, and therefore an increased intake of carbohydrates becomes necessary. "Due to the contact of the cold air, digestive fire is confined, and consequently its vitality (metabolism) is increased ; for this reason in

---

253.(a) तस्याशितादाद्याहाराद्बलं वर्णश्च वर्द्धते ।
तस्यर्त्तुसात्म्यं विदितं चेष्टाहारव्यपाश्रयम् ॥

चरक-संहिता, सूत्रस्थानम्, ६ ।

winter, one can digest much more heavy stuffs (than in the summer)." *Charaka* I. 6. 9 [254].

Not to eat rapidly : Do not eat too rapidly. For if eaten too rapidly, the ingesta does not give adequate savor, nor is it properly fixed (masticated and saturated with salivary ferments), and is abnormal in its course in the alimentary canal, and its normal reactions are not perceived ; therefore one should not eat too rapidly." *Charaka* III. 1. 19 [255].

A lean person has more vitality than a fat person : "To make a fat person lean, indigestible food (which is insufficiently assimilated, but only given to satiate hunger) and fasting should be prescribed. And to make a lean man fat, easily digestible food to satiation should be given." Charaka I. 21. 16 [256]. "But though both leanness and fatness have their inconvenience, between them, leanness is preferable, for in a

---

254. शीते शीतानिलस्पर्शसंरुद्धो बलिनां बली ।

पक्ता भवति हेमन्ते मात्राद्रव्यगुरुक्षमः ॥ चरक-संहिता, सूत्रस्थानम्, ६ ।

255. नातिद्रुतमश्नीयात् । अतिद्रुतं हि भुञ्जानस्य तत्स्नेहनस्वादनभोजनस्याप्रतिष्ठानं भोज्यदोषसाद्गुण्योपलब्धिश्च न नियता, तस्मान्नातिद्रुतमश्नीयात् ।

चरक-संहिता, विमानस्थानम्, १ ।

256. गुरु चातर्पणञ्चेष्टं स्थूलानां कर्षणं प्रति ।

कृशानां वृंहणार्थन्तु लघु सन्तर्पणञ्च यत् ॥ चरक-संहिता, सूत्रस्थानम्, २१ ।

disease, a fat individual suffers more (accumulation of fat in the body is due to fundamentals : (1) Either excess of food is taken, especially carbohydrates, beyond the bodily needs, and with good digestion, the surplus of converted glycogen above the current expenditure is stored in the body as fat ; to a moderate extent, this is very becoming, as it beautifies the form of the body ; but in excess it is apt to interfere with the action of the heart and other vital organs by pressure as well as fatty infiltration. However, the dyspeptics do not get fat and remain lean with excessive amount of food, for the ingesta can be only partly absorbed, due to deficiency, quantitatively and qualitatively, of digestive enzymes. (2) Fatty accumulation and degeneration takes place in hypo-metabolism, due to glandular deficiency as in myxedema. On the other hand, hypermetabolism causes gradual emaciation. As vitality is related with metabolism, so leanness not associated with nutritional insufficiency or wasting diseases, has more resisting power against pathogenic micro-organisms)." *Charaka* I. 21. 13[256a].

---

256. (a) स्थौल्यकार्श्ये वरं कार्श्यं समोपकरणौ हि तौ।
यद्युभौ व्याधिरागच्छेत् स्थूलमेवातिपीड़येत्॥
चरक-संहिता, सूत्रस्थानम्, २१।

Mental excitement interferes with Digestion : "Worry, sorrow, fear, anger, sadness, perplexity and vigilance (sleeplessness) interfere with digestion, even if the food be good and taken in right quantity (mental excitement arrests the digestive secretions, and by raising the blood pressure by excessive secretion of adrenalin, the sympathetic nervous system becomes irritated)." *Charaka* III. 2. 6[257]

Mouth Hygiene : "After eating, one should repeatedly gargle, and wash out the mouth (to wash out the food particles that may be in the buccal cavity, to prevent their harboring of micro-organisms which cause decomposition and foul odor of the mouth)." *Suśruta* I. 46. 520[258]. "Food particles sticking in or within the (crevices of) teeth, should be taken out slowly with tooth-picks ; for otherwise they cause foulness of the mouth (The negligence of these two simple oral hygienic rules, is spreading fast in India, as in

---

257. मात्रयाप्यभ्यवहृतं पथ्यं चान्नं न जीर्य्यति ।
चिन्ताशोकभयक्रोधदुःखमोहप्रजागरैः ॥

चरक-संहिता, विमानस्थानम्, २ ।

258. प्रचालयेदङ्गिरास्यं भुञ्जानस्य मुहुर्म्मुहुः ।

सुश्रुत-संहिता, सूत्रस्थानम्, ४६ ।

Europe, the *Dental Caries*)." *Suśruta* I. 46. 525[259].

Foods to be avoided : "The food that is discolored, contaminated, left over (from the plate of some one else), mixed with pebbles, grass or similar substances, repulsive in appearance, kept over night, insipid, or decomposed, should not be taken ; nor the food that is cooked for a long time (vitamine is destroyed by over-cooking or cooking at a high temperature), is hardened (digestive ferments can not penetrate through hardened masses), cold (the injesta has to be heated to the body temperature before the digestive ferments can act energetically upon them and they can be absorbed), cooked again, porridge having uneven cooked grains, and what is cooked at a high temperature." *Suśruta* I. 46. 518[260].

II.—*General Hygiene*

Not to interfere with the natural call of Nature : "An intelligent person should not

---

259. दन्तान्तरगतश्चान्नं शोधनेनाहरेच्छनैः।
कुर्य्यादनाहृतं तद्धि मुखस्यानिष्टगन्धताम् ॥ ५२५
सुश्रुतसंहिता, सूत्रस्थानम्, ४६।

260. अचोचं दुष्टमुच्छिष्टं पाषाणतृणलोष्ट्रवत्।
द्विष्टं व्युषितमस्वादु पूति चान्नं विवर्ज्जयेत् ॥
सुश्रुत-संहिता, सूत्रस्थानम्, ४६।

retain (interfere with the passage by the voluntary contraction of the muscles) feces, urine, intestinal gas, vomiting, sneezing, yawning, hunger, thirst, tears, sleep or the fatigued breath (carbon dioxide)." *Charaka* I. 7. 2[261].

Periodic Cleaning of the System : "In the spring, in the rainy season, and the autumn, one should cleanse his system. First he should use ointment, then sweating, and after that emetics and purgatives. Later enemata and errhines should be given (The periodic flushing of the intestines by enemata or purgatives, is now recognized by all as a good hygienic prophylaxis. In weakness of the kidney, Turkish bath twice or thrice a year is also very desirable, to throw out of the system the accumulated toxins through the skin, which the kidney has failed to eliminate or as a relief to the over-worked kidneys)." *Charaka* I. 7. 35[262].

---

261. न वेगान् धारयेद्धीमान् जातान् मूत्रपुरीषयोः ।
न रेतसो न वातस्य न वम्याः क्षवथो र्नच ।
नोद्गारस्य न जृम्भाया न वेगान् क्षुत्पिपासयोः ।
न वाष्पस्य न निद्राया निःश्वासस्य श्रमेण च ॥

सुश्रुतसंहिता, सूत्रस्थानम्, ७ ।

262. माधवप्रथमे मासि नभस्य प्रथमे पुनः ।
सहस्य प्रथमे चैव हारयेद्दोषसञ्चयम् ॥

चरक-संहिता, सूत्रस्थानम्, ७ ।

Physical Exercise: Exercise is the exerti to invigorate and to increase the strength of the body; one should take physical exercise measuredly. For it induces lightness, agility, vigor, endurance, removes flatulence, and increases metabolism. But if it be done in excess, it brings about lassitude, fatig spermatorrhea, gastrorrhagia, dyspnea, bronchitis, fever and vomiting". *Charaka* I. 7. 24-26[263].

Excess to be avoided: "An intelligent person, even if necessary, should not indulge in excess of exercise, laughing, speaking, travelling, sexual intercourse and vigilance." *Charaka* I. 7. 27[264].

"A person who takes regular exercise, and eats after his previous meal has been digested, and takes barley and wheat, does not suffer from

---

263. शरीरचेष्टा या चेष्टा स्थैर्यार्था बलवर्द्धिनी ।
देहव्यायामसंख्याता मात्रया तां समाचरेत् ॥
लाघवं कर्म्मसामर्थ्यं स्थैर्यं क्लेशसहिष्णुता ।
दोषक्षयोऽग्निवृद्धिश्च व्यायामादुपजायते ॥
श्रमः क्लमः क्षयस्तृष्णा रक्तपित्तं प्रतामकः ।
अतिव्यायामतः कासो ज्वरश्छर्द्दिश्च जायते ॥
चरक-संहिता, सूत्रस्थानम्, ७ ।

264. व्यायामहास्यभाष्याध्वग्राम्यधर्म्मप्रजागरान् ।
नोचितानपि सेवेत बुद्धिमानतिमात्रया ॥
चरक-संहिता, सूत्रस्थानम्, ७ ।

over-eating, and he loses his adiposis. "*Charaka* I. 23. 10[265].

Purgatives and Purgation : "The best of root purgatives is Ipomœa turpethum, of the barks—Symplocos racemosa, of the fruits—Terminalia chebula, of the oils—Ricinus communis (castor oil), of the juice—Cleome pentaphylla, and of the milky exudations—that of Euphorbiæ antiquorum." *Suśruta* I. 44. 2[266].

"The effectiveness of purgation is marked by subsidence of weakness, emaciation (loss of body weight), fatigue and the course of the disease, the improvement of the heart's action, clearness of complexion, normal appetite and thirst, normal inclination for evacuation of feces and urine, improvement in the sense perceptions and

---

265. व्यायामनित्यो जीर्णाशी यवगोधमभोजनः ।
सन्तर्पणकृतैर्दोषैः स्थौल्यं मुक्त्वा विमुच्यते ॥
चरक-संहिता, सूत्रस्थानम, २३ ।

266. अरुणाभं त्रिवृन्मूलं श्रेष्ठं मूलविरेचने ।
प्रधानं तिल्वकस्त्वक्षु फलेष्वपि हरीतकी ॥
तैलेष्वेरण्डजं तैलं स्वरसे कारवेल्लिका ।
सुधापयः पयःसूक्तमिति प्राधान्यसंग्रहः ॥
सुश्रुत-संहिता, सूत्रस्थानम्, ४४ ।

the mind, passage of the intestinal gas, and the increased metabolism." *Charaka* I. 16. 3[267].

Do not sneeze before covering your mouth: "Without covering your mouth, do not yawn, sneeze or laugh (to prevent the spreading of pathogenic germs, especially the Bacilli tuberculosis)." *Charaka* I. 8. 17[268].

Treatment against Poisoning: In the first poisoning, the patient should be made to vomit (the poison that has been ingested by an emetic) and then after giving cold water (to dissolve the poison that may be sticking to the wall of the alimentary canal), a detoxicant mixed with butter and honey should be given (to neutralize the toxins, and to make them comparatively innocuous by chemical combinations)" *Suśruta* V. 2. 25[269].

Treatment against venomous snake-bite:

---

267. दौर्ब्बल्यं लाघवं ग्लानिर्व्याधीनामल्पता रुचिः ।
हृदयशुद्धिः क्षुत्तृष्णा काले वेगप्रवर्त्तनम् ॥
बुद्धीन्द्रियमनःशुद्धिर्मारुतस्यानुलोमता ।
सम्यग्विरिक्तलिङ्गानि कायाग्नेश्चानुवर्द्धनम् ॥
चरक-संहिता, सूत्रस्थानम्, १५ ।

268. नासंवृतमुखे जृम्भां क्षवथुं हास्यं वा प्रवर्त्तयेत् ।
चरक-संहिता, सूत्रस्थानम्, ८ ।

"If the arm or leg is bitten by a snake (if it be subcutaneous, the poisoning is slow, but if intravascular, it is rapid), a tight ligature should be made about four fingers' breadth above the wound, to prevent the poison flowing upward (with the blood or lymph) by cord, leather-band or tree bark (tourniquet, to compress the blood and the lymphatic vessels). Where tight ligature is not possible, free incisions should be made near the bite (to drain out the poisoned blood and the lymph) and theaffected area cauterized (preferably by a liquid caustic, permanganate of potash—3 p. c. solution—which can penetrate deep into the tissues quickly). Suction (by hygroscopic calcined stones which suck the fluid with the poisonous principles), incision (to drain out the poisoned blood and the lympth) and cauterization (to destroy the poisonous principles and the poisoned area) are always applicable (after tight ligature). *Suśruta* V. 5. 2[270]. Injection of polyvalent antivenom serum has proved very promising.

---

269. प्रथमे विषवेगे तु वान्तं शीताम्बुसेवितम्।
अगदं मधुसर्पिर्भ्यां पाययेत समायुतम्॥
सुश्रुत-संहिता, कल्पस्थानम्, २।

270. सर्व्वैरेवादितः सर्पैः शाखादष्टस्य देहिनः।
दंशस्योपरि बध्नीयादरिष्टाश्चतुरङ्गुले॥

III. Sexual Hygiene.

Physical Maturity · "An intelligent physician should know that man at 25 years of age and woman at 16 attain at their (physical) maturity with full (organic) development." *Suśruta* I. 35. 9[271].

"He who cares for longevity should not have sexual intercourse, before he is 16 years old, or after he is 70 (Though a boy at 16 has his spermatozoa developed and is capable of reproduction, yet he needs to conserve and utilize the spermin up to the age of 25 for the development of his body and mind ; in old age, the tension of copulation is liable to cause rupture of the calcified and friable blood-vessels)." *Charaka* VI. 2. 60[272].

प्रोतचर्म्मान्तवल्कानां मृदुनान्यतमेन च ।
न गच्छति विषं देहमरिष्टाभिर्निवारितम् ॥
दहेद्दंशमथोत्कृत्य यत्र बन्धो न जायते ।
आचूषणच्छेददाहाः सर्व्वत्रैव तु पूजिताः ॥

सुश्रुत-संहिता, कल्पस्थानम्, ५

271. पञ्चविंशे ततो वर्षे पुमान् नारी तु षोड़शे ।
समत्वागतवीर्य्यौ तौ जानीयात् कुशलो भिषक् ॥ ९

सुश्रुत-संहिता, सूत्रस्थानम् , ३५ ।

272. नत्त्वेव षोड़शाद्वर्षात् सप्तत्याः परतो न च ।
आयुष्कामो नरः स्त्रीभिः संयोगं कर्त्तुमर्हति ॥

चरक-संहिता, चिकित्सितस्थानम् , २ ।

Tuberculosis increases sexual desire : "If a tuberculous patient (consumptive) gradually loses his strength, and his expectorations increase, yet he is fond of sexual intercourse, the disease will lead him to his death (It is well known that the tubercular patients become very sexually inclined ; it is very probable that the rich phosphorus contents of the Bacillus tuberculosis become liberated in the disintegration process as a reaction of the organism, and this circulating with the blood acts as an aphrodisiac, and consequently sexual erethism is one of the most distinguished characteristics of this disease)." *Charaka* VI. 3. 5[273].

Sexual intercourse forbidden : "Do not have sexual intercourse with a menstruating woman (there seems to be a universal prejudice against intercourse with a menstruating woman ; it is possible that the presence of blood has been regarded by the primitive man as impure, or unesthetic ; it is probable, however, that the motive is more utilitarian, as many of the religious observances, regulations and injunctions are certainly based on principles of

---

273. बलञ्च हीयते यस्य प्रतिश्यायश्च वर्द्धते ।
तस्य नारीप्रसक्तस्य शोषोऽन्तायोपजायते ॥

चरक-संहिता, इन्द्रियस्थानम्, ५

hygiene or economic considerations; in apparently cured and neglected old gonorrhea, the gonococci might still live in the upper tract, and may be dislodged with the flow of the menstrual blood, and cause urethritis to the man with whom she may have copulation, while in other times it might remain entirely innocuous; a menstruating woman on her part is rather sexually inclined during that period, and would be much relieved of turgescence by the embrace), with a diseased, or unclean woman (for hygienic reasons) or with one whose vagina is narrow (vaginismus), whose beauty does not appeal (rouse the senses), or whose conduct is repulsive or who is artless, homely, or one who goes with other men (thus can be infected and spread the disease); nor go with another man's wife; nor practise bestiality, or unnatural vices (sodomy and pederasty)." *Charaka* I. 8. 25[274].

Aphrodisiac: "A pretty, youthful, well-formed, charmingly attired, willing and well-educated

---

274. न रजस्वलां नातुरां नामेध्यां नाशस्तां नानिष्टरूपाचारोपचारां नादक्षां नाकामां नान्यकामां नान्यस्त्रियं नान्ययोनिं नायोनौ अभिगच्छेत्।

चरक-संहिता, सूत्रस्थानम्, ८।

woman (wife) is the best aphrodisiac (in impotence)." *Charaka* VII. 2. 5[275].

Impregnation: "In the (sexual) congress of man and woman, by the nervous tension heat (tumescence) is generated. The heat and (vaginal) secretion provoke the discharge of the semen, and which unites with the ovum (*ārttava* is a vague expression; but it is certain that it meant more than menstruation blood, as it could not exist after menstrual flow ceased; perhaps it was an indistinct conception of the ovule which when it becomes ripe, ruptures the Graafian follicle in which it is enclosed and causes menstruation). Then the united sperm and the ovum (the fecundated ovum) reach the uterus." *Suśruta* III. 3. 3[276].

"As the germination (of a seed) takes place by the combination of proper season, field, moisture and seed, so pregnancy is developed

---

275. सुरूपा यौवनस्था या लक्षणैर्या विभूषिता ।
या वश्या शिक्षिता या च सा स्त्री वृष्यतमा मता ॥

चरक-संहिता, चिकित्सितस्थानम्, २ ।

276. तत्र स्त्रीपुंसयोः संयोगे तेजः शरीराद्वायुरुदीरयति । ततस्तेजोऽनिलसन्निपाताच्छुक्रं च्युतं योनिमभिप्रतिपद्यते संसृज्यते चार्त्तवेन । ततोऽग्निषोमसंयोगात् संसृज्यमानो गर्भो गर्भाशयमनुप्रतिपद्यते ।

सुश्रुत-संहिता, शारीरस्थानम्, २ ।

by their proper combination (*ṛtu* = proper season standing for the first 12 days after menstruation ; *kṣetra* = field for uterus ; *amvu* = moisture for ovum ; *vïja* = seed, for sperm, i. e. for spermatozoon)." *Suśruta* III. 2. 33[277].

Heredity : "The child inherits the characteristics of the parents acquired by them under the influence of diet, behaviour and (physical and mental) exertions, during their copulation (in which the impregnation takes place. Though hereditary transmission can not be explained by such a simple formula, yet it is undeniable that the germplasms must be under profound impression of the physical and the mental state of the parents in the time of fertilization. An irritable spermatozoon either by alcohol, or by the morbid condition of blood, is very apt to create the same diathesis in the offspring)." *Suśruta* III. 9. 63[279].

"He who abstains from meat and wine, and

---

277. ध्रुवं चतुर्णां सान्निध्याद्गर्भः स्याद्विधिपूर्व्वकः ।
ऋतुक्षेत्राम्बुवीजानां सामग्र्यादङ्कुरो यथा ॥

सुश्रुत-संहिता, शारीरस्थानम्, २ ।

278. आहाराचारचेष्टाभिर्यादृशीभिः समन्वितौ ।
स्त्रीपुंसौ समुपेयातां तयोः पुत्रोऽपि तादृशः ॥ ४६

सुश्रुत-संहिता, शारीरस्थानम्, ४६ ।

takes only beneficial food, and leads a pure (hygienic) life, he and his descendants do not suffer from insanity." *Charaka* VI. 9. 63 [279].

"If a man copulates with a menstruating woman on the first day of her course, he shortens his life, and there is embryonic abortion of the fruit of conception ; if on the second day, there is still-birth ; if on the third day, the child is of incomplete development and becomes short-lived ; but if on the fourth day, the child is well-developed and possesses good vitality (a long life). As a thing (floating substance) thrown in a river can not ascend up-stream against the course of the current, so when the menstrual blood flows, the seed (spermatozoon) can not enter in and become active (during the copulative act, the forward and the backward movement, especially of the glans-penis, acts almost like a valve of the suction-pump, creating a kind of vacuum state, widening the mouth of the womb, deflating it and drawing it forward, so that when the semen is discharged, it shoots like a jet of spray and is sucked by the womb with

---

279. निवृत्तामिषमद्यो यो हिताशी प्रयत: शुचि: ।
निजागन्तुभिरुन्मादै: सत्त्ववान् न स युज्यते ॥
चरक-संहिता, चिकित्सितस्थानम्, ९ ।

the ovum ; in case the vagina is filled with menstrual blood or fluid, this suction can not but be incomplete ; the vaginal secretions at the entrance of the penis or in strong sexual desire serve simply to lubricate the passage, so that the delicate mucous membrane can not be hurt). Therefore one should not indulge in the sexual union during the first three days of menstruation, nor (after twelve days) in the month (in the second week the ovum begins to degenerate, and either it is incapable of fertilization, or if fecundated, it is apt to reproduce a weakling)." *Suśruta* III. 2. 31[280].

Sex-determination of the offspring : "If a male child is desired, the husband should practise continence for a month (to increase sexual erethism and vigor), and after fattening himself with clarified butter, milk-fat, milk and rice, shall copulate with his wife after music, endearments (to excite the senses) and assurance of

280. तत्र प्रथमे दिवसे ऋतुमत्यां मैथुनगमनमनायुष्यं पुंसां भवति। यश्च तत्राधीयते गर्भः, स प्रसवमानो विमुच्यते। द्वितीयेऽप्येवं सूतिकागृहे वा। तृतीयेऽप्येवम्-सम्पूर्णाङ्गोऽल्पायुर्वा भवति। चतुर्थे तु सम्पूर्णाङ्गो दीर्घायुश्च भवति। न च प्रवर्त्तमाने रक्ते वीजं प्रविष्टं गुणकरं भवति, यथा नद्यां प्रतिस्रोतः प्लावि द्रव्यं प्रक्षिप्तं प्रतिनिवर्त्तते नोर्द्ध्वं गच्छति तद्वदेव द्रष्टव्यम्। तस्मान्नियमवतीं त्रिरात्रं परिहरेत्, अतः परं मासादुपेयात् ॥ ३१ सुश्रुत-संहिता, शारीरस्थानम्, २।

love to her, on the fourth, sixth, eighth, tenth or twelfth day of menstruation, and she likewise should have lived a continent life for a month, fattened herself with clarified butter and fed on oily and nitrogenous foods.

If the conjugal duty is performed on these days, it conduces to (the promotion of) wisdom, longevity, health, increase of population, wealth and strength.

If a girl is desired , sexual union should take place on the fifth, seventh, ninth or eleventh day. From the thirteenth day (up to the new monthly cycle ; from the second week after menstruation, the ovum begins to deteriorate and is usually incapable of impregnation) cohabitation is blameworthy (as the union is fruitless, it is only for the sensual gratification and indulgence, and not for the welfare of the race)". *Suśruta* III. 2. 28-30[281].

---

281. ततोऽपराह्णे पुमान् मासं ब्रह्मचारी सर्पिःस्निग्धः सर्पिःक्षीराभ्यां शाल्योदनं भुक्त्वा मासं ब्रह्मचारिणीं तैलस्निग्धां तैलमाषोत्तराहारां नारीमुपेयाद्रात्रौ सामादिभिरभिविश्वास्य विकल्प्यैवं चतुर्थ्यां षष्ठ्यामष्टम्यां दशम्यां द्वादश्याञ्चोपेयादिति पुत्रकामः ॥ २८

एषूत्तरोत्तरं विद्यादायुरारोग्यमेव च ।
प्रजासौभाग्यमैश्वर्य्यं बलञ्च दिवसेषु वै ॥ २९

अतः परं पञ्चम्यां सप्तम्यां नवम्यामेकादश्याञ्च स्त्रीकामः । त्रयोदशीप्रभृतयो निन्द्याः ॥ ३०
सुश्रुत-संहिता, शारीरस्थानम्, २ ।

Sex-determination is still speculative. It was believed a few years ago that there were two kinds of ovum, male and female, the former produced by the right ovary and the latter by the left. By animal experimentation and human ovariotomy, it has been found to be erroneous. The egg produced by the ovary is still bi-sexual, hermaphroditic in nature, and its sex is not determined like all its mono-cellular prototypes, before it phylogenetically ascends the scale of evolution, that is before amphimixis is started through the process ef fertilization by the male reproductive cell. That is the starting point of sexual differentiation which begins with the impregnation of the ovum. The question then arises whether the sex-determinant resides in the spermatozoon or in the ovum. In the Hymenoptera an accessory chromosome has been found in nearly half the spermatozoa, and it was regarded by McClung as the sex-determining factor. It may be simply an '*idant*'—bearer of arrested hereditary trait. But the experiments of Loeb have demonstrated that the spermatozoon, at least in the lower scale of evolution, only acts as a stimulant to start the amphimixis, and it can be substituted by artificial chemical stimulus. And in the aphids, parthenogenetic generations